Diagnosis and Treatment of Metabolic Diseases

Diagnosis and Treatment of Metabolic Diseases

Editor: Bryan Glover

AMERICAN
MEDICAL PUBLISHERS
www.americanmedicalpublishers.com

AMERICAN
MEDICAL PUBLISHERS
www.americanmedicalpublishers.com

Cataloging-in-Publication Data

Diagnosis and treatment of metabolic diseases / edited by Bryan Glover.
p. cm.
Includes bibliographical references and index.
ISBN 978-1-63927-721-6
1. Metabolism--Disorders. 2. Metabolism--Disorders--Diagnosis.
3. Metabolism--Disorders--Treatment. I. Glover, Bryan.
RC627.54 .D53 2023
616.39--dc23

American Medical Publishers,
41 Flatbush Avenue,
1st Floor, New York,
NY 11217, USA

ISBN 978-1-63927-721-6 (Hardback)

Contents

Preface

Metabolism refers to the body's mechanism through which it converts food into energy on a cellular level. It is carried out by thousands of enzymes, taking part in numerous interdependent metabolic pathways to perform this process. Metabolic diseases refer to diseases that disrupt the normal metabolism of a person. These diseases affect the capability of the cells to carry out crucial biochemical reactions, including the transport and processing of carbohydrates, lipids and proteins. The causes of metabolic diseases are usually hereditary. However, the majority of people affected with any metabolic disease may seem healthy for several months or years. The initial symptoms generally occur once the body's metabolism becomes stressed, such as during a febrile illness or after long fasting. These diseases can be treated through nutritional management if detected initially. This book aims to explain the diagnosis and treatment of metabolic diseases. It presents researches and studies performed by experts across the globe. This book will help new researchers by foregrounding their knowledge in this condition.

This book has been the outcome of endless efforts put in by authors and researchers on various issues and topics within the field. The book is a comprehensive collection of significant researches that are addressed in a variety of chapters. It will surely enhance the knowledge of the field among readers across the globe.

It gives us an immense pleasure to thank our researchers and authors for their efforts to submit their piece of writing before the deadlines. Finally in the end, I would like to thank my family and colleagues who have been a great source of inspiration and support.

Editor

1

Effects of Daily Raspberry Consumption on Immune-Metabolic Health in Subjects at Risk of Metabolic Syndrome

Maximilien Franck [1,2], Juan de Toro-Martín [1], Véronique Garneau [1], Valérie Guay [1], Michèle Kearney [1], Geneviève Pilon [1,3], Denis Roy [1], Patrick Couture [1,4], Charles Couillard [1,2], André Marette [1,3] and Marie-Claude Vohl [1,2,*]

1 Centre Nutrition, Santé et Société (NUTRISS) and Institut sur la Nutrition et les Aliments Fonctionnels (INAF), Université Laval, Québec, QC G1V 0A6, Canada; maximilien.franck.1@ulaval.ca (M.F.); juan.de-toro-martin.1@ulaval.ca (J.d.T.-M.); veronique.garneau@fsaa.ulaval.ca (V.G.); valerie.guay@fsaa.ulaval.ca (V.G.); michele.kearney@fsaa.ulaval.ca (M.K.); genevieve.pilon@criucpq.ulaval.ca (G.P.); denis.roy@fsaa.ulaval.ca (D.R.); patrick.couture@fmed.ulaval.ca (P.C.); charles.couillard@fsaa.ulaval.ca (C.C.); andre.marette@criucpq.ulaval.ca (A.M.)
2 School of Nutrition, Université Laval, Québec, QC G1V 0A6, Canada
3 Quebec Heart and Lung Institute (IUCPQ) Research Center, 2725 Chemin Sainte-Foy, Québec, QC G1V 4G5, Canada
4 Endocrinology and Nephrology Unit, CHU de Québec-Université Laval, Québec, QC G1V 4G2, Canada
* Correspondence: marie-claude.vohl@fsaa.ulaval.ca

Abstract: Consumption of red raspberries has been reported to exert acute beneficial effects on postprandial glycemia, insulinemia, triglyceridemia, and cytokine levels in metabolically disturbed subjects. In a two-arm parallel-group, randomized, controlled trial, 59 subjects with overweight or abdominal obesity and with slight hyperinsulinemia or hypertriglyceridemia were randomized to consume 280 g/day of frozen raspberries or to maintain their usual diet for 8 weeks. Primary analyses measured metabolic differences between the groups. Secondary analyses performed with omics tools in the intervention group assessed blood gene expression and plasma metabolomic changes following the raspberry supplementation. The intervention did not significantly affect plasma insulin, glucose, inflammatory marker concentrations, nor blood pressure. Following the supplementation, 43 genes were differentially expressed, and several functional pathways were enriched, a major portion of which were involved in the regulation of cytotoxicity, immune cell trafficking, protein signal transduction, and interleukin production. In addition, 10 serum metabolites were found significantly altered, among which β-alanine, trimethylamine N-oxide, and bioactive lipids. Although the supplementation had no meaningful metabolic effects, these results highlight the impact of a diet rich in raspberry on the immune function and phospholipid metabolism, thus providing novel insights into potential immune-metabolic pathways influenced by regular raspberry consumption.

Keywords: berry fruits; metabolic syndrome; multi-omics; immunity; gene expression; sphingolipids; phenolic compounds

1. Introduction

Both clinical and epidemiological studies highlight the contribution of a plant-food-predominant diet in the maintenance, or even the improvement, of metabolic homeostasis owing to its fiber and phytochemical contents [1]. Long-term consumption of a diet poor in these components constitutes the main predisposing factor to metabolic homeostasis dysregulation [2,3]. Metabolic dysregulations can be seen as a broad range of intermediate phenotypes, all converging with time toward metabolic syndrome, a cluster of interrelated immune-metabolic abnormalities increasing the risk of developing type 2 diabetes or atherosclerotic diseases [4]. Although public health authorities promote plant-food-predominant diets [5], efforts to increase vegetable and fruit consumption have been hardly efficient. Accordingly, it has been demonstrated that dietary habits are difficult to change over the long term [6], highlighting the need to identify simple nutritional interventions that increase the fiber and phytochemical contents of the diet. In this regard, growing evidence has supported the role of berry fruits in the prevention and management of metabolic disorders [7]. Among the most commonly consumed berries, red raspberry (Rb; *Rubus idaeus* L.) is low in sugar and particularly rich in both fiber and phenolic compounds, mostly anthocyanins, and ellagitannins [8].

Collectively, in vitro and ex vivo research conducted with Rb extracts or purified components have revealed various antioxidative, anti-inflammatory, and metabolic properties through which Rb components may help treat or improve immune-metabolic abnormalities [9,10]. Several animal studies have confirmed these beneficial effects with both Rb components and the entire fruit [11–13]. Moreover, some of these studies brought to light the immunomodulatory effects of Rb phenolic compounds [14,15]. Altogether, these results are consistent with those observed with black raspberry (*Rubus occidentalis*), although of reduced amplitude for an equal amount, presumably attributable to its lower phenolic content [16,17]. Unlike the black raspberry, for which the health-promoting effects have been confirmed in numerous human studies [18,19], very few human randomized controlled intervention studies have been undertaken to assess the health impact of whole Rb or its components, and most of them looked only at the short-term metabolic impact [20–25].

In that respect, the aims of this randomized controlled clinical trial were to investigate the health effects of Rb consumption on immune-metabolic features in subjects at risk of developing metabolic syndrome and to delineate the mechanisms underlying these effects through transcriptomics and metabolomics. In the context of personalized nutrition, this holistic approach is part of the efforts undertaken to further understand the impact of foods or nutrients on metabolic syndrome.

2. Materials and Methods

2.1. Study Participants and Eligibility Criteria

A two-arm parallel-group, randomized, controlled trial of the effects of Rb consumption on immune-metabolic parameters was conducted at the Institute of Nutrition and Functional Foods (INAF) at Université Laval between January 2018 and August 2019. Study participants from the greater Quebec City metropolitan area were recruited through emails, newspapers, and media advertisements. A total of 468 individuals contacted our research team for information related to the study, among which 119 were scheduled for a screening visit at the clinical investigation unit, and 59 were found to be eligible to participate in the study (Figure 1).

The age and medical history of participants were assessed at week 0, before the beginning of the intervention. To be included in the study, subjects had to be men or pre-menopausal women, Caucasian, aged between 18 to 60 years, have a body-mass index (BMI) between 25 and 40 kg/m^2 or a waist circumference $\geq$ 94 cm for men and $\geq$80 cm for women, as well as meet at least one of the following criteria: Plasma triglycerides (TG) > 1.35 mmol/L, or insulin concentration > 42 pmol/L, using our new analytic method and corresponding to a threshold value of 60 pmol/L with the former method that was predictive of a higher risk of cardiovascular disease in the Quebec population [26]. Subjects were excluded if they had a diagnosis for diabetes, hypercholesterolemia, or hypertension, had a taste aversion for or were allergic or intolerant to Rb, were taking medication known to affect study parameters, had taken antibiotics, supplements, or natural health products on a regular basis over the past 3 months, had undergone surgery in the last 3 months, or had planned surgery during the duration of the study. Nicotine usage, non-conventional dietary patterns (e.g., vegan, gluten-free or ketogenic diets), bodyweight loss or gain greater than 5% in the last 3 months, or daily alcohol consumption greater than 2 drinks were also considered exclusion criteria. The study was approved by the Université Laval Ethics Committee in January 2018 (CER-Université 2017–218). Upon recruitment, written informed consent was obtained from all subjects prior to the beginning of the study procedures. This trial was registered at clinicaltrials.gov as NCT03620617. Changes in anthropometric and metabolic variables in response to the Rb supplementation were defined as the primary outcomes, whereas pre- and post-supplementation changes in metabolomics and transcriptomics were considered as the secondary outcomes.

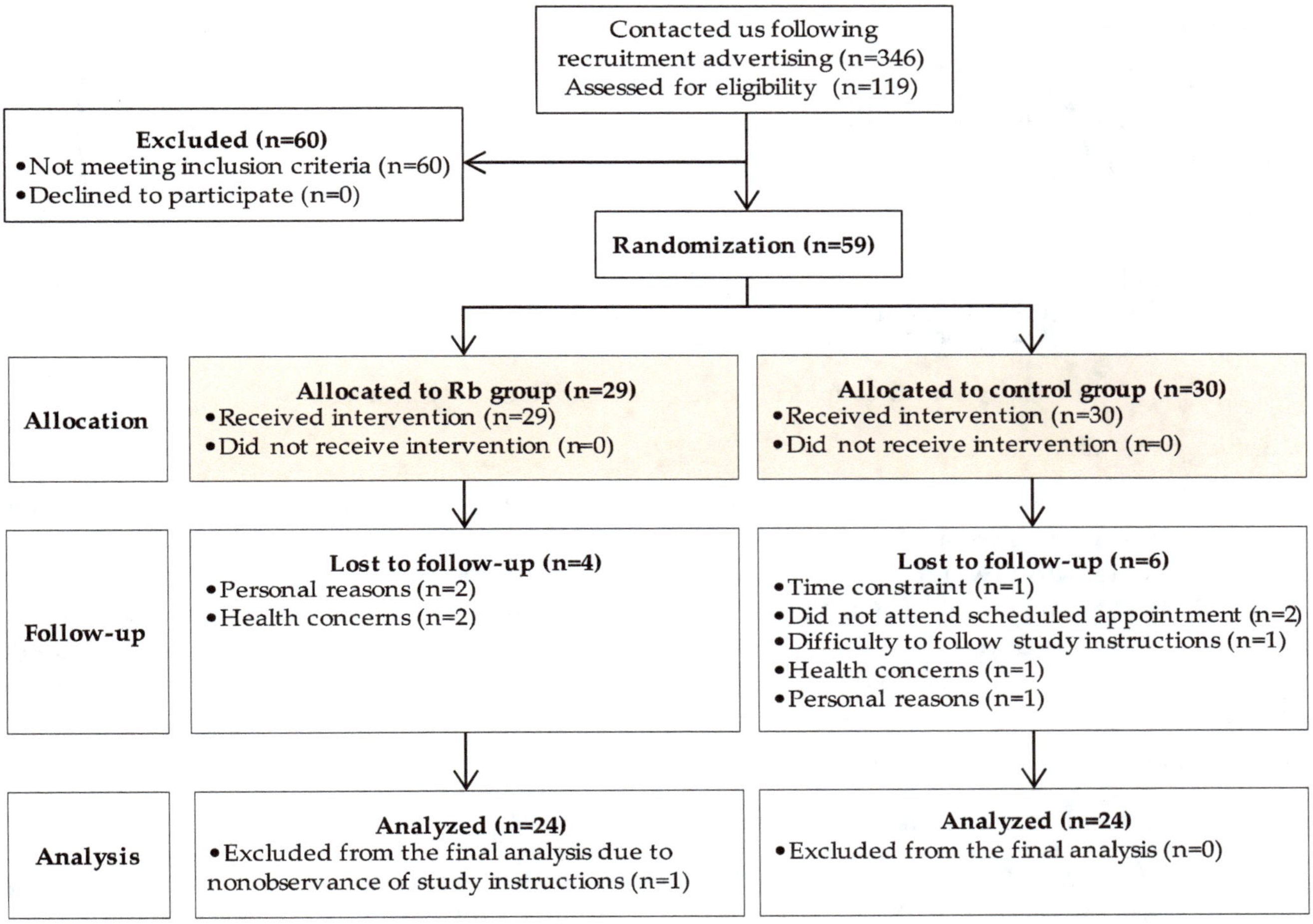

Figure 1. Patient flow diagram for recruitment, randomization, and data collection.

2.2. *Nutritional Intervention*

The randomization occurred after eligibility was confirmed. Participants were randomized to study arms using an in-house electronic management platform. A sex-stratified block randomization ensuring a 2:2 treatment allocation for each sex to either the intervention group consuming frozen Rb, or the control group was used (Figure 2). The randomization process was under the responsibility of the lead study coordinator. Three clinical coordinators and one graduate student were responsible for the recruitment and follow-up of participants in this study. None of the participants dropped out when they found out which group they had been assigned to. After a 2-week run-in period, participants assigned to the intervention group were invited to consume 280 g of frozen Rb daily (roughly 2 cups) for 8 weeks. Control group participants were invited to maintain their health and food habits stable for an 8-week period. Participants of both groups were scheduled for clinical visits after the run-in period (week 0), during the intervention (week 4), and at the end of the protocol (week 8). During the protocol, including the run-in period, participants were asked to avoid the use of supplements, natural health products, wine, or products with a polyphenolic profile similar to that of Rb and to limit the consumption of berries other than those provided, and any other products containing berries, to 2 portions per week. They were also instructed to limit coffee and tea consumption to 1 serving/day, and alcohol to 2 drinks/week. Participants had to complete a journal reporting any deviation from the dietary instructions listed above, as well as the Rb quantity consumed for the intervention group. The count of empty Rb packages returned by the participants was used to assess their compliance with the study protocol. Participants received regular emails to follow-up on any issues that may arise and to enhance adherence to the protocol.

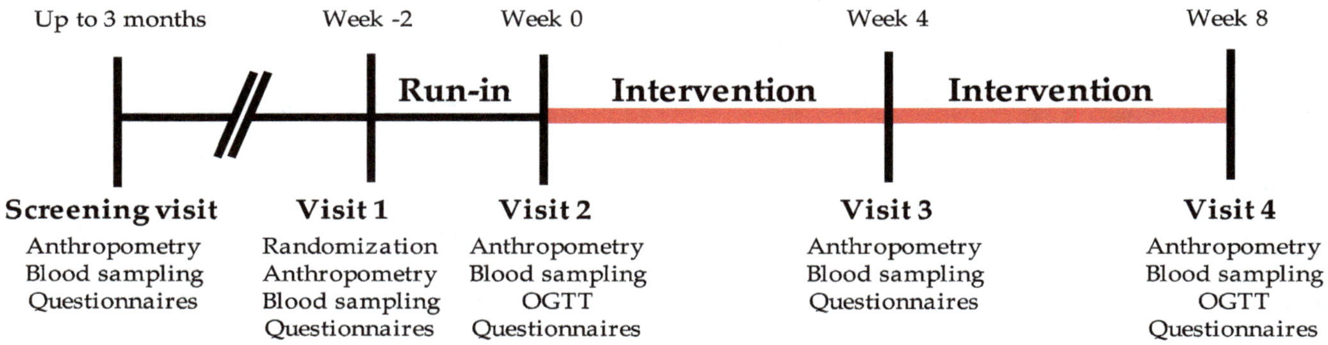

Figure 2. Graphical representation of the study protocol.

2.3. *Anthropometric Measurements*

At each clinical visit, waist and hip circumferences were measured to the nearest millimeter according to procedures recommended at the Airlie conference [27]. Height was also measured to the nearest millimeter. Bodyweight was measured using a BWB-800 electronic scale (Tanita, Arlington Heights, IL, USA) to an accuracy of 0.1 kg. For weight measurements, participants were asked to wear light indoor clothes and to remove their shoes. BMI was calculated as weight in kilograms divided by height in meters squared (kg/m^2). Systolic (SBP) and diastolic (DBP) blood pressure measurements were assessed while sitting on a chair after a 10 min rest. The mean of 3 measurements performed at 3 min intervals was used for the analyses.

2.4. *Nutritional and Physical Activity Assessments*

Nutritional habits were assessed at each clinical visit to the clinical investigation unit through the use of a web-based and self-administered Food Frequency Questionnaire (FFQ), validated for French-speaking Canadian adults [28]. The FFQ was based on 136 items grouped into the 8 following categories: Dairy products, fruits, vegetables, meat and alternatives, cereals and grain products, beverages, other foods, and supplements. Participants reported how often they consumed each item per day, per week, per month, or none at all in the last month. Finally, pictures with examples of portion sizes were used to reflect a better estimation of the portion consumed by the participant. Physical activity habits were evaluated using the Leisure Time Activity questionnaire, which was completed by participants at the beginning and at the end of the intervention [29].

2.5. *Biochemical Analyses*

Fasting plasma samples were collected on weeks 0, 4, and 8, and used to measure total-cholesterol (Total-C), LDL-cholesterol (LDL-C), HDL-cholesterol (HDL-C), TG, glucose, and insulin levels. Total-C and TG concentrations were measured using enzymatic assays [30]. Apolipoprotein B (ApoB) was measured by immunonephelometry assay using a Siemens Dimension Vista™ 1500 Analyzer. The HDL-C fraction was obtained after precipitation of VLDL and LDL particles in the infranatant with heparin manganese chloride. LDL-C was calculated with the Friedewald formula [31]. High-sensitivity C-reactive protein (CRP) levels were measured by immunoassay [32]. Fasting glycated hemoglobin

(HbA1c) was measured in plasma by immunoturbidimetry (Biorad HPLC D-100). Oral glucose tolerance tests (OGTTs) using a 75 g glucose solution were conducted twice during the intervention period (weeks 0 and 8). Blood samples were drawn at −15, 0, 15, 30, 60, 90, and 120 min during the OGTT to assess plasma insulin and glucose levels. Glucose concentrations were enzymatically measured [33], while insulin concentrations were measured by chemiluminescence (Siemens Advia Centaur XPT). The homeostatic model assessment of insulin resistance (HOMA-IR) index and the Matsuda index were calculated from OGTT values [34,35].

2.6. Transcriptomic Analyses

Gene expression profiling before and after the supplementation was conducted in whole blood, commonly used to assess the effects of dietary interventions in human trials [36]. The effects of Rb supplementation on the gene expression profile was examined in blood samples collected into PAXgene preparation tubes (Qiagen, Valencia, CA, USA) at week 0 and 8, and stored at −80 °C until the analyses. Total RNA was extracted, and samples were sent to the Génome Québec Innovation Centre (McGill University, Montreal, Canada) for sequencing. The purity and integrity of RNA samples were assessed using a 2100 Bioanalyzer (Agilent, Santa Clara, CA, USA). RNA samples were converted to cDNA with the Illumina NEB stranded mRNA library preparation kit (Illumina, San Diego, CA, USA) based on the manufacturer's protocol. The prepared libraries were then sequenced on an Illumina NovaSeq6000 S4 sequencer using paired-end, 100 bp reads. Quality trimming of the raw reads was carried out to remove bases with a Phred33 score < 30 and reads with less than 50 bases using Trim Galore (v0.6.5), a wrapper tool around Cutadapt (v1.15) and FastQC (v0.11.9). Kallisto (0.46.2) with 100 bootstraps and default parameters was run for alignment and normalization. Reads were aligned to the GRCh38 human reference transcriptome [37]. Transcriptomic data reported as counts per million (cpm), were filtered based on a worthwhile number of counts in a minimum number of samples in the edgeR v3.28.1 package [38]. The differential expression analysis was conducted using a generalization of a paired t-test implemented in the quasi-likelihood functionality of edgeR. Differentially expressed transcripts between pre- vs. post-intervention at a nominal p-value < 0.05 were considered for further analysis. The functional significance of genes showing at least a 25% difference (1.25-fold change) between pre- and post-supplementation states was explored by pathway enrichment analysis using the clusterProfiler v3.16.0 R package [39]. The clusterProfiler package implements statistical methods to analyze and visualize functional profiles of genes and gene clusters and produces adjusted p-values using the Benjamini–Hochberg procedure (BH-p) to indicate pathways that were significantly enriched. The following pathway databases were used for functional enrichment analysis: Gene Ontology Biological Processes (GO-BP) and the Kyoto Encyclopedia of Genes and Genomes (KEGG). Transcriptomic data analysis was implemented in R v3.6.3.

2.7. Metabolomic Analyses

The quantitative analysis of 630 metabolites from 26 biochemical classes was performed in paired plasma samples from 24 participants before and after the Rb supplementation with the MxP® Quant 500 kit (Biocrates Life Sciences AG, Innsbruck, Austria). The targeted metabolomic profiling was performed by the Analytical Facility for Bioactive Molecules at the Hospital for Sick Children (Toronto, Canada). Metabolite data from 24 matched participants were processed using the MetaboAnalystR package (v3.0) [39]. First, 117 features with a constant or single value across samples were found and deleted. Non-informative signals were further filtered out based on the interquartile range estimate, and samples were normalized by quantile normalization. Metabolite data were log-transformed and scaled by Pareto scaling. After quantile normalization, one more feature with a constant value was found and deleted. From the original 630 metabolites analyzed, a total of 382 were finally retained for statistical analysis. Paired t-tests were used to analyze within-subject changes in plasma metabolite levels between pre- and post-supplementation states. A volcano plot associated with paired t-tests was further used to identify the most differentially abundant metabolites between pre- and post-supplementation groups.

A p-value < 0.05, along with a count of significant pairs higher than 50% showing at least 25% difference (1.25-fold change), were the criteria used to consider metabolite plasma levels differing significantly between pre- and post-supplementation states. The dimensional reduction was conducted by using the partial least squares discriminant analysis (PLS-DA), a supervised algorithm able to reduce the number of metabolites in high-dimensional metabolomics data to produce robust and easy-to-interpret models. This method was able to differentiate the class membership through multivariate regression of a given set of metabolites. In the present study, we used a variation of PLS-DA, the multilevel PLS-DA (mPLS-DA), given its ability to exploit the paired structure of the multivariate data obtained before and after the Rb supplementation in the same group of participants [39,40]. Concretely, a sparse mPLS-DA (smPLS-DA) was used to identify the most important metabolites helping to discriminate matched study groups [41]. The smPLS-DA algorithm was implemented using the mixOmics R package (v6.12.1) [42]. Variable importance in projection (VIP) coefficients were computed as a weighted sum of squares of the smPLS-DA loadings to depict the relative importance of each metabolite in the classification model. Predictors with large VIP were the most relevant for discriminating class membership [43].

2.8. Statistical Analyses

The normality of distribution of all variables was assessed using skewness and kurtosis, and none of the variables needed transformation before analysis. Descriptive characteristics between the Rb and the control group were presented as means (±SD) or frequencies. Chi-square tests for categorical variables and analyses of variance (general linear model, type III sum of squares) for continuous variables were used to seek for inter-group differences in baseline characteristics and in changes between follow-up and baseline. The mixed procedure in SAS with special provisions for repeated measures that incorporated data from all visits was used to examine the effects of time, treatment, and their interaction on clinical variables. Data were adjusted for age, sex, BMI, and baseline values. For all analyses, a p-value < 0.05 was considered for statistical significance. Statistical analyses were performed using SAS version 3.8 (SAS Institute, Cary, NC, USA).

3. Results

3.1. Trial Flow, Baseline Characteristics, and Compliance

Of the 119 subjects screened for eligibility, 59 were enrolled in the study, 29 were randomized to the Rb group, and 30 to the control group (Figure 2). Eleven participants (6 and 5 from the Rb and control group, respectively) withdrew during follow-up by the inability to comply with study procedures or schedule conflict. Therefore, 48 subjects were included in the per-protocol analysis.

According to BMI values, 22 subjects had obesity (BMI > 30 kg/m^2), 19 were overweight (BMI between 25 and 30 kg/m^2), and 7 were in the normal weight range (BMI < 25 kg/m^2). The mean BMI of participants was 29.9 kg/m^2 (ranging from 22.3–43.7), and the mean age was 32.2 years (ranging from 22 to 57). Upon randomization, baseline characteristics were well-distributed at baseline and, therefore, no significant differences between the Rb group and the control group were observed for age, sex, anthropometric, physiologic, or metabolic variables (Table 1). However, although not statistically significant, the HOMA-IR difference between groups may be considered as clinically meaningful. No adverse events related to Rb supplementation were reported during the study. Adherence to the study protocol was good, with an overall compliance of 92.8%.

Table 1. Clinical and laboratory baseline characteristics of study participants.

Variable	N	Control			N	Rb			*p*-value
Sex (men/women)	24		9/15		24		7/17		0.54
Age (years)	24	31.92	±	8.05	24	32.46	±	10.12	0.83
BMI (kg/m^2)	24	29.38	±	3.94	24	30.42	±	5.00	0.43
Waist circumference (cm)	24	98.10	±	11.81	24	98.53	±	13.32	0.90
Fasting glucose (mmol/L)	24	4.84	±	0.47	23	4.98	±	0.59	0.38
Fasting insulin (pmol/L)	22	73.91	±	33.57	19	83.11	±	43.54	0.21
HbA1C (%)	24	5.05	±	0.29	24	5.03	±	0.31	0.85
Plasma TG (mmol/L)	24	1.56	±	0.78	24	1.46	±	0.80	0.66
ApoB-100 (g/L)	24	0.88	±	0.17	24	0.92	±	0.24	0.48
HDL-C (mmol/L)	24	1.33	±	0.23	24	1.32	±	0.40	0.94
LDL-C (mmol/L)	24	2.55	±	0.74	24	2.65	±	0.86	0.69
CRP (mg/L)	24	2.72	±	2.82	23	2.68	±	2.34	0.95
HOMA-IR	13	1.78	±	0.76	11	2.84	±	1.73	0.06
MATSUDA	13	5.79	±	2.43	11	4.54	±	2.24	0.21

Data are means ± standard deviations. Sex is presented as counts. *p*-values were obtained by a general linear model, type III sum of squares, and chi-square tests (sex). BMI, body mass index. HbA1C, glycated hemoglobin. TG, triglycerides. ApoB-100, Apolipoprotein B. HDL-C, high-density lipoprotein cholesterol. LDL-C, low-density lipoprotein cholesterol. CRP, C-reactive protein. HOMA-IR, homeostatic model assessment of insulin resistance.

3.2. *Food Intake and Physical Activity*

There was no significant difference in energy intake between groups at any time point during the protocol. Accordingly, no significant treatment by time interactions was found in macronutrients or other nutritional compounds, with the exception of those deriving directly from Rb composition, namely glucose, fructose, soluble and insoluble fiber (Table 2). According to the FFQ data, adding 2 cups/day of Rb accounted, respectively, for 17.6%, 17.1%, 13.3%, and 25.5% of total dietary glucose, fructose, soluble, and insoluble fibers intakes. Moreover, when analyzing dietary intakes based on food groups (bread and cereals, fruits, vegetables, dairy products, animal proteins), there were no significant differences between groups except for fruit consumption ($p < 0.0001$, a mean of 2, 3 portions for the control group vs. 6 portions for the Rb group during the intervention). The intervention resulted in a nutritionally significant shift (around 3 servings) in fruit consumption in the Rb group. Physical activity remained stable throughout the protocol (Table 2).

3.3. *Primary Outcomes*

We found no significant differences between follow-up and baseline values between control and intervention groups for any of the parameters analyzed (Table 3). The statistical adjustment for age, sex, and BMI had no effect on the lack of differences between the Rb and control groups (data not shown).

Repeated measures analysis revealed a significant treatment by time interaction effect on SBP ($p = 0.03$) and plasma ApoB levels ($p = 0.03$) (Table 4). Indeed, in the control group, we found a significant increase in plasma ApoB concentrations from the beginning of the intervention (0.86–0.16 g/L) to the mid-point visit (0.95–0.17 g/L), before regaining its initial level at the end of the study (0.87–0.19 g/L). Again, a significant effect of time was observed for both HDL-C ($p = 0.03$) and LDL-C ($p = 0.01$) in the control group. There was no other singular or interaction effect of time and treatment for any other metabolic or anthropometric variable. In accordance to the lack of change in fasting and postprandial plasma insulin and glucose concentrations in response to the intervention, both HOMA-IR and MATSUDA indexes derived from OGGT were not found to differ significantly.

Table 2. Daily dietary intakes by nutrients and by food group over time within and between groups.

Time	Week 0		Week 4		Week 8		*p*-Values		
Treatment	**Control**	**Rb**	**Control**	**Rb**	**Control**	**Rb**	**Time**	**tx**	**tx*Time**
Energy (kcal)	2132.8 ± 823.2	2059.7 ± 662.1	1992.7 ± 692.4	1983.3 ± 682.1	2060.7 ± 638.7	2075.8 ± 623.2	0.32	0.70	0.83
Lipids (g)	93.5 ± 44.9	82.7 ± 28.6	87.7 ± 40.9	76.4 ± 31.8	91.4 ± 37.7	80.9 ± 28.7	0.25	0.60	0.99
Proteins (g)	90.1 ± 37.3	87.2 ± 30.9	87.4 ± 32.1	84.0 ± 30.1	91.9 ± 28.6	88.3 ± 30.8	0.53	0.68	1.00
Soluble Fiber (g)	8.3 ± 4.1	7.7 [a] ± 3.3	7.3 [x] ± 3.4	8.5 [y] ± 3.1	7.5 [x] ± 3.1	8.9 [by] ± 3.1	0.69	0.01	0.02
Insoluble Fiber (g)	15.6 ± 7.8	15.0 [x] ± 6.8	13.8 [a] ± 6.9	23.1 [by] ± 6.6	14.4 [x] ± 6.2	23.8 [by] ± 6.3	<0.0001	<0.0001	<0.0001
Fructose (g)	24.1 [a] ± 14.4	24.9 [a] ± 9.9	19.3 [bx] ± 8.9	29.7 [by] ± 9.4	22.2 [x] ± 9.0	29.9 [by] ± 8.9	0.41	<0.0001	0.002
Glucose (g)	23.7 [a] ± 13.3	25.1 [a] ± 8.9	19.8 [bx] ± 8.8	30.2 [by] ± 7.9	22.2 [x] ± 8.8	30.9 [by] ± 7.8	0.18	<0.0001	0.0005
Alcohol (g)	3.2 ± 3.6	2.8 ± 2.8	2.5 ± 2.1	1.9 ± 1.7	2.8 ± 2.5	2.3 ± 1.4	0.07	0.37	0.95
Caffeine (mg)	147.7 ± 148.9	103.6 ± 114.9	147.9 ± 142.7	95.2 ± 126.9	150.0 ± 149.7	106.6 ± 142.7	0.59	0.65	0.73
Bread and cereals (serving)	3.9 ± 2.2	4.6 ± 2.3	4.0 ± 2.0	4.1 ± 2.6	4.1 ± 2.3	4.1 ± 1.9	0.45	0.36	0.26
Fruits (serving)	2.9 [a] ± 2.6	3.1 [a] ± 1.6	2.2 [bx] ± 1.7	6.0 [by] ± 1.3	2.9 [x] ± 1.9	5.9 [by] ± 1.3	<0.0001	<0.0001	<0.0001
Vegetables (serving)	3.6 ± 1.9	3.6 ± 2.3	3.3 ± 1.6	2.6 ± 1.6	3.4 ± 1.6	3.2 ± 2.1	0.02	0.10	0.41
Dairy products (serving)	2.0 ± 1.7	2.2 ± 1.1	2.0 ± 1.3	2.3 ± 1.3	1.8 ± 0.9	2.2 ± 1.4	0.69	0.51	0.74
Animal proteins (serving)	2.3 ± 1.2	1.8 ± 0.9	2.2 ± 1.2	1.8 ± 0.8	2.5 ± 1.2	2.0 ± 1.1	0.13	0.39	0.93
Physical activity (AMI)	298.1 ± 147.0	259.0 ± 131.9			280.8 ± 190.5	218.3 ± 159.9	0.13	0.34	0.54

Data are means ± standard deviations. A mixed model adjusted for age, sex, BMI, and baseline values was used to obtain *p*-values. Time effect, treatment effect, and the interaction of treatment by time were significant at $\alpha = 0{,}05$. Significant *p*-values are in bold. Letters stand for significant differences (a,b for time effect and x,y for treatment effect). $N = 24$ for both Rb and control. tx, treatment. AMI, Activity Metabolic Index. tx*Time stands for the interaction between treatment and time effects.

Table 3. Differences between follow-up and baseline.

Variable	N	Control	*N*	Rb	*p*-Value
BMI (kg/m^2)	24	−0.01 ± 0.60	24	+0.10 ± 0.57	0.43
Waist circumference (cm)	24	−0.18 ± 2.18	24	+0.39 ± 3.12	0.46
Fasting glucose (mmol/L)	23	+0.01 ± 0.35	22	−0.09 ± 0.29	0.27
Fasting insulin (pmol/L)	19	+3.10 ± 22.98	16	+3.12 ± 26.49	0.99
HbA1C (%)	23	−0.03 ± 0.13	23	+0.03 ± 0.14	0.13
Plasma TG (mmol/L)	22	−0.04 ± 0.53	23	−0.17 ± 0.68	0.48
ApoB-100 (g/L)	23	+0.01 ± 0.09	23	−0.03 ± 0.12	0.30
HDL-C (mmol/L)	23	−0.04 ± 0.10	23	−0.01 ± 0.18	0.43
LDL-C (mmol/L)	22	+0.01 ± 0.42	23	+0.03 ± 0.42	0.89
CRP (mg/L)	20	+0.90 ± 2.33	22	−0.04 ± 1.59	0.14
HOMA-IR	13	+0.11 ± 0.74	11	−0.16 ± 0.53	0.33
Matsuda index	13	−0.60 ± 2.08	11	+0.14 ± 1.43	0.33

Data are means ± standard deviations. *p*-values were obtained by a general linear model, type III sum of squares. BMI, body mass index. HbA1C, glycated hemoglobin. TG, triglycerides. ApoB-100, Apolipoprotein B. HDL-C, high-density lipoprotein cholesterol. LDL-C, low-density lipoprotein cholesterol. CRP, C-reactive protein. HOMA-IR, homeostatic model assessment of insulin resistance.

Table 4. Variations of anthropometrics, body composition, and blood pressure parameters over time within and between groups.

Time	Week 0				Week 4		Week 8		*p*-Values		
Treatment	**N**	**Control**	**N**	**Rb**	**Control**	**Rb**	**Control**	**Rb**	**Time**	**tx**	**tx*Time**
SBP (mmHg)	24	110.8 ± 11.2	24	112.8 ± 11.0	110.7 ± 12.9	113.1 ± 10.4	112.8 ± 11.9	110.9 ± 11.0	0.99	0.37	0.03
DBP (mmHg)	24	68.9 ± 8.7	24	71.9 ± 8.9	68.8 ± 10.4	71.8 ± 9.0	69.6 ± 11.1	70.3 ± 9.3	0.86	0.67	0.34
BMI (kg/m2)	24	29.4 ± 3.9	24	30.4 ± 4.9	29.5 ± 3.9	30.5 ± 5.0	29.4 ± 3.9	30.5 ± 5.1	0.44	0.69	0.69
Waist circumference (cm)	24	98.1 ± 11.8	24	98.5 ± 13.3	98.5 ± 12.1	98.4 ± 13.3	97.9 ± 12.9	98.9 ± 14.1	0.93	0.73	0.23
Hips circumference (cm)	24	108.9 ± 7.5	24	112.1 ± 10.2	109.5 ± 8.4	112.3 ± 10.5	109.3 ± 8.4	112.1 ± 10.5	0.63	0.59	0.77
CRP	20	2.50 ± 2.50	21	2.1 ± 1.64	2.65 ± 2.60	2.86 ± 2.59	2.46 ± 2.42	3.28 ± 2.67	0.30	0.16	0.26
ApoB-100	23	0.86 [a] ± 0.16	23	0.92 ± 0.24	0.95 [b] ± 0.17	0.92 [y] ± 0.21	0.87 [a] ± 0.19	0.89 ± 0.25	0.002	0.02	0.03
Total-C (mmol/L)	23	4.53 [a] ± 0.79	23	4.60 ± 0.91	4.85 [b] ± 0.81	4.70 ± 0.84	4.51 [a] ± 0.88	4.54 ± 0.86	0.001	0.14	0.22
HDL-C (mmol/L)	23	1.33 ± 0.23	23	1.30 ± 0.40	1.39 [a] ± 0.29	1.32 ± 0.35	1.29 [b] ± 0.27	1.30 ± 0.33	0.03	0.49	0.17
LDL-C (mmol/L)	22	2.44 [a] ± 0.67	23	2.62 ± 0.87	2.78 [b] ± 0.68	2.74 ± 0.78	2.45 [a] ± 0.55	2.65 ± 0.82	0.001	0.42	0.14
TG (mmol/L)	22	1.42 ± 0.61	23	1.47 ± 0.82	1.32 ± 0.60	1.39 ± 0.64	1.38 ± 0.61	1.29 ± 0.61	0.37	0.59	0.72
Fasting glucose (mmol/L)	23	4.82 ± 0.47	22	5.00 ± 0.59	4.85 ± 0.49	5.11 ± 0.57	4.83 ± 0.52	4.91 ± 0.57	0.12	0.99	0.25
Fasting insulin (pmol/L)	17	65.3 ± 29.0	16	80.1 ± 37.4	65.9 ± 29.1	77.5 ± 33.2	64.0 ± 23.2	83.3 ± 44.2	0.77	0.59	0.10
HbA1C (%)	23	5.02 ± 0.27	23	5.04 ± 0.32	4.98 ± 0.29	5.03 ± 0.30	5.00 ± 0.27	5.07 ± 0.29	0.11	0.22	0.23

Data are means ± standard deviations. A mixed model adjusted for age, sex, BMI, and baseline values was used to obtain *p*-values (except for BMI and waist circumference, which were adjusted for age, sex, and baseline values only). Time effect, treatment effect, and the interaction of treatment by time were significant at $\alpha = 0.5$. Significant *p*-values are in bold. Letters stand for significant differences (a,b for time effect and x,y for treatment effect). tx, treatment. SPB, systolic blood pressure. DBP, diastolic blood pressure. BMI, body mass index. CRP, C-reactive protein. ApoB-100, Apolipoprotein B. Total-C, total cholesterol. HDL-C, high-density lipoprotein cholesterol. LDL-C, low-density lipoprotein cholesterol. TG, triglycerides. HbA1C, glycated hemoglobin. HOMA-IR, homeostatic model assessment insulin resistance. tx*Time stands for the interaction between treatment and time effects.

3.4. *Secondary Outcomes*

3.4.1. Effects of Rb Supplementation on Gene Expression

The study of differential gene expression in blood cells in the Rb group revealed a total of 1384 genes differentially expressed following Rb supplementation ($p < 0.05$), from which 119 showed a fold change greater than 1.25. Following multiple testing correction, none of these genes reached the significance threshold of FDR-$p < 0.05$. We then relaxed the significance criteria in order to identify those genes differentially expressed at $p < 0.001$ (Table 5). A total of 43 genes were identified, among which 9 were found to be upregulated and 34 downregulated, with fold changes ranging from −1.5 (*ADGRG1*) to 1.4 (*PNPLA4*), with 8 of the 43 genes demonstrating at least a 1.25-fold change (Figure 3A). Individual changes in gene expression levels for the top differentially up- and down-regulated genes presented in Figure 3B illustrate the inter-individual variability of gene expression changes among participants.

The pathway enrichment analysis was conducted with all of the 119 genes showing at least a p-value < 0.05 and a fold change > 1.25 in response to the Rb supplementation (Figure 3C). Most differentially expressed genes were clustered into intracellular signal transduction pathways, as shown by the top-12 significantly enriched GO-BP categories, including those involved in the regulation of Ras and Rho signal transduction and several pathways related to the production of interleukins IL-6 and IL-1β. A relevant signal transduction pathway related to MAPK signaling was also found to be significantly enriched in the KEGG database.

3.4.2. Effects of Rb Supplementation on Metabolite Levels

Paired t-test analysis brought out that, following Rb supplementation, a total of 14 metabolites had significantly different plasma levels (paired t-test p-value < 0.05), as compared to pre-supplementation levels. This number was reduced to 10 metabolites after applying more restricted statistical significance criteria (fold-change >1.25 and significant metabolite counts > 50%) (Figure 4A and Table 6). Plasma metabolites showing a significant reduction following Rb supplementation are shown on the top-left corner of the paired volcano plot, and those showing a significant increase are shown on the top-right corner (Figure 4A). Top-three under- and over-abundant metabolites are shown in paired boxplots in Figure 4B. More specifically, we identified β-alanine, deoxycholic acid glycine conjugate (GDCA), and trimethylamine N-oxide (TMAO) among the metabolites showing the most significant increase following Rb supplementation. On the other hand, three TG species, TG (16:1/32:1), TG (18:2/32:2) and TG (18:0/32:0), were among the metabolites undergoing a significant decrease (respectively -0.96 ± 1.83, -1.04 ± 1.99 and -0.93 ± 2.17 μmol/L, $p = 0.02$, 0.02 and 0.04). The score plot derived from smPLS-DA shows the complete separation of pre- and post-supplementation groups, without overlap (Figure 4C). Component 1 was the main one responsible for group discrimination, accounting for 5% of the variance, with component 2 accounting for 2.4%, respectively. The 10 metabolites associated with the first component and underlying the discrimination between pre- and post-supplementation groups are shown in the loadings panel of the first component (Figure 4D). Most of these metabolites were also identified as differentially abundant between pre- and post-supplementation groups (Figure 4B).

Table 5. List of the most significant differentially expressed genes in Rb group after 8 weeks of Rb supplementation.

RefSeq	Gene Symbol	Gene Name	Nominal p-Value	FDR	FC
NM_001114759	*ZNF683*	Zinc finger protein 683	4.5×10^{-6}	0.07	−1.28
NM_001470	*GABBR1*	Gamma-aminobutyric acid type B receptor subunit 1	7.4×10^{-6}	0.07	1.22
NM_033423	*GZMH*	Granzyme H	2.5×10^{-5}	0.12	−1.19
NM_031950	*FGFBP2*	Fibroblast growth factor binding protein 2	2.6×10^{-5}	0.12	−1.20
NM_030760	*S1PR5*	Sphingosine-1-phosphate receptor 5	4.8×10^{-5}	0.18	−1.21
NM_139355	*MATK*	Megakaryocyte-associated tyrosine kinase	8.4×10^{-5}	0.26	−1.16
NM_020395	*INTS12*	Integrator complex subunit 12	9.5×10^{-5}	0.26	1.39
NM_001144884	*SLC30A7*	Solute carrier family 30 member 7	1.7×10^{-4}	0.28	1.23
NM_005170	*ASCL2*	Achaete-scute family bHLH transcription factor 2	1.8×10^{-4}	0.28	−1.16
NM_025069	*ZNF703*	Zinc finger protein 703	1.9×10^{-4}	0.28	−1.14
NM_001083116	*PRF1*	Perforin 1	2.1×10^{-4}	0.28	−1.25
NM_138360	*CARMIL3*	Capping protein regulator and myosin 1 linker 3	2.1×10^{-4}	0.28	−1.29
NM_005601	*NKG7*	Natural killer cell granule protein 7 (1)	2.2×10^{-4}	0.28	−1.20
NM_001024401	*SBK1*	SH3 domain binding kinase 1	2.2×10^{-4}	0.28	−1.12
NM_006653	*FRS3*	Fibroblast growth factor receptor substrate 3	2.2×10^{-4}	0.28	1.17
NR_110601	*PGS1*	Phosphatidylglycerophosphate synthase 1	2.9×10^{-4}	0.33	1.20
NR_110030	*LINC01215*	Long intergenic non-protein coding RNA 1215	3.0×10^{-4}	0.33	1.24
NM_001363693	*NKG7*	Natural killer cell granule protein 7 (2)	3.2×10^{-4}	0.33	−1.24
NM_001145770	*ADGRG1*	Adhesion G protein-coupled receptor G1	3.5×10^{-4}	0.34	−1.52
NR_024618	*LINC02035*	Long intergenic non-protein coding RNA 2035	3.6×10^{-4}	0.34	1.14
NM_000234	*LIG1*	DNA ligase 1	3.9×10^{-4}	0.34	−1.23
NM_001122630	*CDKN1C*	Cyclin dependent kinase inhibitor 1C	3.9×10^{-4}	0.34	-1.18
NM_170783	*ZNRD1*	Zinc ribbon domain containing 1	4.1×10^{-4}	0.34	−1.22
NM_013432	*TONSL*	Tonsoku like, DNA repair protein	4.8×10^{-4}	0.36	−1.15
NM_001145777	*FKBP5*	FKBP prolyl isomerase 5	4.9×10^{-4}	0.36	1.19
NM_198053	*CD247*	CD247 molecule	5.1×10^{-4}	0.36	−1.10
NM_032737	*LMNB2*	Lamin B2	5.2×10^{-4}	0.36	−1.09
NM_004650	*PNPLA4*	Patatin like phospholipase domain containing 4 (1)	6.2×10^{-4}	0.37	−1.30
NM_001271822	*SERPINB6*	Serpin family B member 6	6.2×10^{-4}	0.37	−1.17
NM_001358511	*PRDX5*	Peroxiredoxin 5	6.4×10^{-4}	0.37	−1.29
NM_005686	*SOX13*	SRY-box transcription factor 13	6.4×10^{-4}	0.37	−1.14
NM_017931	*TTC38*	Tetratricopeptide repeat domain 38	6.4×10^{-4}	0.37	−1.12
NM_001142389	*PNPLA4*	Patatin like phospholipase domain containing 4 (2)	6.8×10^{-4}	0.37	1.43
NM_012483	*GNLY*	Granulysin	6.9×10^{-4}	0.37	−1.18
NM_001004310	*FCRL6*	Fc receptor like 6	6.9×10^{-4}	0.37	−1.20
NM_024310	*PLEKHF1*	Pleckstrin homology and FYVE domain containing 1	7.2×10^{-4}	0.37	−1.16
NM_013351	*TBX21*	T-box transcription factor 21	7.3×10^{-4}	0.37	−1.18
NM_007182	*RASSF1*	Ras association domain family member 1	7.6×10^{-4}	0.37	−1.14
NM_006056	*NMUR1*	Neuromedin U receptor 1	7.7×10^{-4}	0.37	−1.13
NM_001110556	*FLNA*	Filamin A	8.9×10^{-4}	0.42	−1.12
NM_004669	*CLIC3*	Chloride intracellular channel 3	9.3×10^{-4}	0.42	−1.22
NM_001136044	*TMUB1*	Transmembrane and ubiquitin-like domain containing 1	9.3×10^{-4}	0.42	−1.11
NM_001335	*CTSW*	Cathepsin W	9.5×10^{-4}	0.42	−1.14

RefSeq stands for the reference sequence accession number. A negative fold change stands for a decrease in gene expression levels following Rb supplementation. FDR stands for False Discovery Rate-adjusted p-values obtained by paired t-test. FC stands for fold change. Numbers in parentheses in the Gene name column stand for transcript variants.

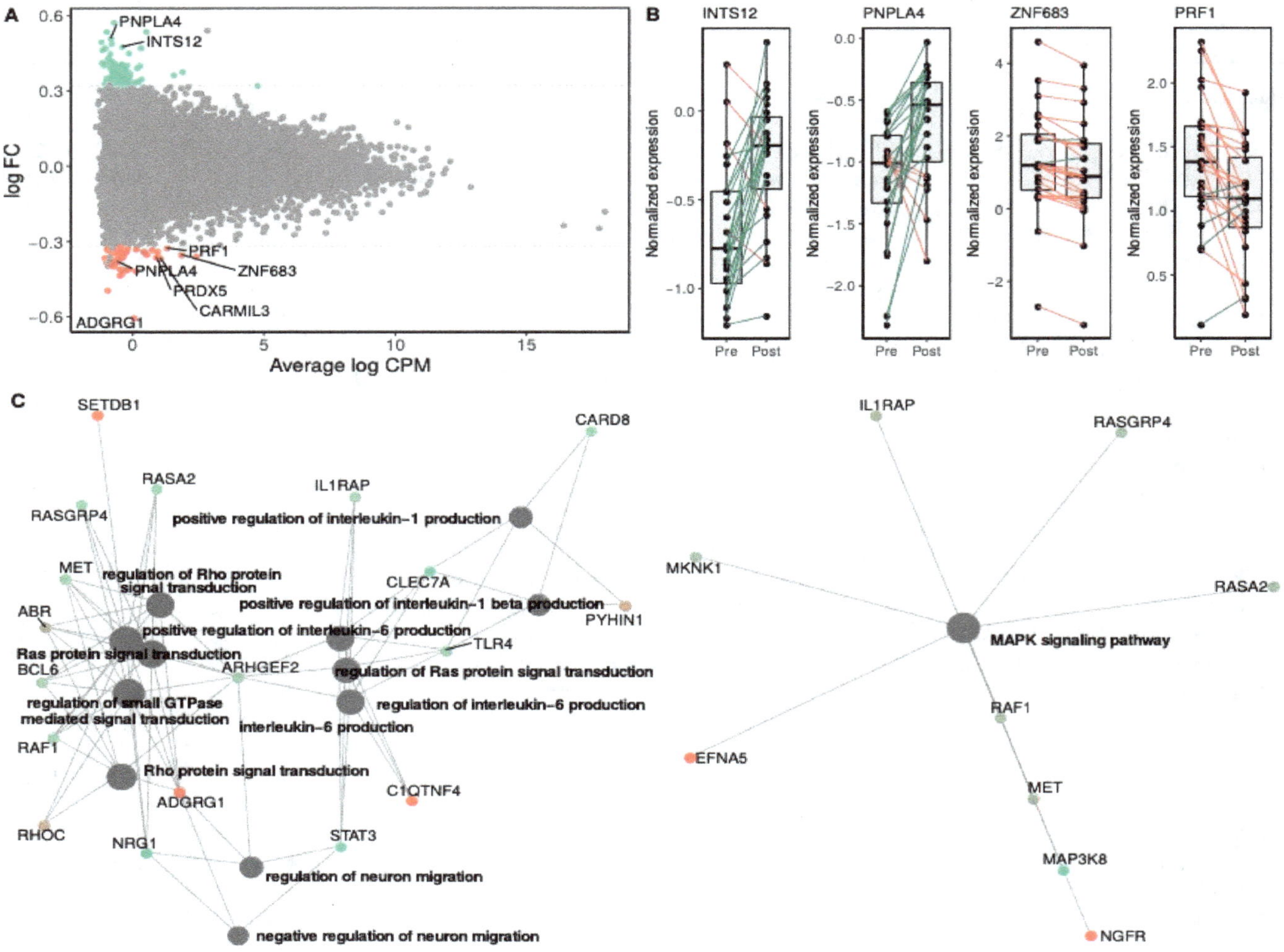

Figure 3. Gene expression change between pre- and post-supplementation states in the Rb group. Panel (**A**) shows the log2 average abundance of transcripts in counts per million mapped reads (log CPM) on the x-axis and the log2 fold-change (log FC) on the y-axis. Non-significant genes are represented by grey dots. Over- and under-expressed genes (FC > 1.25) with unadjusted significant differences (paired t-test p-value < 0.05) are colored in green and red, respectively. Significant differentially expressed genes from paired t-tests (p-value < 0.001) and showing at least a 1.25 FC are labeled with gene names. The dashed lines represent 1.25 FC. Panel (**B**) shows the top differentially expressed genes between pre- and post-supplementation states in the Rb group. Box and whisker plots show median, first, and third quartiles, and maximum and minimum values for the 24 sample pairs before (Pre) and after (Post) the Rb supplementation. The three transcripts, which exhibited the most significant (p-value < 0.001) over- and under-expression derived from paired t-tests (post vs. pre), are shown on the top and bottom rows, respectively. Green and red lines stand for increasing or decreasing gene expression levels between pre- and post-supplementation states within individual paired samples. Panel (**C**) shows network plots of enriched terms following the Rb supplementation. Network plots depict the linkages among differentially regulated gene clusters and functional enriched terms in the Gene Ontology Biological Processes (GO-BP) (left) and Kyoto Encyclopedia of Genes and Genomes (KEGG) (right) pathway databases. The size of the grey dots is proportional to the number of genes in the enriched pathway (from 7 to 13 genes), and the red-to-green color gradient of gene dots represents the direction of the gene expression fold-change following the Rb supplementation.

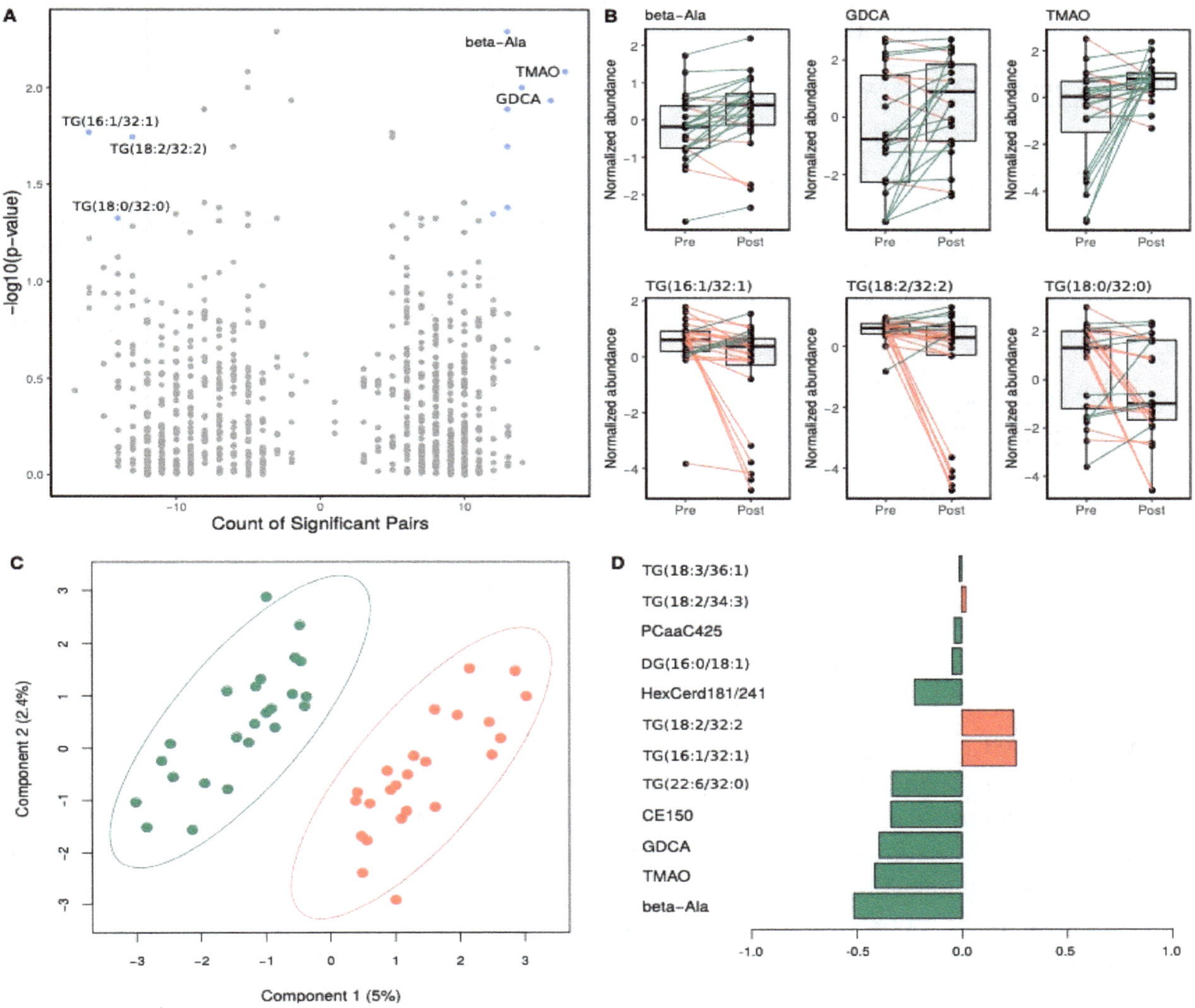

Figure 4. Impact of Rb supplementation on plasma metabolite levels. Panel (**A**) shows a volcano plot of paired comparisons between metabolite plasma levels in pre- and post-supplementation groups. On the x-axis, a count of significant sample pairs is shown. On the y-axis, the minus logarithm of paired t-test p-values is shown. Metabolites showing statistically significant changes following the Rb supplementation (p-value < 0.05 and fold change > 1.25) are depicted as blue dots on the right (increase) and left (decrease) top corners. Top-three significantly different metabolites of both increasing and decreasing values are labeled. Panel (**B**) shows top metabolites showing significant changes following Rb supplementation. Box and whisker plots show median, first, and third quartiles, and maximum and minimum values for the 24 sample pairs before (Pre) and after (Post) the Rb supplementation. The three metabolites, which exhibited the most significant decrease and increase following the supplementation, are shown on the top and bottom rows, respectively. Green and red lines stand for increasing or decreasing plasma metabolite levels between pre- and post-supplementation states within individual paired samples. Panel (**C**) shows a bi-dimensional score plot depicting the distinct plasma metabolomic profile between pre- (red dots) and post-supplementation (green dots) paired participants. The two principal components of the smPLS-DA model along with their corresponding variance in group discrimination are shown on y- and x-axis, respectively. Panel (**D**) shows a loading plot representing the top 10 metabolites selected on the first component of the smPLS-DA model. Most important metabolites in group discrimination are ordered according to their loading weights (horizontal bars), from bottom to top. Bar color indicates the group for which the mean value is the highest for each feature (orange and green stand for pre- and post-supplementation groups, respectively).

Table 6. List of the plasma metabolites showing significant changes in plasma levels in Rb group after 8 weeks of Rb supplementation.

Metabolite Name	Common Name	Super Pathway	p-Value	HMDB
beta-Ala	β-Alanine	Biogenic Amines	0.005	HMDB0000056
TMAO	Trimethylamine N-oxide	Amine Oxides	0.008	HMDB0000925
GDCA	Deoxycholic acid glycine conjugate	Bile Acids	0.01	HMDB00631
CE15:0	Cholesterol 1-pentadecanoate	Cholesterol Esters	0.01	HMDB0060057
TG (22:6/32:0)	1-Palmitoyl-2-palmitoyl-3-docosahexaenoyl-glycerol	Triacylglycerols	0.01	HMDB10418
TG (16:1/32:1)	1-Octadecanoyl-2-(9Z-hexadecenoyl)-3-(9Z-tetradecenoyl)-glycerol	Triacylglycerols	0.02	HMDB0044888
TG (18:2/32:2)	1-Palmitoleoyl-2-palmitoleoyl-3-linoleoyl-glycerol	Triacylglycerols	0.02	HMDB05435
HexCer(d18:1/24:1)	Hexosylceramide	Glucosylceramides	0.02	-
PC aa C42:5	1-Arachidonyl-2-docosapentaenoyl-sn-glycero-3-phosphocholine	Glycerophospholipids	0.04	HMDB0008287
TG (18:0/32:0)	1-Octadecanoyl-2-octadecanoyl-3-(9Z-tetradecenoyl)-glycerol	Triacylglycerols	0.04	HMDB0044753

p-values stand for paired t-tests. HMDB, Human Metabolome Database.

4. Discussion

To our knowledge, this is the first randomized controlled trial to investigate immune-metabolic changes in response to Rb supplementation over such a long timescale. Briefly, the present intervention resulted in the modulation of the expression of numerous genes and circulating levels of some plasma metabolites being potential biomarkers of metabolic syndrome. Despite the effect of Rb supplementation at transcriptomic and metabolomic levels, its impact on traditional metabolic syndrome features was relatively modest, with no significant effects observed on relevant metabolic outcomes. However, very few clinical trials have looked at the health effects of Rb, and most of them were based on acute postprandial interventions with small numbers of subjects. That way, findings from two recent studies indicated that acute Rb supplementation, with daily consumptions of 125 and 250 g, may lower postprandial hyperglycemia, hypertriglyceridemia, and inflammatory response (IL-6 and TNF-α), as well as SBP when extended for four weeks, in diabetic or prediabetic individuals [20,21]. By contrast, two other acute postprandial studies conducted on healthy subjects offered less conclusive results, with no lowering effects on glycemic and insulinemic responses [23,24]. Overall, results from clinical trials suggest that Rb consumption can acutely attenuate metabolic syndrome features in subjects with a pre-existing metabolic condition, lowering postprandial glucose, plasma TG and inflammatory biomarkers levels. The mild clinical impact of the present Rb supplementation is, therefore, not surprising and may be attributable to the fact that participants were at risk of developing metabolic syndrome but displayed limited metabolic alterations. Thus, it appears that Rb effects may be clinically noticeable on individuals whose homeostatic set points have shifted to altered states. However, the significant increase in glucose and fructose intake observed in the Rb group, and attributable to the reported increase in fruit servings, might have masked the effects of Rb on cardiometabolic health.

We further used transcriptomics and metabolomics to reveal the effects of Rb at a molecular level. Two of the most significantly down-regulated genes, *ZNF683* and *ADGRG1*, are both linked to immune system functioning. *ZNF683* encodes for a key regulatory transcription factor of natural killer (NK) cell differentiation [44] that also drives the expression of *ADGRG1* [45]. Furthermore, *ADGRG1* is down-regulated upon NK cell activation, controls NK cell effector functions, and is thus closely associated with the production of cytolytic proteins, such as perforin and granzyme, which are major players of the cytolytic process of NK cells and T lymphocytes [45]. Accordingly, *PRF1*, *GZMH*, *GNLY*, *FGFBP2*, and two transcript variants of *NKG7*, which code, respectively, for the perforin-1 protein, granzyme H, granulysin, fibroblast growth factor-binding protein 2, and NK cell granule protein 7 were down-regulated. In addition, the gene encoding for the sphingosine-1-phosphate receptor 5 (*S1PR5*), which is implicated in monocyte trafficking and the exit of mature NK cells from the bone marrow and lymph nodes into blood and lymph circulation, was also significantly downregulated [46,47]. S1PR5 belongs to the G protein-coupled receptor family S1PR1-5, known to mediate the effects of sphingosine-1-phosphate (S1P), a bioactive phospholipid, which exerts pleiotropic effects. S1P stems from the phosphorylation by sphingosine kinases of sphingosine that is derived from the hydrolysis of ceramide species [48]. With the class of hexosylceramides (HexCer) being involved in the extensive network of sphingolipids metabolism [49], it is worth highlighting the potential connection between S1P and HexCer(d18:1/24:1), a ceramide whose plasma levels significantly increased in response to the intervention. Similarly, GDCA, another metabolite undergoing a significant increase following the intervention, has been shown, amongst other conjugated bile acids, to activate S1PR2, which belongs to the receptor family mentioned above [50].

Several signaling pathways related to IL-1β and IL-6 production, as well as to Ras, Rho, and MAPK protein signal transduction, were found to be significantly enriched in response to Rb supplementation. Interestingly, Ras, Rho, and MAPK are part of the signal transduction pathways on which S1PR1-5 action relies [51], suggesting a link with the downregulation of *S1PR5*, as well as with the increase of plasma HexCer(d18:1/24:1) and GDCA. Taken together, this points toward a slight modulation of the "inside-out signaling" process of immune cells. Of interest, animal studies have demonstrated beneficial effects of black raspberry on colorectal and pancreatic cancer, in conjunction with enhanced infiltration of NK cells into the colon and modulations of cytotoxic NK and T cell subsets [16,52]. Part of Rb effects has been linked to its richness in ellagitannins and anthocyanins. Previous research has shown that ellagitannins can modulate mice and human leucocytes activity and cytokine production [14,53]. Based on these findings, part of the transcriptional variations observed herein could be attributed to the high ellagitannins content of Rb.

Amongst metabolites tested, β-alanine exhibited the largest increase following Rb supplementation. It is the intermediate between glycine and gamma-aminobutyric acid (GABA), and acts as a partial GABA receptor antagonist. GABAergic signaling is known to play a role in gastrointestinal motility through vagus nerve stimulation [54]. Components of the GABA signaling machinery are also expressed in immune cells and are involved in the regulation of cytokine production, immune cell proliferation, and chemotaxis [55]. Moreover, we found that *GABBR1*, which is coding for the subunit 1 of GABA type B receptor, was the most upregulated gene in response to Rb. Interestingly, an agonist of the GABAB receptor has been shown to reduce the secretion of cytokines, including TNF-α and IL-6, in blood mononuclear cells and to interfere with their chemotaxis [56]. Based on these findings, one may speculate that the significant increase in plasma β-alanine concentration is causally related to *GABBR1* upregulation, as well as to IL-6 pathways enrichment. Surprisingly, TMAO, a gut microbiota-derived metabolite from dietary choline, choline-containing phospholipids, betaine, and carnitine, also underwent a large increase. It has been previously found that TMAO increases monocyte recruitment and activation, leading to the upregulation of inflammatory cytokine genes, monocyte adhesion, and to the formation of foam cells [57]. TMAO is then considered as a pro-atherogenic metabolite associated with an increased risk of cardiovascular disease. This increase in TMAO may be owed to an increase in animal protein consumption of the participants, which was not the case in the present study. More startling is that the reverse trend is generally observed with small fruit extract supplementation, which suggests the effect of an unknown factor that remains to be identified [58,59]. Finally, in addition to GDCA and HexCer (d18:1/24:1), other lipids belonging to cholesterol esters and glycerophospholipids pathways significantly increased, whilst triacylglycerols increased for some and decreased for others. Similarly, in a randomized controlled trial conducted on individuals with metabolic syndrome who consumed 300 g/day of berries comprising 100 g of Rb for 8 weeks, serum lipidomic profiling revealed several lipids discriminating berry consumers from controls, notably cholesterol esters, phosphatidylethanolamines, phosphatidylcholines, and TGs [24]. Of note here, are the shared biochemical pathways undergoing modulations following both interventions, first the cholesterol ester and triacylglycerols pathways, but also the functional connections between the phosphatidylcholines, TMAO, sphingosine and hexosylceramides. Our findings, together with those of Puupponen-Pimiä et al. [24], point toward sphingolipids and choline metabolism. Accordingly, studies linked sphingolipid metabolism dysregulation to insulin resistance and ceramide accumulation to insulin signaling inhibition [60]. In addition, an interconnection between polyphenols intake and sphingolipid metabolism has been established [61]. Specifically, anthocyanins were reported to attenuate insulin resistance by modulating sphingomyelin conversion and ceramide de novo synthesis [62], while ellagic acid has been identified as a potential inhibitor of sphingosine kinase [63].

Taken together, clinical, transcriptional, and metabolomical prisms have shed some light on the potential mechanisms underlying the health effects of Rb. A non-negligible part of these transcriptional results points toward slight modulations in the tight interplay between the cytotoxicity of lymphocytes and immune cell trafficking. This phenomenon may be viewed in relation to changes in phospholipid metabolism, *S1PR5* downregulation being potentially linked to the modulation of sphingolipid and choline metabolism, reflected in the upregulation of HexCer (d18:1/24:1) and TMAO, respectively. In addition, according to the heterogeneity observed in the response of genes and metabolites, these results point to the need for further research on the determinants of the inter-individual variability in response to foods and nutrients.

Strengths and Limitations

This study has several limitations. First, participants were Caucasians at risk of metabolic syndrome, which limits the generalization of the results. Second, the use of a crossover instead of a parallel design could have reduced the inter-individual variability in baseline characteristics. In addition, freezing small fruits could alter their content in phenolic compounds and, therefore, reduce their effects. For instance, it has been reported that the anthocyanin content of Haskap berries was reduced by nearly 60% after being frozen at −18 °C for 6 months [64]. Due to high hemolysis in some plasma samples, which prevents adequate measurement of plasma insulin levels, HOMA-IR and Matsuda indexes have been calculated for only a limited number of subjects in each group. Finally, the free-living design of the present study led to a significant increase in fruits consumption in the Rb group. Accordingly, glucose and fructose intakes were significantly higher in the Rb group, as compared to the control group, thus limiting the possibilities of clearly delineating the effects of raspberries on cardiometabolic health. Nonetheless, this study has strengths such as its randomization, which prevents selection bias in allocating intervention to participants. Compliance to the treatment was high, with no differences observed between groups in withdrawals from the study. Thus, although a per protocol analysis was used, exclusion of data are unlikely to have introduced bias.

5. Conclusions

In conclusion, clinical results are in line with those previously reported in human studies [24,25], as it appears that Rb health effects are clinically noticeable only in subjects with advanced metabolic disorders [20,21]. Omics profiling provided an overview of Rb health effects at the molecular level. Future investigations should be deepened to increase our understanding of the impact of Rb consumption on phospholipid metabolism and immune system and the links in-between.

Author Contributions: Conceptualization, V.G. (Véronique Garneau), D.R., C.C., A.M., and M.-C.V.; data curation, J.d.T.-M. and V.G. (Véronique Garneau); formal analysis, M.F. and J.d.T.-M.; funding acquisition, D.R., C.C., A.M., and M.C.-V.; investigation, M.F., V.G. (Véronique Garneau), V.G. (Valérie Guay), M.K. and P.C.; methodology, J.d.T.-M. and M.C.-V.; project administration, V.G. (Véronique Garneau) and M.C.-V.; resources, M.C.-V.; software, J.d.T.-M.; visualization, M.F. and J.d.T.-M.; writing—original draft, M.F.; writing—review and editing, J.d.T.-M., V.G. (Véronique Garneau), V.G. (Valérie Guay), M.K., G.P., D.R., P.C., C.C., A.M., and M.C.-V., M.F., J.d.T.-M. and M.C.-V. have primary responsibility for final content. All authors have read and agreed to the published version of the manuscript.

Acknowledgments: The authors thank the study participants for their excellent collaboration and acknowledge the work of the clinical investigation unit staff. M.-C.V. is a Tier 1 Canada Research Chair in Genomics Applied to Nutrition and Metabolic Health. M.F. received a studentship from the Centre Nutrition, Santé et Société (NUTRISS).

References

1. Eichelmann, F.; Schwingshackl, L.; Fedirko, V.; Aleksandrova, K. Effect of plant-based diets on obesity-related inflammatory profiles: A systematic review and meta-analysis of intervention trials. *Obes. Rev.* **2016**, *17*, 1067–1079. [CrossRef] [PubMed]
2. Reynolds, A.; Mann, J.; Cummings, J.; Winter, N.; Mete, E.; Morenga, L.T. Carbohydrate quality and human health: A series of systematic reviews and meta-analyses. *Lancet* **2019**, *393*, 434–445. [CrossRef]
3. O'Keefe, S.J. The association between dietary fibre deficiency and high-income lifestyle-associated diseases: Burkitt's hypothesis revisited. *Lancet Gastroenterol. Hepatol.* **2019**, *4*, 984–996. [CrossRef]
4. Alberti, K.; Eckel, R.H.; Grundy, S.M.; Zimmet, P.Z.; Cleeman, J.I.; Donato, K.A.; Fruchart, J.-C.; James, W.P.T.; Loria, C.M.; Smith, S.C. Harmonizing the Metabolic Syndrome. *Circulation* **2009**, *120*, 1640–1645. [CrossRef]
5. Health Canada. Canada's Dietary Guidelines. 2019. Available online: https://food-guide.canada.ca/en/guidelines (accessed on 31 October 2020).
6. Shepherd, R. *Resistance to Changes in Diet. Proceedings of the Nutrition Society*; CABI Publishing: Wallingford, UK, 2002; Volume 61, pp. 267–272.
7. Luís, Â.; Domingues, F.; Pereira, L. Association between berries intake and cardiovascular diseases risk factors: A systematic review with meta-analysis and trial sequential analysis of randomized controlled trials. *Food Funct.* **2018**, *9*, 740–757. [CrossRef]
8. Rao, A.V.; Snyder, D.M. Raspberries and Human Health: A Review†. *J. Agric. Food Chem.* **2010**, *58*, 3871–3883. [CrossRef]
9. Seeram, N.P.; Adams, L.S.; Zhang, Y.; Lee, R.; Sand, D.; Scheuller, H.S.; Heber, D. Blackberry, Black Raspberry, Blueberry, Cranberry, Red Raspberry, and Strawberry Extracts Inhibit Growth and Stimulate Apoptosis of Human Cancer Cells In Vitro. *J. Agric. Food Chem.* **2006**, *54*, 9329–9339. [CrossRef]
10. Wang, P.-W.; Cheng, Y.-C.; Hung, Y.-C.; Lee, C.-H.; Fang, J.-Y.; Li, W.-T.; Wu, Y.-R.; Pan, T.-L. Red Raspberry Extract Protects the Skin against UVB-Induced Damage with Antioxidative and Anti-inflammatory Properties. *Oxidative Med. Cell. Longev.* **2019**, *2019*, 1–14. [CrossRef]
11. Tu, L.; Sun, H.; Tang, M.; Zhao, J.; Zhang, Z.; Sun, X.; He, S. Red raspberry extract (Rubus idaeus L shrub) intake ameliorates hyperlipidemia in HFD-induced mice through PPAR signaling pathway. *Food Chem. Toxicol.* **2019**, *133*, 110796. [CrossRef]
12. Noratto, G.; Chew, B.P.; Atienza, L.M. Red raspberry (Rubus idaeus L.) intake decreases oxidative stress in obese diabetic (db/db) mice. *Food Chem.* **2017**, *227*, 305–314. [CrossRef]
13. Kirakosyan, A.; Seymour, E.M.; Kondoleon, N.; Gutierrez-Albanchez, E.; Wolforth, J.; Bolling, S. The intake of red raspberry fruit is inversely related to cardiac risk factors associated with metabolic syndrome. *J. Funct. Foods* **2018**, *41*, 83–89. [CrossRef]
14. Allen, C.T.; Peden-Adams, M.M.; Eudaly, J.; Keil, D.E. Subchronic Exposure to Ellagic Acid Impairs Cytotoxic T-Cell Function and Suppresses Humoral Immunity in Mice. *Immunopharmacol. Immunotoxicol.* **2003**, *25*, 409–422. [CrossRef]
15. Nowak, A.; Sójka, M.; Klewicka, E.; Lipińska, L.; Klewicki, R.; Kołodziejczyk, K. Ellagitannins from Rubus idaeus L. Exert Geno- and Cytotoxic Effects against Human Colon Adenocarcinoma Cell Line Caco-2. *J. Agric. Food Chem.* **2017**, *65*, 2947–2955. [CrossRef] [PubMed]
16. Pan, P.; Kang, S.; Wang, Y.; Liu, K.; Oshima, K.; Huang, Y.-W.; Zhang, J.; Yearsley, M.; Yu, J.; Wang, L.-S. Black Raspberries Enhance Natural Killer Cell Infiltration into the Colon and Suppress the Progression of Colorectal Cancer. *Front. Immunol.* **2017**, *8*, 997. [CrossRef] [PubMed]
17. Knobloch, T.; Ryan, N.M.; Bruschweiler-Li, L.; Wang, C.; Bernier, M.C.; Somogyi, Á.; Yan, P.; Cooperstone, J.L.; Mo, X.; Brüschweiler, R.; et al. Metabolic Regulation of Glycolysis and AMP Activated Protein Kinase Pathways during Black Raspberry-Mediated Oral Cancer Chemoprevention. *Metabolites* **2019**, *9*, 140. [CrossRef] [PubMed]

18. Jeong, H.S.; Kim, S.; Hong, S.J.; Choi, S.C.; Choi, J.-H.; Kim, J.-H.; Park, C.-Y.; Cho, J.Y.; Lee, T.-B.; Kwon, J.-W.; et al. Black Raspberry Extract Increased Circulating Endothelial Progenitor Cells and Improved Arterial Stiffness in Patients with Metabolic Syndrome: A Randomized Controlled Trial. *J. Med. Food* **2016**, *19*, 346–352. [CrossRef]
19. Sardo, C.; Kitzmiller, J.P.; Apseloff, G.; Harris, R.B.; Roe, D.J.; Stoner, G.D.; Jacobs, E.T. An Open-Label Randomized Crossover Trial of Lyophilized Black Raspberries on Postprandial Inflammation in Older Overweight Males. *Am. J. Ther.* **2016**, *23*, e86–e91. [CrossRef]
20. Xiao, D.; Zhu, L.; Edirisinghe, I.; Fareed, J.; Brailovsky, Y.; Burton-Freeman, B.M. Attenuation of Postmeal Metabolic Indices with Red Raspberries in Individuals at Risk for Diabetes: A Randomized Controlled Trial. *Obesity* **2019**, *27*, 542–550. [CrossRef]
21. Schell, J.; Betts, N.M.; Lyons, T.J.; Basu, A. Raspberries Improve Postprandial Glucose and Acute and Chronic Inflammation in Adults with Type 2 Diabetes. *Ann. Nutr. Metab.* **2019**, *74*, 165–174. [CrossRef]
22. Istas, G.; Feliciano, R.P.; Weber, T.; Garcia-Villalba, R.; Tomás-Barberán, F.A.; Heiss, C.; Rodriguez-Mateos, A. Plasma urolithin metabolites correlate with improvements in endothelial function after red raspberry consumption: A double-blind randomized controlled trial. *Arch. Biochem. Biophys.* **2018**, *651*, 43–51. [CrossRef]
23. Clegg, M.E.; Pratt, M.; Meade, C.M.; Henry, C.J.K. The addition of raspberries and blueberries to a starch-based food does not alter the glycaemic response. *Br. J. Nutr.* **2011**, *106*, 335–338. [CrossRef] [PubMed]
24. Puupponen-Pimiä, R.; Seppänen-Laakso, T.; Kankainen, M.; Maukonen, J.; Törrönen, R.; Kolehmainen, M.; Leppänen, T.; Moilanen, E.; Nohynek, L.; Aura, A.-M.; et al. Effects of ellagitannin-rich berries on blood lipids, gut microbiota, and urolithin production in human subjects with symptoms of metabolic syndrome. *Mol. Nutr. Food Res.* **2013**, *57*, 2258–2263. [CrossRef] [PubMed]
25. Törrönen, R.; Kolehmainen, M.; Sarkkinen, E.; Poutanen, K.; Mykkänen, H.; Niskanen, L. Berries Reduce Postprandial Insulin Responses to Wheat and Rye Breads in Healthy Women. *J. Nutr.* **2013**, *143*, 430–436. [CrossRef]
26. Scarsella, C.; Alméras, N.; Mauriège, P.; Blanchet, C.; Sauvé, L.; Dewailly, E.; Bergeron, J.; Després, J.-P. Prevalence of metabolic alterations predictive of cardiovascular disease risk in the Québec population. *Can. J. Cardiol.* **2003**, *19*, 51–57. [PubMed]
27. Norgan, N.G. A Review of: Anthropometric Standardization Reference Manual Edited by T. G. LOHMAN, A.F. ROCHE and R. MARTORELL. (Champaign, IL.: Human Kinetics Books, 1988.) ISBN 087322 121 4. *Ergonomics* **1988**, *31*, 1493–1494. [CrossRef]
28. Labonté, M.-È.; Cyr, A.; Baril-Gravel, L.; Royer, M.-M.; Lamarche, B. Validity and reproducibility of a web-based, self-administered food frequency questionnaire. *Eur. J. Clin. Nutr.* **2011**, *66*, 166–173. [CrossRef]
29. Taylor, H.L.; Jacobs, D.R.; Schucker, B.; Knudsen, J.; Leon, A.S.; Debacker, G. A questionnaire for the assessment of leisure time physical activities. *J. Chronic Dis.* **1978**, *31*, 741–755. [CrossRef]
30. Burstein, M.; Samaille, J. Sur un dosage rapide du cholesterol lié aux α-et aux β-lipoprotéines du sérum. *Clin. Chim. Acta* **1960**, *5*, 609. [CrossRef]
31. Friedewald, W.T.; Levy, R.I.; Fredrickson, D.S. Estimation of the Concentration of Low-Density Lipoprotein Cholesterol in Plasma, Without Use of the Preparative Ultracentrifuge. *Clin. Chem.* **1972**, *18*, 499–502. [CrossRef]
32. LeDue, T.B.; Weiner, D.L.; Sipe, J.D.; Poulin, S.E.; Collins, M.F.; Rifai, N. Analytical evaluation of particle-enhanced immunonephelometric assays for C-reactive protein, serum amyloid A and mannose-binding protein in human serum. *Ann. Clin. Biochem. Int. J. Lab. Med.* **1998**, *35*, 745–753. [CrossRef]
33. Richterich, R.; Dauwalder, H. [Determination of plasma glucose by hexokinase-glucose-6-phosphate dehydrogenase method]. *Schweiz. Med. Wochenschr.* **1971**, *101*, 615–618. [PubMed]
34. Matthews, D.R.; Hosker, J.P.; Rudenski, A.S.; Naylor, B.A.; Treacher, D.F.; Turner, R.C. Homeostasis model assessment: Insulin resistance and β-cell function from fasting plasma glucose and insulin concentrations in man. *Diabetologia* **1985**, *28*, 412–419. [CrossRef] [PubMed]
35. Matsuda, M.; DeFronzo, R.A. Insulin sensitivity indices obtained from oral glucose tolerance testing: Comparison with the euglycemic insulin clamp. *Diabetes Care* **1999**, *22*, 1462–1470. [CrossRef] [PubMed]
36. Reynés, B.; Priego, T.; Cifre, M.; Oliver, P.; Palou, A. Peripheral Blood Cells, a Transcriptomic Tool in Nutrigenomic and Obesity Studies: Current State of the Art. *Compr. Rev. Food Sci. Food Saf.* **2018**, *17*, 1006–1020. [CrossRef]

37. Bray, N.L.; Pimentel, H.; Melsted, P.; Pachter, L. Near-optimal probabilistic RNA-seq quantification. *Nat. Biotechnol.* **2016**, *34*, 525–527. [CrossRef]
38. McCarthy, D.J.; Chen, Y.; Smyth, G.K. Differential expression analysis of multifactor RNA-Seq experiments with respect to biological variation. *Nucleic Acids Res.* **2012**, *40*, 4288–4297. [CrossRef]
39. Chong, J.; Xia, J. MetaboAnalystR: An R package for flexible and reproducible analysis of metabolomics data. *Bioinformatics* **2018**, *34*, 4313–4314. [CrossRef] [PubMed]
40. Cao, M.D.; Giskeødegård, G.F.; Bathen, T.F.; Sitter, B.; Bofin, A.M.; Lønning, P.E.; Lundgren, S.; Gribbestad, I.S. Prognostic value of metabolic response in breast cancer patients receiving neoadjuvant chemotherapy. *BMC Cancer* **2012**, *12*, 39. [CrossRef]
41. Westerhuis, J.A.; Van Velzen, E.J.J.; Hoefsloot, H.C.J.; Smilde, A.K. Multivariate paired data analysis: Multilevel PLSDA versus OPLSDA. *Metabolomics* **2010**, *6*, 119–128. [CrossRef]
42. Le Cao, K.-A.; Boitard, S.; Besse, P. Sparse PLS discriminant analysis: Biologically relevant feature selection and graphical displays for multiclass problems. *BMC Bioinform.* **2011**, *12*, 253. [CrossRef]
43. Rohart, F.; Gautier, B.; Singh, A.; Le Cao, K.-A. mixOmics: An R package for 'omics feature selection and multiple data integration. *PLoS Comput. Biol.* **2017**, *13*, e1005752. [CrossRef] [PubMed]
44. Post, M.; Cuapio, A.; Osl, M.; Lehmann, D.; Resch, U.; Davies, D.M.; Bilban, M.; Schlechta, B.; Eppel, W.; Nathwani, A.; et al. The Transcription Factor ZNF683/HOBIT Regulates Human NK-Cell Development. *Front. Immunol.* **2017**, *8*, 535. [CrossRef] [PubMed]
45. Chang, G.-W.; Hsiao, C.-C.; Peng, Y.-M.; Braga, F.A.V.; Kragten, N.A.; Remmerswaal, E.B.; Van De Garde, M.D.; Straussberg, R.; König, G.M.; Kostenis, E.; et al. The Adhesion G Protein-Coupled Receptor GPR56/ADGRG1 Is an Inhibitory Receptor on Human NK Cells. *Cell Rep.* **2016**, *15*, 1757–1770. [CrossRef] [PubMed]
46. Debien, E.; Mayol, K.; Biajoux, V.; Daussy, C.; De Agüero, M.G.; Taillardet, M.; Dagany, N.; Brinza, L.; Henry, T.; Dubois, B.; et al. S1PR5 is pivotal for the homeostasis of patrolling monocytes. *Eur. J. Immunol.* **2013**, *43*, 1667–1675. [CrossRef]
47. Drouillard, A.; Mathieu, A.-L.; Marçais, A.; Belot, A.; Viel, S.; Mingueneau, M.; Guckian, K.; Walzer, T. S1PR5 is essential for human natural killer cell migration toward sphingosine-1 phosphate. *J. Allergy Clin. Immunol.* **2018**, *141*, 2265–2268.e1. [CrossRef]
48. Maceyka, M.; Milstien, S.; Spiegel, S. Sphingosine kinases, sphingosine-1-phosphate and sphingolipidomics. *Prostaglandins Other Lipid Mediat.* **2005**, *77*, 15–22. [CrossRef]
49. Iqbal, J.; Walsh, M.T.; Hammad, S.M.; Cuchel, M.; Tarugi, P.; Hegele, R.A.; Davidson, N.O.; Rader, D.J.; Klein, R.L.; Hussain, M.M. Microsomal Triglyceride Transfer Protein Transfers and Determines Plasma Concentrations of Ceramide and Sphingomyelin but Not Glycosylceramide. *J. Biol. Chem.* **2015**, *290*, 25863–25875. [CrossRef]
50. Studer, E.; Zhou, X.; Zhao, R.; Wang, Y.; Takabe, K.; Nagahashi, M.; Pandak, W.M.; Dent, P.; Spiegel, S.; Shi, R.; et al. Conjugated bile acids activate the sphingosine-1-phosphate receptor 2 in primary rodent hepatocytes. *Hepatology* **2011**, *55*, 267–276. [CrossRef]
51. Bryan, A.M.; Del Poeta, M. Sphingosine-1-phosphate receptors and innate immunity. *Cell. Microbiol.* **2018**, *20*, e12836. [CrossRef]
52. Pan, P.; Zhu, Z.; Oshima, K.; Aldakkak, M.; Tsai, S.; Huang, Y.-W.; Dong, W.; Zhang, J.; Lin, C.-W.; Wang, Y.; et al. Black raspberries suppress pancreatic cancer through modulation of NKp46 + CD8 +, and CD11b + immune cells. *Food Front.* **2020**, *1*, 70–82. [CrossRef]
53. Bessler, H. On the Link between Ellagic Acid and the Immune Balance between Human Mononuclear and Colon Carcinoma Cells. *Immunol Curr Res* **2017**, *1*, 1.
54. Wu, F.-S.; Gibbs, T.T.; Farb, D.H. Dual activation of GABAA and glycine receptors by β-alanine: Inverse modulation by progesterone and 5α-pregnan-3α-ol-20-one. *Eur. J. Pharmacol. Mol. Pharmacol.* **1993**, *246*, 239–246. [CrossRef]
55. Jin, Z.; Mendu, S.K.; Birnir, B. GABA is an effective immunomodulatory molecule. *Amino Acids* **2013**, *45*, 87–94. [CrossRef] [PubMed]
56. Duthey, B.; Hübner, A.; Diehl, S.; Boehncke, S.; Pfeffer, J.; Boehncke, W.-H. Anti-inflammatory effects of the GABAB receptor agonist baclofen in allergic contact dermatitis. *Exp. Dermatol.* **2010**, *19*, 661–666. [CrossRef]
57. Geng, J.; Yang, C.; Wang, B.; Zhang, X.; Hu, T.; Gu, Y.; Li, J. Trimethylamine N-oxide promotes atherosclerosis via CD36-dependent MAPK/JNK pathway. *Biomed. Pharmacother.* **2018**, *97*, 941–947. [CrossRef] [PubMed]

58. Annunziata, G.; Maisto, M.; Schisano, C.; Ciampaglia, R.; Narciso, V.; Tenore, G.C.; Novellino, E. Effects of Grape Pomace Polyphenolic Extract (Taurisolo®) in Reducing TMAO Serum Levels in Humans: Preliminary Results from a Randomized, Placebo-Controlled, Cross-Over Study. *Nutrients* **2019**, *11*, 139. [CrossRef] [PubMed]
59. Bresciani, L.; Dall'Asta, M.; Favari, C.; Calani, L.; Del Rio, D.; Brighenti, F. An in vitro exploratory study of dietary strategies based on polyphenol-rich beverages, fruit juices and oils to control trimethylamine production in the colon. *Food Funct.* **2018**, *9*, 6470–6483. [CrossRef]
60. Mandal, N.; Grambergs, R.; Mondal, K.; Basu, S.K.; Tahia, F.; Dagogo-Jack, S. Role of ceramides in the pathogenesis of diabetes mellitus and its complications. *J. Diabetes Complicat.* **2020**, *10*, 107734. [CrossRef]
61. Cas, M.D.; Ghidoni, R. Cancer Prevention and Therapy with Polyphenols: Sphingolipid-Mediated Mechanisms. *Nutrients* **2018**, *10*, 940. [CrossRef]
62. Si, X.; Tian, J.; Shu, C.; Wang, Y.; Gong, E.S.; Zhang, Y.; Zhang, W.; Cui, H.; Li, B. Serum Ceramide Reduction by Blueberry Anthocyanin-Rich Extract Alleviates Insulin Resistance in Hyperlipidemia Mice. *J. Agric. Food Chem.* **2020**, *68*, 8185–8194. [CrossRef]
63. Gupta, P.; Mohammad, T.; Khan, P.; Alajmi, M.F.; Hussain, A.; Rehman, T.; Hassan, I. Evaluation of ellagic acid as an inhibitor of sphingosine kinase 1: A targeted approach towards anticancer therapy. *Biomed. Pharmacother.* **2019**, *118*, 109245. [CrossRef] [PubMed]
64. Khattab, R.; Celli, G.B.; Ghanem, A.; Brooks, M.S.-L. Effect of frozen storage on polyphenol content and antioxidant activity of haskap berries (Lonicera caerulea L.). *J. Berry Res.* **2015**, *5*, 231–242. [CrossRef]

2

Garlic Derived Diallyl Trisulfide in Experimental Metabolic Syndrome: Metabolic Effects and Cardioprotective Role

Jovana N. Jeremic [1], Vladimir Lj. Jakovljevic [2,3], Vladimir I. Zivkovic [2], Ivan M. Srejovic [2], Jovana V. Bradic [1], Isidora M. Milosavljevic [1], Slobodanka Lj. Mitrovic [4], Nemanja U. Jovicic [5], Sergey B. Bolevich [3], Andrey A. Svistunov [6], Suresh C. Tyagi [7] and Nevena S. Jeremic [1,7,*]

1 Department of Pharmacy, Faculty of Medical Sciences, University of Kragujevac, Svetozara Markovica 69, 34 000 Kragujevac, Serbia; jovana.jeremic@medf.kg.ac.rs (J.N.J.); jovanabradickg@gmail.com (J.V.B.); isidora.stojic@medf.kg.ac.rs (I.M.M.)

2 Department of Physiology, Faculty of Medical Sciences, University of Kragujevac, Svetozara Markovica 69, 34 000 Kragujevac, Serbia; drvladakgbg@yahoo.com (V.L.J.); vladimirziv@gmail.com (V.I.Z.); ivan_srejovic@hotmail.com (I.M.S.)

3 Department of Human Pathology, I.M. Sechenov First Moscow State Medical University, Trubetskaya Street 8, 119991 Moscow, Russia; bolevich2011@yandex.ru

4 Department of Pathology, Faculty of Medical Sciences, University of Kragujevac, Svetozara Markovica 69, 34 000 Kragujevac, Serbia; smitrovic@medf.kg.ac.rs

5 Department of Histology and Embryology, Faculty of Medical Sciences, University of Kragujevac, Svetozara Markovica 69, 34 000 Kragujevac, Serbia; nemanjajovicic.kg@gmail.com

6 Research Institute of Pharmacy, I.M. Sechenov First Moscow State Medical University, Trubetskaya Street 8-2, 119991 Moscow, Russia; svistunov@sechenov.ru

7 Department of Physiology, School of Medicine, University of Louisville, 500 S Preston Street, Louisville, KY 40202, USA; suresh.tyagi@louisville.edu

* Correspondence: nbarudzic@hotmail.com

Abstract: This study aimed to examine the effects of diallyl trisulfide (DATS), the most potent polysulfide derived from garlic, on metabolic syndrome and myocardial function in rats with metabolic syndrome (MetS). For that purpose, we used 36 male *Wistar albino* rats divided into control rats, rats with MetS and MetS rats treated with 40 mg/kg of DATS every second day for 3 weeks. In the first part, we studied the impact of DATS on MetS control and found that DATS significantly raised H_2S, decreased homocysteine and glucose levels and enhanced lipid and antioxidative, while reducing prooxidative parameters. Additionally, this polysulfide improved cardiac function. In the second part, we investigated the impact of DATS on ex vivo induced ischemia/reperfusion (I/R) heart injury and found that DATS consumption significantly improved cardiodynamic parameters and prevented oxidative and histo-architectural variation in the heart. In addition, DATS significantly increased relative gene expression of eNOS, SOD-1 and -2, Bcl-2 and decreased relative gene expression of NF-κB, IL-17A, Bax, and caspases-3 and -9. Taken together, the data show that DATS can effectively mitigate MetS and have protective effects against ex vivo induced myocardial I/R injury in MetS rat.

Keywords: diallyl trisulfide; garlic; metabolic syndrome; isolated rat heart

1. Introduction

Cardiovascular diseases (CVDs) are a leading cause of premature death and a major chronic disability worldwide [1]. One of the serious CVDs, a growing health problem, is myocardial infarction (MI), which is commonly followed by extended ischemia and heart failure. Ischemia causes cardiac dysfunction, arrhythmias, myocardial infarction and sudden death, mediated by low pH values, low oxygen levels and disruption of K^+ and Ca^{2+} concentrations [1]. Strategy in salvaging damaged myocardium in ischemia involves restoration of blood flow. However, the most common, activation of the complex inflammatory response in the reperfusion period leads to irreversible damage called reperfusion injury [2]. Therefore, ischemia/reperfusion (I/R) injury is typically occurring as a result of vessel occlusion followed by a set of stresses during the recovery of blood flow. The factors contributing to I/R injury are very complex and besides already mentioned include microvascular dysfunction, the release of reactive oxygen species (ROS), and activation of mitochondrial apoptosis and necrosis [3]. However, these mediators are common in the pathology of metabolic syndrome (MetS) as well. Namely, modified metabolism, damaged microvasculature and weakened immune system are the major MetS-related adverse effects on the cardiac system [4,5]. The number of MetS patients with ischemic heart disease is alarmingly increasing and long-term prognosis, as well as control of complications, remain poor. Therefore, it is necessary to improve cardioprotective strategies and find new agents against I/R injury (so-called preconditioning agents) to preserve myocardial capacity and reduce the risk of cardiovascular events in patients with MetS [3,4].

Garlic (*Allium sativum* L.) is a traditional food recognized as beneficial for numerous diseases since ancient times. Although the precise protective mechanisms are still unclear and require further explanation, many authors hypothesize that *Allium* species caused the most beneficial effects by sulfur compounds [6]. It is a well-known fact that abundant organosulfur compounds found in the garlic interact with thiol groups or thiol-containing compounds from biological systems and augments bioavailability of hydrogen sulfide (H_2S) [6,7]. Additionally, numerous studies have found that as a gasotransmitter, H_2S is key modulators of I/R injury and could alleviate heart damage probably by activating of adenosine triphosphate-sensitive potassium channels (K-ATP) [7], affecting several pro-inflammatory cytokines [8] and decreasing hydrogen peroxide in parallel with increasing GSH levels [9]. Raw intact garlic bulbs contain high amounts of γ-glutamylcysteine, which can undergo hydrolysis or oxidation and at the end decompose to sulfur-containing compounds. The most important organosulfur compound isolated from garlic is diallyl trisulfide (DATS) also known as allitridin or 4,5,6-trithia-1,8-nonadiene. DATS, as one of the most stable and safe naturally occurring polysulfide, is an attractive H_2S donor for in vivo studies with an eye to clinical relevance [10,11].

Findings from our previous study referring to blood-glucose-lowering and cardioprotective effects of DATS in chemically induced type 1 diabetes mellitus [12] encouraged us to examine the effect of DATS on the more complex disease, which involve a group of pathophysiological abnormalities, such as MetS. To our best knowledge, there are no available reports that explain the role of DATS consumption in MetS, which provide the precise association between blood pressure, glycemia and lipid profile, as well functional and morphological properties of the heart after DATS administration. Therefore, the present study aimed to examine the effects of DATS on MetS and its potential cardioprotective role in ex vivo-induced cardiac I/R injury in rats with MetS.

2. Results

2.1. Anti-Metabolic Syndrome Effects of DATS

2.1.1. Biochemical Parameters

All measured lipid parameters were significantly increased except high-density lipoprotein (HDL), which was decreased in rats with MetS compared to CTRL. DATS consumption in MetS rats significantly reduced triglycerides (TG) and low-density lipoprotein (LDL) and significantly increased HDL levels (Figure 1a).

Three weeks of DATS consumption resulted in a statistically significant increase of serum H_2S levels in rats with metabolic syndrome compared to untreated rats. In contrast to these results, homocysteine levels were significantly higher in the MS group, compared with the CTRL and MS+DATS groups (Figure 1b).

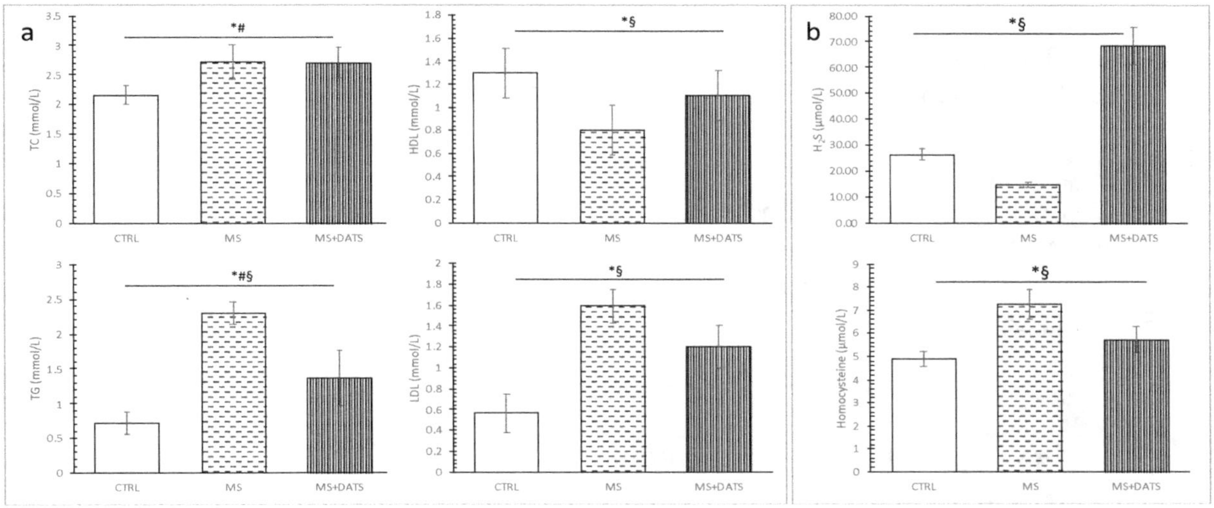

Figure 1. Effects of diallyl trisulfide (DATS) consumption on (**a**) lipid parameters: TC—total cholesterol, TG—triglycerides, HDL—high-density lipoprotein and LDL—low-density lipoprotein; (**b**) H_2S—hydrogen sulfide and homocysteine levels. Values are presented as mean ± SD, n = 12, per group. * $p < 0.05$ CTRL vs. MS, # $p < 0.05$ CTRL vs. MS+DATS, § $p < 0.05$ MS vs. MS+DATS.

2.1.2. Insulin and Glucose Levels during Oral Glucose Tolerance Test (OGTT)

Fasting blood glucose levels were significantly increased in both groups of MetS rats (MS and MS+DATS) compared to the CTRL group. Furthermore, DATS consumption significantly decreased glucose level (fasting blood glucose, as well as 120 and 180 min after an oral glucose loading) (Figure 2a).

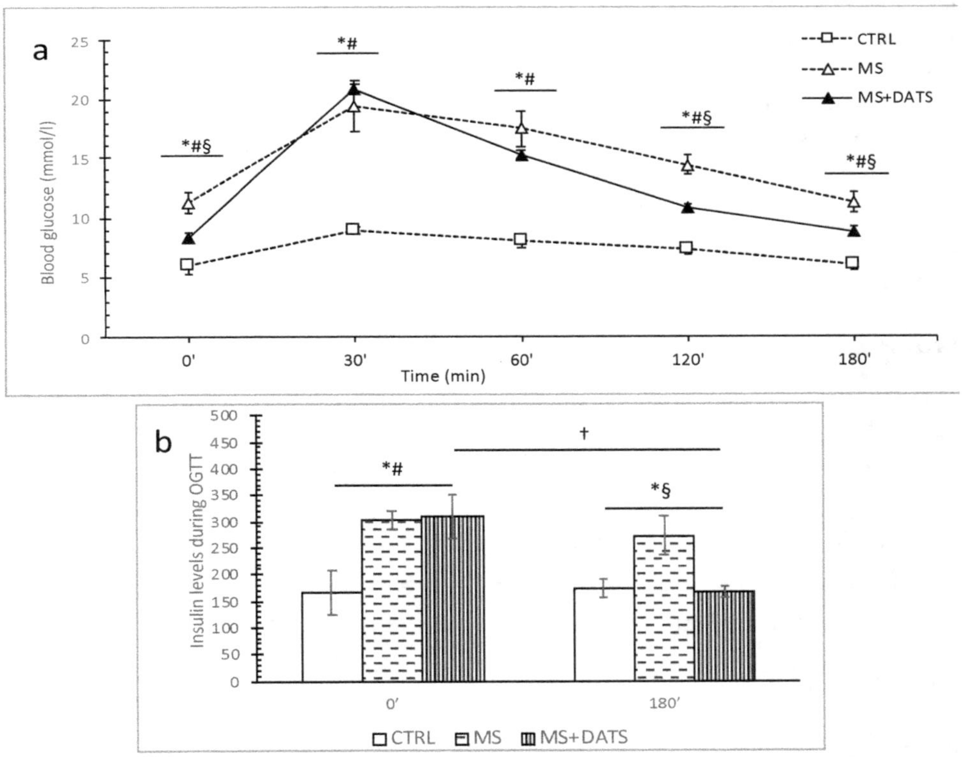

Figure 2. Effect of DATS consumption on glucose and insulin level during oral glucose tolerance test (OGTT). (**a**) Fasting blood glucose level (0′) and blood glucose levels 30′, 60′, 120′ and 180′ after an oral glucose loading (2 g/kg body weight); (**b**) fasting insulin levels and 180′ after an oral glucose loading. Values are presented as mean ± SD, n = 6, per group. * $p < 0.05$ CTRL vs. MS, # $p < 0.05$ CTRL vs. MS+DATS, § $p < 0.05$ MS vs. MS+DATS, † $p < 0.05$ MS at 0′ vs. MS at 180′.

Similar, fasting insulin concentrations were significantly increased in MetS rats (MS and MS+DATS) compared with CTRL; meanwhile, 180 min after an oral glucose loading, insulin level was significantly increased in MS both when compared to CTRL and MS+DATS groups (Figure 2b).

2.1.3. Redox Status

TBARS was significantly decreased, while nitrites (NO_2^-) were significantly increased in DATS treated rats with MetS compared with untreated rats (CTRL and MS groups). Besides, the superoxide anion radical (O_2^-) level was significantly increased in the MS group in comparison with CTRL and MS+DATS (Figure 3a).

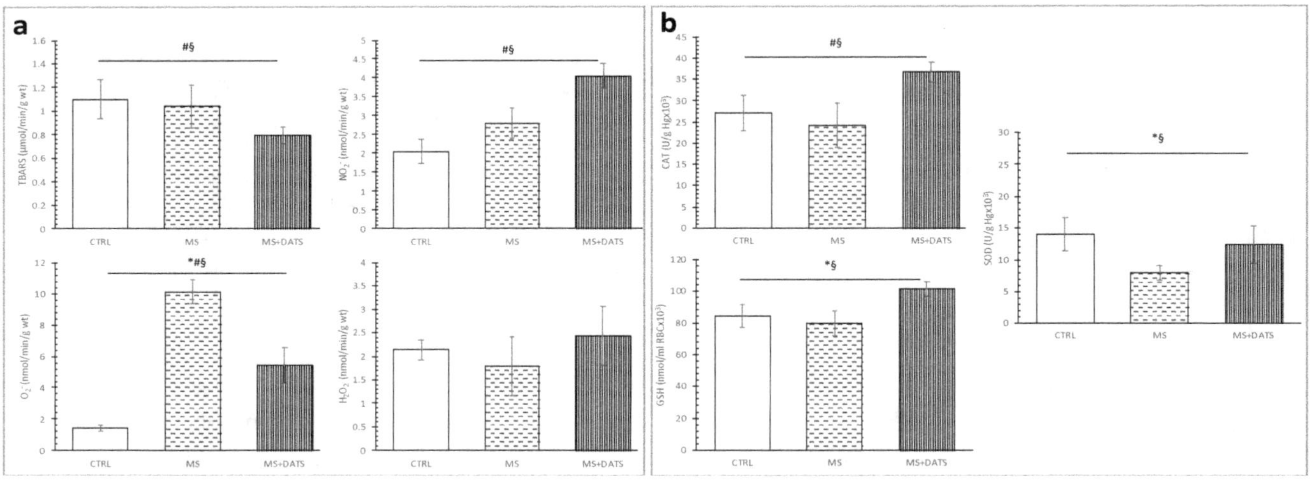

Figure 3. Effects of DATS consumption on oxidative stress parameters; (**a**) pro-oxidants: TBARS—index of lipid peroxidation, O_2^-—superoxide anion radical, NO_2^-—nitrite, H_2O_2—hydrogen peroxide; (**b**) antioxidants: CAT—catalase, GSH—reduced glutathione peroxide and SOD—superoxide dismutase. Values are presented as mean ± SD, n = 12, per group. * $p < 0.05$ CTRL vs. MS, # $p < 0.05$ CTRL vs. MS+DATS, § $p < 0.05$ MS vs. MS+DATS.

On the other hand, superoxide dismutase (SOD) and reduced glutathione (GSH) were significantly decreased in MS group compared to CTRL. Importantly, treatment with DATS resulted in a significant enhancement of catalase (CAT), SOD activity and increased GSH amount (Figure 3b).

2.1.4. In Vivo Cardiac Function

MetS rats had significantly changed echocardiographic parameters (decreased diastolic and systolic interventricular septal wall thickness (IVS), as well as increased left ventricular internal diameter (LVIDd)), but DATS treatment prevented these alterations (Figure 4a). Similar, percentages of fractional shortening and ejection fraction were decreased in rats with MetS, while DATS consumption significantly improved these parameters (Figure 4b).

Blood pressure and heart rate were significantly increased in rats with MetS compared with CTRL, while 3 weeks of DATS consumption significantly decreased only diastolic blood pressure (Figure 4c).

2.2. *Efficiency of DATS Preconditioning in Rats with MetS*

2.2.1. Cardiodynamic and Oxidative Stress Parameters

Parameters of left ventricular contractile force (dp/dt max and dp/dt min, at all points of interest) and parameters of left ventricular pressure (SLVP and DLVP) were significantly altered as follows MS+DATS > CTRL > MS. Moreover, heart rate (HR) was higher in MS+DATS then in the CTRL group at the last minute of reperfusion (Figure 5a).

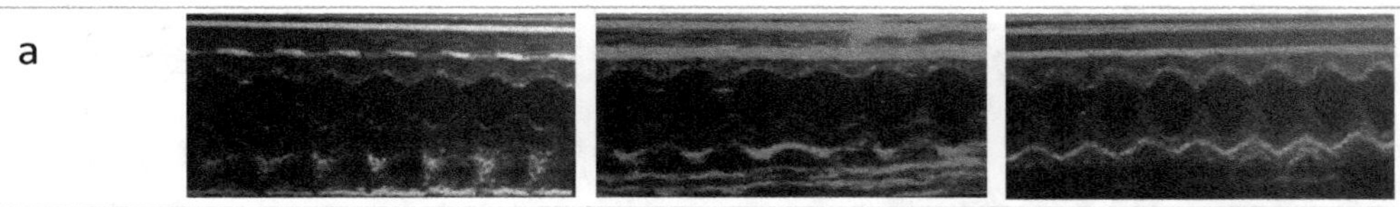

	CTRL	MS	MS+DATS
IVSd (cm)	0.165 ± 0.03	0.128 ± 0.032*	0.159 ± 0.034§
LVIDd (cm)	0.631 ± 0.04	0.623 ± 0.073	0.619 ± 0.032
LVPWd (cm)	0.201 ± 0.05	0.220 ± 0.009	0.203 ± 0.037
IVSs (cm)	0.305 ± 0.03	0.233 ± 0.047*	0.322 ± 0.048§
LVIDs (cm)	0.265 ± 0.06	0.324 ± 0.010*	0.218 ± 0.032§
LVPWs (cm)	0.318 ± 0.08	0.316 ± 0.006	0.342 ± 0.103

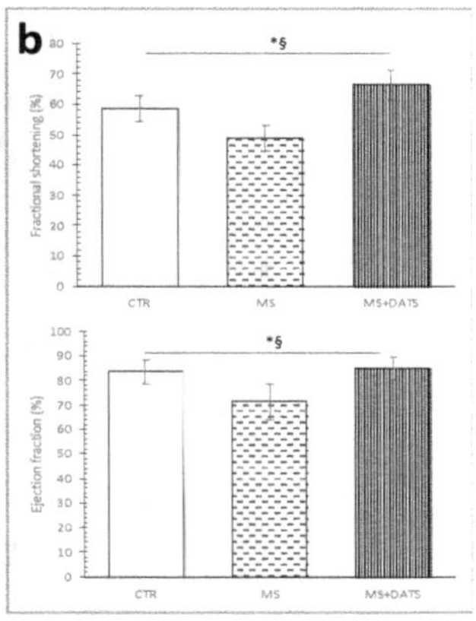

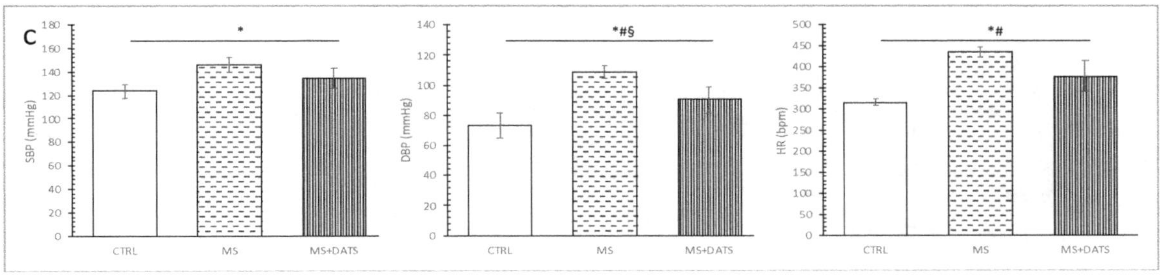

Figure 4. Effects of DATS consumption on in vivo cardiac function: (**a**) cardiodynamic parameters, representative M-mode echocardiography findings; (**b**) fractional shortening and ejection fraction; (**c**) SBP—systolic blood pressure, DBP—diastolic blood pressure and HR—heart rate. Values are presented as mean ± SD, n = 12, per group. * $p < 0.05$ CTRL vs. MS, # $p < 0.05$ CTRL vs. MS+DATS, § $p < 0.05$ MS vs. MS+DATS.

Furthermore, MetS rats had significantly increased values of the index of lipid peroxidation (measured as TBARS) and O_2^- in coronary venous effluent, while DATS treatment significantly decreased levels of TBARS, O_2^- and hydrogen peroxide (H_2O_2), an increased level of NO_2^- (Figure 5b).

2.2.2. Pathohistological Evaluation of Myocardial Tissue

I/R-induced cardiac histo-architectural variation was analyzed using hematoxylin/eosin staining that confirms the perturbed structure in MetS rat heart. Namely, in MS group extensive edema, cell swelling, and tissue necrosis (infarcted) zone with separation of muscle fibers were found. On the other hand, histological alterations were considerably reduced in DATS-treated group where mild edema, reduced inflammatory process and reduced necrotic area were obtained (Figure 6a). These ultrastructural changes were further confirmed with cardiac troponin T (cTnT) staining. As shown in Figure 6b in MS group there was an obvious loss of cTnT staining and slightly positive (brown) staining, while in the MS+DATS group, there was a decrease in staining with more intense (brown color) remaining found.

More importantly, DATS treatment decreased the incidence of cardiomyocytes with and terminal deoxynucleotidyl transferase dUTP nick end labeling (TUNEL) positive nucleus, DNA fragment and apoptosis activity compared to untreated rats (MS+DATS vs. MS) (Figure 7a). Additionally, analysis of Picrosirius red and vimentin content using ImageJ revealed a significant increase in the amount of fibrosis in rats with MetS compared to the CTRL group. On the other hand, DATS consumption significantly decreased fibrosis (MS+DATS vs. MS) (Figure 7b,c).

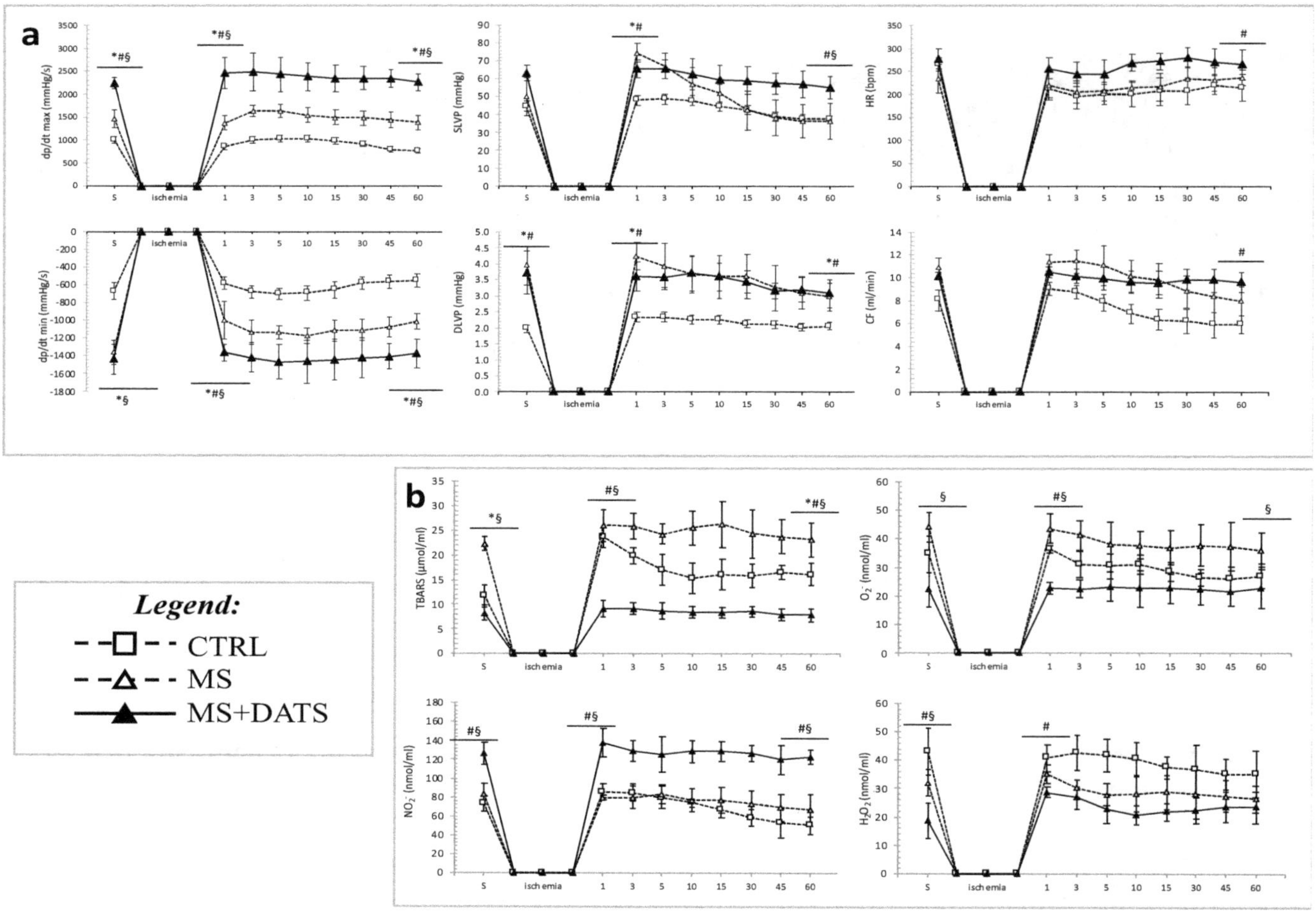

Figure 5. Preconditioning effects of DATS on (**a**) cardiodynamic parameters: dp/dt max—the maximum rate of LV pressure development, dp/dt max—minimum rate of LV pressure development, SLVP—systolic LV pressure, DLVP—diastolic LV pressure, HR—heart rate and CF—coronary flow; (**b**) pro-oxidants: TBARS—index of lipid peroxidation, O_2^-—superoxide anion radical, NO_2^-—nitrite, H_2O_2—hydrogen peroxide. Values are presented as mean ± SD, n = 12, per group. * $p < 0.05$ CTRL vs. MS, # $p < 0.05$ CTRL vs. MS+DATS, § $p < 0.05$ MS vs. MS+DATS.

Immunohistochemical analysis showed that in rats with MetS, Bax and Caspase-3 protein expression were significantly increased, while Bcl2 and HSP70 protein expression were significantly decreased in myocardium when compared to CTRL rats. By the DATS consumption, alteration of the expression of all mentioned protein was prevented and more similar to CTRL than to MS group (Figure 8a–d).

Relative gene expression of endothelial nitric oxide synthetase (eNOS), SOD-1 and SOD-2 were significantly decreased in MS group compared to CTRL, while DATS consumption significantly increased relative gene expression of these parameters (Figure 9a).

On the other hand, relative gene expression of Bax, caspase-3 and caspase-9 were significantly increased, while Bcl-2 was significantly decreased in MS compared to the CTRL group. Contrarily, DATS consumption significantly decreased relative gene expression of Bax and both determined caspases and increased relative gene expression of Bcl-2 (Figure 9b).

Relative gene expression of NF-κB and TNF-α were significantly increased in MS compared to CTRL, while DATS treatment significantly decreased the relative gene expression of NF-κB and IL-17A (Figure 9c).

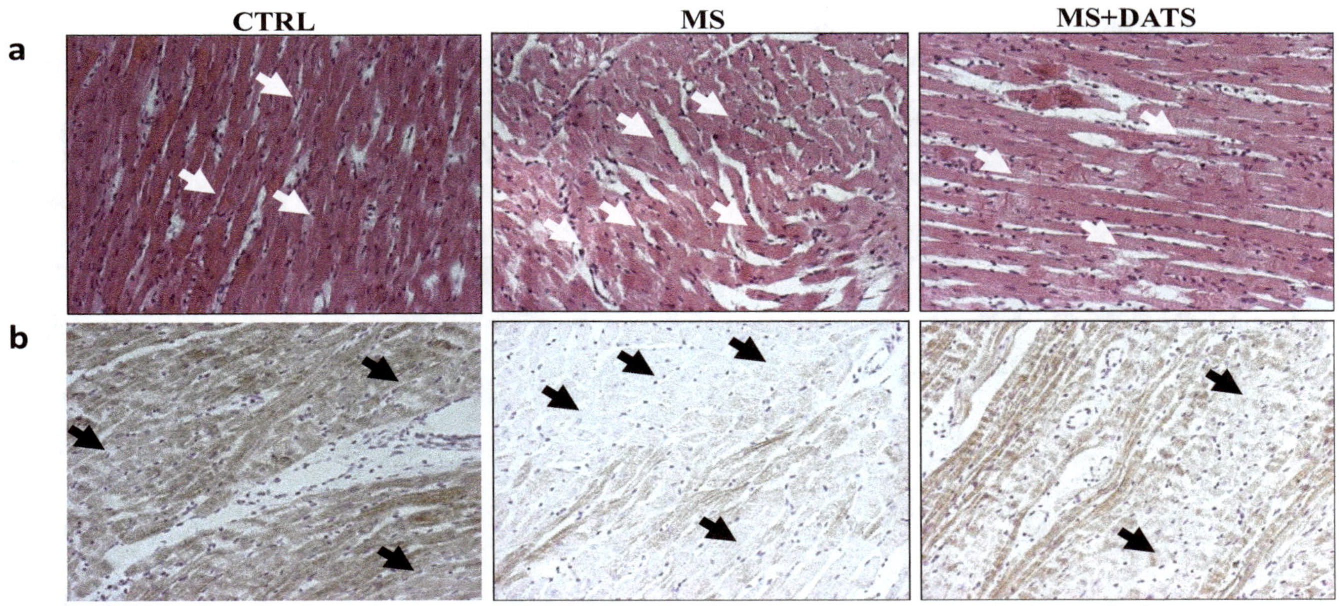

Figure 6. Representative heart tissue sections of (**a**) hematoxylin/eosin-staining (white arrows indicate representative changes in the heart tissue); (**b**) cTnT-immunostaining (black arrows indicate the area with the least colored cTnT in the heart tissue). Original magnification 20×.

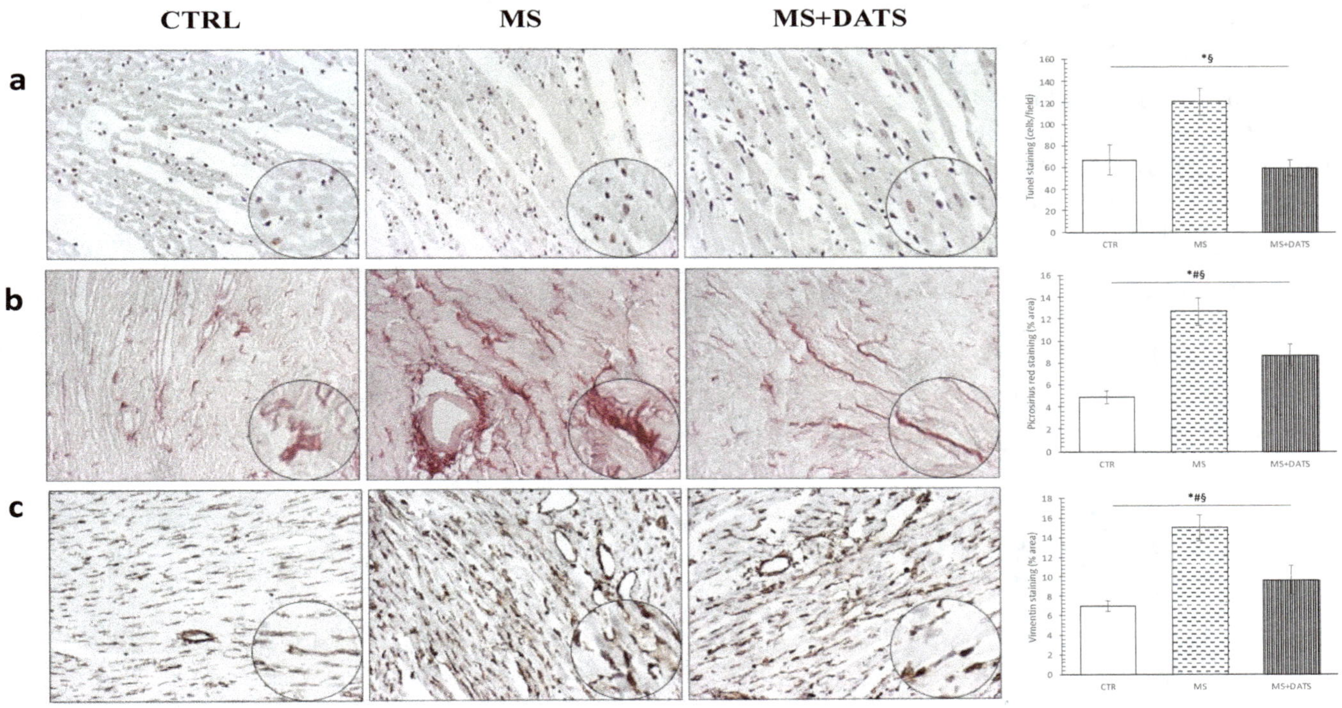

Figure 7. Representative heart tissue sections of (**a**) immunostaining of myocytes with terminal deoxynucleotidyl transferase dUTP nick end labeling (TUNEL) positive nucleus; (**b**) picrosirius red staining; (**c**) vimentin content. Values are presented as mean ± SD. * $p < 0.05$ CTRL vs. MS, # $p < 0.05$ CTRL vs. MS+DATS, § $p < 0.05$ MS vs. MS+DATS. Original magnification 20× and 40×.

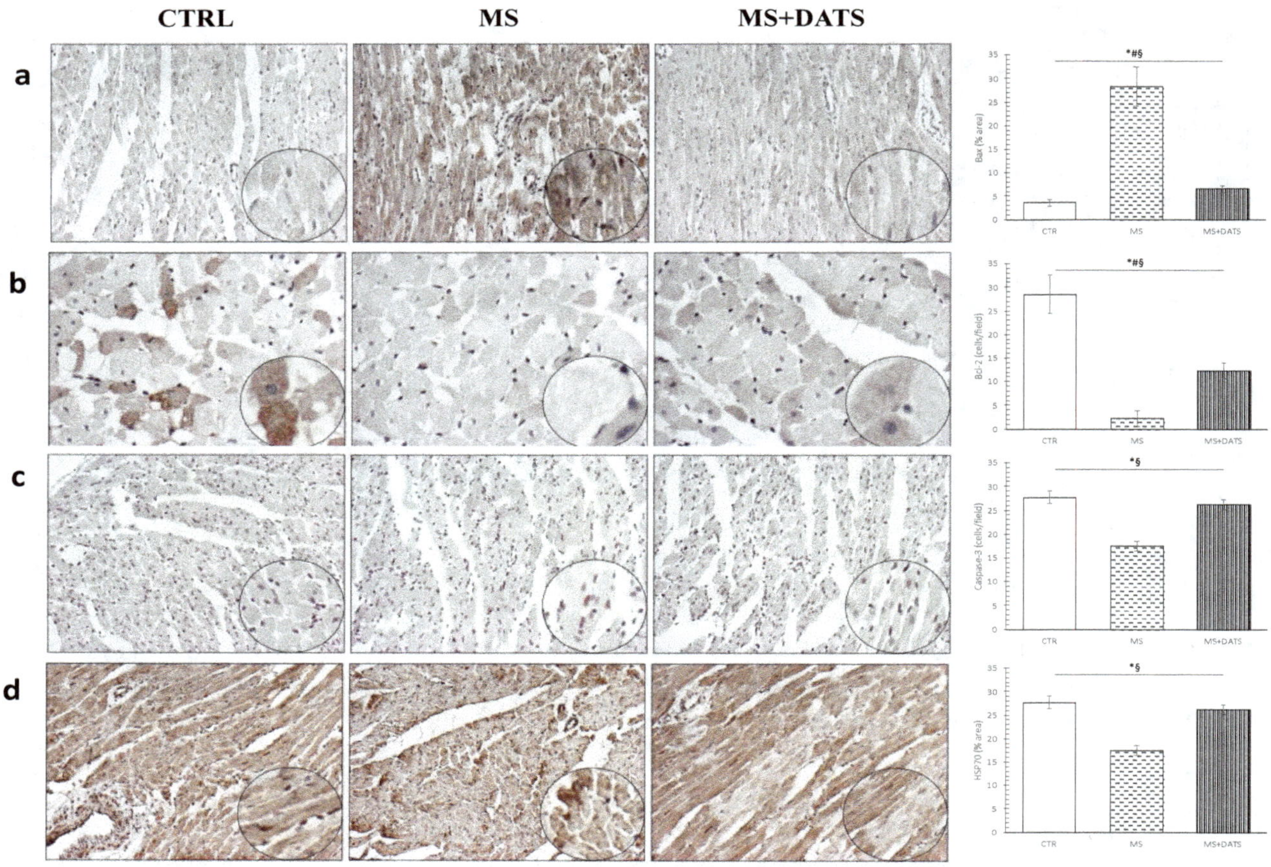

Figure 8. Representative heart tissue sections of immunohistochemical staining of (**a**) Bax; (**b**) Bcl-2; (**c**) Caspase-3; (**d**) heat shock protein 70. Values are presented as mean ± SD. * $p < 0.05$ CTRL vs. MS, # $p < 0.05$ CTRL vs. MS+DATS, § $p < 0.05$ MS vs. MS+DATS. Original magnification 20× and 40×.

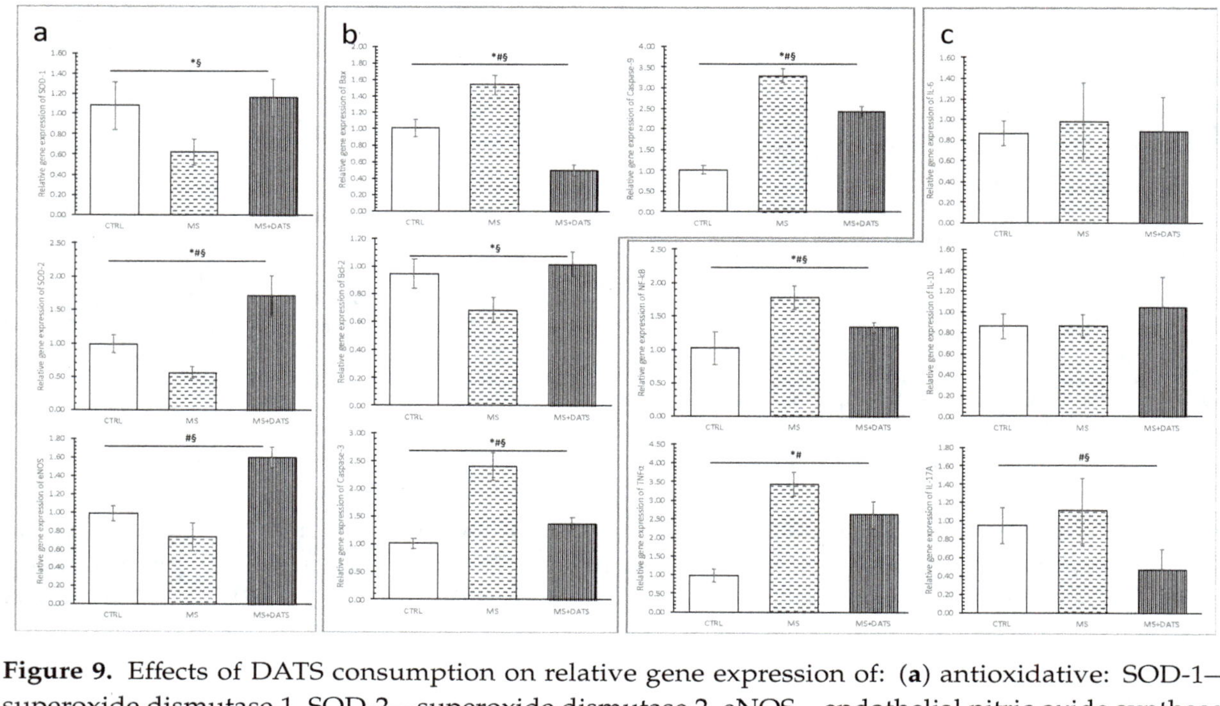

Figure 9. Effects of DATS consumption on relative gene expression of: (**a**) antioxidative: SOD-1—superoxide dismutase 1, SOD-2—superoxide dismutase 2, eNOS—endothelial nitric oxide synthase; (**b**) (anti)apoptotic: Bcl-2—B-cell lymphoma 2, Bax, caspase-3, caspase-9; (**c**) (anti)inflammative parameters: NF-κB, TNF-α, IL-6, IL-10, IL-17A. Values are presented as mean ± SD, n = 12, per group. * $p < 0.05$ CTRL vs. MS, # $p < 0.05$ CTRL vs. MS+DATS, § $p < 0.05$ MS vs. MS+DATS.

3. Discussion

Although DATS as a H_2S donor has been described several decades ago, many aspects of its effects on the cardiovascular system and metabolic disorders remain poorly known. In the present study, it was demonstrated for the first time that DATS can effectively mitigate MetS and have protective effects against ex vivo induced myocardial I/R injury in MetS rat.

MetS as a heterogeneous disorder is characterized by insulin resistance, pancreatic beta-cell dysfunction, hypertension, obese and hyperlipidemia [13]. To stimulate MetS in rats we used an animal model which involves a high-fat diet (HFd) for 4 weeks, followed by single, low-dose of streptozotocin (STZ) injection. Based on literature data, these two stressors in combination are great for experimental model because they mimic the pathology of MetS and T2DM in humans [14,15]. Besides, consumption of HFd is prevalent all over the world, which also supports the fact that used model is suitable because it is comparable to MetS in humans [14].

In the first part of our study, we were focused on the impact of DATS on metabolic control of disease, such as lipidemic and glycemic profile. In our experimental model, MetS rats displayed elevated levels of glucose, TC, TG, LDL and declined levels of HDL compared to healthy rats which are in correlation with manifestations of MetS described in the literature. On the other hand, 3 weeks of DATS consumption had a strong influence on metabolic parameters, which was manifested in a decrease of TG and LDL as well increase of HDL (Figure 1a). These results agree with those described by other authors who have examined different garlic-based extracts and reported an improved lipid profile [16,17]. The possible protective effects of garlic and DATS may be due to indirect or direct inhibition of endogenous cholesterol synthesis and/or due to changes in the portions of lipoprotein cholesterol fractions [18]. Previous studies indicate that ingestion of garlic is linked with inhibition of hepatic fatty acid synthesis mainly by lowering activities of the crucial enzymes and consequently by reducing lipid accumulation in the liver and TG in the plasma [19]. This agrees with other research which showed that supplementation with garlic extracts significantly inhibit the increment of lipid levels in serum due to inhibition of hydroxyl methyl glutaryl coenzyme A (HMG-CoA) reductase, which plays one of crucial role in controlling lipid levels in plasma and various tissues [20]. A recent study shows that NaHS (inorganic H_2S donor) extremely reduces TG serum levels in mice fed with HFd through stimulation of 5′ adenosine monophosphate protein kinase (AMPK) and subsequent autophagic responses. NaHS by increasing H_2S activates the flux of autophagy in the liver, AMPK blocks mTOR which in turn activates the autophagy pathway [21]. DATS as an H_2S donor probably may influence TG level via the same pathways. The garlic consumption in MetS also leads to a decrease in glucose levels with reduced insulin resistance and increased insulin sensitivity [22], which was obtained as well in our study after the introduction of DATS (Figure 2). Furthermore, several papers reported the hypoglycemic activity of garlic is attributed to sulfur compounds, such as DATS and others: diallyl disulfide (DADS), diallyl sulfide (DAS), alliin, allicin and ajoene, due to their free -SH group [23,24]. Decreased blood glucose levels after garlic consumption might be explained by the diminution of glucose absorption from the gastrointestinal tract by garlic and its active compounds [25].

Increasing evidence in animal and human studies shows that oxidative stress plays a central role in the pathogenesis and complications of MetS. Free radicals generated by glucose oxidation in combination with the loss of endogenous antioxidants can lead to damage of organelles in the cells and the development of insulin resistance [26]. Since, in a previously published paper, we noticed that DATS could enhance antioxidative parameters in rats with chemically induced diabetes mellites type 1 [12], we hypothesized that DATS as a powerful antioxidant may also help in alleviating MetS and MetS-related complications. We obtained a significant reduction of prooxidants and increment of antioxidants (Figure 3), which is in agreement with the previous data describing the effects of whole garlic, garlic oil, extracts and its active compounds [23,27,28]. DATS consumption was effective in the reduction of TBARS and O_2^- in plasma of MetS rats (Figure 3a), which was supported by an increase in the activities of all measured antioxidative parameters (Figure 3b). DATS treatment in our study was able to restore GSH levels which are known to be reduced in MetS due to deficiency in GSH precursor amino acids [29]. Furthermore, studies have shown that hyperglycemia can induce c-Jun N-terminal kinase (JNK) dependent nuclear factor (NF-κB) activation through the generation of ROS and cause cell apoptosis. The DATS treatment can suppress cardiomyocyte apoptosis by inhibiting JNK/NF-κB signaling via attenuating ROS generation [11].

Another aspect of our study was based on the determination of cardiac function as an important pathogenic feature of MetS. In some studies, Hcy is described as an independent risk factor, while in others it is defined as merely a risk marker. Regardless of the current controversies, Hcy and hyperhomocysteinemia (HHcy) are the new-multifactorial risk factors which interact with CVD [30]. Therefore, we attempted to discover the Hcy and HHcy relationship during the chronic consumption of DATS in rats with MetS. In our study, there was a significant increase in the level of Hcy which was expected since the rise of Hcy is linked to non-insulin-dependent diabetes mellitus. These results are in correlation with the findings referring to antioxidative stress markers since is been reported that auto-oxidation of Hcy contributes to the additional generation of ROS [31]. On the contrary, DATS intake was capable of reducing the Hcy levels thus exerting protective effects on the cardiovascular system (Figure 1b). Mechanisms by which DATS mediates beneficial effects on Hcy include modulation of variety intracellular signaling process but details remain unclear. It has been previously proved that elevated plasma levels of Hcy, are followed by a drop of endogenous production of H_2S [31]. In our study, decreased Hcy supports an increase of H_2S and might explain our results. By increasing the level of H_2S, lipid hydroperoxides in the oxidized LDL are destroyed and the atherogenic potential of LDL decreases [32]. This also may be one of the possible explanations for the hypolipidemic effects of DATS consumption. Reducing homocysteine levels and increasing H_2S in the serum directly reduces both the risk of cardiovascular disease and the extent of damage to other organs. Chronic administration of DATS significantly decreased DBP and HR in rats with MetS (MS+DATS vs. MS) (Figure 4c), which is consistent with the previous researchers. Blood pressure-lowering effects can be explained by H_2S production [33] and a decrease in peripheral vascular resistance [34]. Moreover, data suggest that NO and H_2S endothelium-dependent and K^+-ATP-dependent vasodilatory effects [35,36]. In that sense, increased production of NO as well as H_2S by DATS intake might be an explanation for obtained hypotensive effects. Furthermore, an echocardiographic examination, performed after chronic consumption of DATS on rats with MetS (MS+DATS), illustrated a significant increase of IVSd, IVSs, FS and decrease of LVIDs, compared to MS group (Figure 4a,b). Increase in FS and EF in combination with a decrease in systemic blood pressure (BP) manifests the improvement in systolic and contractile functions in rat heart from the MS+DATS group.

Since MetS is a significant risk factor for heart diseases and myocardial ischemia [37], in the second part of our study special focus was given to examine the effects of DATS on ex vivo induced I/R injury. We found markedly decreased values of SLVP, DLVP and CF during the reperfusion period in metabolic conditions. On the other hand, the values of these parameters in DATS-treated group remain almost constant over 30 min of reperfusion (Figure 4a,b), which thus indicated undisturbed heart function. Due to the accumulation of endogenous metabolites in the heart during I/R, there is a series of complex cellular and humoral reactions which induce arrhythmias, morphological changes in the myocardial tissue and harmful effects. Blockade of endogenous H_2S synthesis may also induce the modulation of cellular electrophysiology and arrhythmias, especially at the level of ion channels [38]. Therefore, the absence of significant fluctuations in cardiodynamic parameters directly shows the beneficial effects of DATS consumption in rats with MetS. Mechanisms involved in cardioprotection probably include the opening of the K-ATP channels, activation of PKC [39] and ROS scavenging [40], which together reduce the Ca^{2+} influx and shorten the action potential [38]. Among them, cardioprotection provided by activation of K-ATP and PKC most probably plays a central role [41].

The underlying mechanisms of ex vivo I/R injured heart include many reactive processes, such as oxidative stress, inflammation and apoptosis. These biological reactions stimulate each other and cause anatomical and functional changes [38–41]. In our study, we confirmed that chronic DATS administration protects against the I/R injury in the heart. Specifically, the improvement of cardiodynamic parameters was accompanied by antioxidative, anti-inflammatory and anti-apoptotic effects. Our results have shown that DATS consumption inhibits ROS in effluent and increase relative gene expression of antioxidative parameters in LV of rat heart with MetS. As it is presented in Figure 5b, DATS consumption significantly decreased levels of TBARS, O_2^- and H_2O_2 in the stabilization period and during the whole reperfusion period. These results were quite expected because DATS can induce the generation of H_2S, in a thiol-dependent manner, which is well known as an activator of endogenous antioxidant defenses and inhibitor of pro-oxidants. Calvert and coworkers suggested that these effects are provided through the Nrf-2-dependent pathway [42]. In correlation with these, our results highlighted that DATS consumption increased the relative gene expression of SOD-1 and SOD-2 in LV (Figure 7a). Additionally, the increment of SOD directly affects the reduction of cardiomyopathy. These findings are in correlation with previous, which confirmed both exogenous and endogenous derived H_2S exhibit powerful cytoprotective effects in different models of heart failure [11]. Consequently, excessive ROS production and decrement of antioxidative parameters through modulation of the heart structure and stimulation of numerous inflammatory and apoptotic markers can underline pathological processes associated with I/R injured MetS heart. Besides the already mentioned roles of DATS in ROS balancing, we additionally examined its effects on HSP70 (Figure 8d). This is of great interest since it is well known that free radicals especially the superoxide anion radical directly triggers an early increase of this protein in the I/R injured isolated rat heart. These findings suggest that although ROS may cause necrosis of myocytes at the same time may mediate HSP70, which prevents apoptosis and plays a role in the second window of protection [43,44]. On the other hand, in our study of 3 weeks, DATS consumption prevented necrosis in rats with MetS (Figure 6a), while HSP70-expression in heart tissue was slightly higher in this group of rats compared to the untreated group of rats (Figure 8d).

In our study, DATS consumption significantly reduced edema, inflammatory process and necrotic area (Figure 6) in heart tissues of MetS rats. Bearing in mind our results, DATS has the potential to preserve both function and structure of the heart under ischemic conditions. While examining the effects of DATS on (anti)inflammatory markers in LV, we found significantly reduced expression of NF-κB and IL-17A (Figure 9c). There is strong evidence supporting that garlic and garlic compounds inhibit the expression of cell adhesion molecules through downregulation of intracellular transduction pathways, such as AP-1 and JNK or NF-κB [11]. Preconditioning with NaHS preserved heart and kidney from degradation and translocation of NF-κB. In the literature data, there is great uncertainty whether H_2S has pro-inflammatory or anti-inflammatory properties. However, based on our results, DATS as an H_2S donor provides anti-inflammatory effects [7,45]. Inflammation with elevated immunocompetent cells in the cardiac tissue plays a pivotal role in the pathophysiology of cardiomyopathy and it is usually governed by several regulatory genes mediated by apoptosis signals. Therefore, we aimed to access the impact of DATS on (anti)apoptotic markers in LV of the heart. In the hearts of MetS rats subjected to I/R injury, relative gene expression of Bax, caspase-3 and caspase-9 were significantly increased, while Bcl-2 was significantly decreased compared to I/R group. On the other hand, chronic DATS consumption significantly decreased relative gene expression of Bax and both determined caspases, while the relative gene expression of Bcl-2 was increased (Figure 9b). TUNEL assay also confirmed the antiapoptotic effect of DATS (Figure 7a). We found that results of relative gene expression are in correlation with protein expression (Figure 8) and taken together, our results collectively demonstrate that DATS can protect the heart against ex vivo induced I/R injury in MetS hearts, probably by its ability to ameliorate oxidative stress, apoptosis and inflammation in the heart. Our results are in line with previous reports [46] suggesting antiapoptotic effects of DATS have been attributed to H_2S and its possibility to phosphorylate few survival proteins, such as ERK, PI3K and Akt [42].

This study shows that the cardioprotective effects of DATS might be mediated through different cell responses. Although endothelial reticulum and oxidative stress are considered as two independent cellular pathways it is like to be, they are related. Stress responses protein such as HSP70 is required for mediating antioxidant mechanisms against Hcy induced cell damage. In this study, we showed that DATS mediate promotion of HSP70 and couple of pathways probably are responsible for overall cardioprotective effects of DATS. As a strong antioxidant DATS diminishes ROS production and together with an increment of HSP70 prevents cell damage leading to inhibition of caspase-3 activation, with consequent reducing of apoptosis [47].

4. Materials and Methods

4.1. Ethical Statement

Procedures used in this research were approved by the Ethics Committee for experimental animal well-being of the Faculty of Medical Sciences, University of Kragujevac (Kragujevac, Serbia), number: 01-1811 and were carried out following European Directive for the welfare of laboratory animals number: 2010/63/EU (22 September 2010) and principles of Good Laboratory Practice. Additionally, all experimental procedures have performed following the prescribed regulations of European Union Directive for the Protection of the Vertebrate Animals used for Experimental and other Scientific Purposes 86/609/EES and the principles of ethics.

4.2. Experimental Animals

Wistar albino rats used in this study have obtained from the Military Medical Academy, Belgrade, Serbia and housed under controlled regular environmental conditions: temperature (22 ± 2 °C), humidity and illumination (light/darkness cycle, 12/12 h). To adapt to the new environment, rats were caged seven days before the study began. Appropriate diets, standard (9% fat, 20% protein, 53% starch) or HFd (25% fat, 15% protein and 51% starch), and water have provided ad libitum.

All *Wistar albino* rats used in this study were male and were 13 weeks old at the time of sacrifice. At the beginning of the study 36 rats were randomly divided into healthy (CTRL, n = 12) and rats with MetS (n = 24). To induce MetS rats (6 weeks old, bodyweight 180 ± 20 g) were for four weeks fed with HFd and after 12-h starvation intraperitoneal single injection of STZ in the dose of 25 mg/kg was administrated. Three days (72 h) later, fasting blood glucose and insulin as well as blood pressure are measured. Animals with fasting blood glucose level over 7 mmol/L, fasting insulin level above 6 mmol/L and blood pressure level over 130/90 mmHg were included in the study and were considered as rats with MetS [48]. After successful MetS-induction rats were randomly divided into two subgroups: MS (untreated MetS rats) and MS+DATS (MetS rats treated with DATS) and both groups continued with HFd consumption.

4.3. DATS Treatment

To mimic the most common and the easiest administration route, DATS was applied by oral gavage (*per os*), every second day, at a dose of 40 mg/kg of body weight for three weeks [49].

DATS (purity ≥ 98%) was purchased from Sigma-Aldrich Chemie GmbH Eschenstrase 5, 82024 Taufkirchen, Germany. DATS was stored at −20 °C in dark, original bottles, according to the manufacturer's recommendations.

4.4. Biochemical Parameters

The following lipid parameters: total cholesterol (TC), triglycerides (TG), high- and low-density lipoprotein (HDL and LDL) were analyzed spectrophotometrically on a programmed biochemical analyzer (Dimension Xpand, Siemens, IL, USA) in serum using commercial kits (Siemens Healthcare Diagnostics, Frimley, Camberley, Surrey, UK).

The methylene blue method was used for measuring total sulfide levels in the plasma. The supernatant was collected and total sulfide using a standard calibration NaHS curve was determined at a wavelength of 670 nm [50]. For determination, we used a microplate reader (Zenyth, Anthos, UK).

Homocysteine (Hcy) concentration was measured in serum with high-performance liquid chromatography (HPLC) procedure with reverse-phase separation and fluorescence detection, as described earlier. The fluorescence was measured at 390 nm, while emission was measured at 470 nm [51].

4.5. Oral Glucose Tolerance Test (OGTT), Insulin and Glucose Levels Determination

At the end of experimental treatment with DATS, OGTT was performed. After an overnight (12 h) fasting, the blood samples were collected from the tail-tip of the rats to determine the blood glucose and insulin levels (marked as 0). Next, glucose in a dose of 2 g/kg body weight was administered orally, and blood samples were taken by tail bleeding at 30, 60, 120 and 180 min after glucose loading. Glucose levels were immediately estimated at 0, 30, 60, 120 and 180 min, using the Accu-Chek (Roche Diagnostics, Indianapolis, IN, USA) glucometer with its comparing strips. Insulin levels were evaluated in plasma samples by the enzyme-linked immunosorbent assay (ELISA) method, as previously explained at 0 and 180 min [12,48].

4.6. Redox Status

Assessments of systemic pro-oxidant and antioxidant parameters were carried out in blood samples collected in the moment of animals sacrificing. Firstly, whole blood samples were centrifugated to separate the red blood cells (RBCs) from the plasma. In brief, during the centrifugation process, the RBCs are deposited at the bottom of the Vacutainer tubes (red layer), while plasma remains on the surface as an upper phase (yellow layer). After separation of the plasma, the RBCs were washed and stored in lysed forms.

In plasma samples, the levels of prooxidative parameters index of lipid peroxidation (measured as thiobarbituric acid reactive substances (TBARS)), nitrites (NO_2^-), superoxide anion radical (O_2^-), and hydrogen peroxide (H_2O_2) were measured, while in the lysate of erythrocytes, the activity of enzymatic defense system by evaluating of catalase (CAT) and superoxide dismutase (SOD), as well as amount of non-enzymatic antioxidant, reduced glutathione (GSH), were determined.

To determine lipid peroxidation in the plasma, we used an indirect method of determining the concentration of thiobarbituric acid reaction product (thiobarbituric acid reactive substances (TBARS)). The used method is based on the determination of lipid peroxidase level in the reaction of the malondialdehyde with thiobarbituric acid. Distilled water instead of plasma sample was used for the blind test.

To determine nitrite, we used an indirect method for determining the number of released nitrites. Actually, in 0.1 mL perchloric acid we pipetted 0.4 mL ethylenediaminetetraacetic acid (20 mM) and 0.2 mL of plasma samples. Then, we vortexed and incubated 15 min on ice and centrifugated 15 min (6000 rpm). Next, in sludge, we added 220 μL potassium carbonate. From there we took 220 μL samples and added 250 μL of freshly prepared Griess reagent and 125 μL of buffer for NO. After 15 min, we measured on 550 nm wavelength. Instead of plasma samples, the corresponding quantity of distilled water was used as a blind test.

The quantification of superoxide anion radical is based on the reaction of O_2^- with nitro blue tetrazolium until nitro formazan blue. The determination was performed in plasma samples in the following steps: in 50 μL of plasma samples, we added extempore 950 μL of assay mixture and measured on 550 nm three times every 60 s. Instead of plasma samples, the comparing amount of distilled water was utilized as a blind test. Reaction responsible to H_2O_2 is based on the oxidation of phenol red by the reaction of hydrogen peroxide catalyzed by enzyme peroxidase from horseradish (HRPO).

To determine the hydrogen peroxide (H_2O_2) in 200 μL of plasma samples we added 800 μL of phenol red solution and 10 μL peroxidase (POD). And after incubation at room temperature for 10 min we measured the concentration of H_2O_2 at 610 nm. Instead of plasma, for a blind test, we used distilled water. Measurement must be in the time interval from 5 to 60 min because that is a period of generation and release of H_2O_2.

In our study, the catalase was determined in lysate RBCs by dissolving lysate with distilled water in a 1:7 ratio, followed by the addition of ethanol in a 0.1:1 ratio (mixture). Then, in a 50 μL CAT buffer, we added 100 μL of the mixture and 1 mL of 10 mM H_2O_2 into the test tube. For the blind test, we used distilled water instead of sample. Every sample was measured six consecutive times at a wavelength of 360 nm. The final values were obtained based on a calculation scheme that involves subtraction and then the arithmetic means of the obtained values.

To determine SOD activity in 100 μL lysate RBCs we pipetted 1000 μL of carbonate buffer and then vortexed and added 100 μL of adrenaline. This method is based on the epinephrine method by Beutler. For the blind test, we used just mentioned solutions, and all samples, as well as a blind test, were measured at 470 nm wavelength. To measure the activity of GSH in the erythrocyte lysate, we used the spectrophotometric method based on the oxidation reaction of glutathione with 5.5-dithiobis-6.2-nitrobenzoic acid, according to Beutler. In 50 μL of lysate RBCs, we added 200 μL 0.1% ethylenediaminetetraacetic and 385 μL precipitated buffer. After 15 min incubation on ice and 10 min centrifugation on 4000 rpm, an extract was obtained. In 300 μL of the extract, we added 750 μL of sodium phosphate dibasic and 100 μL 5.5-dithiobis-6.2-nitrobenzoic acid. Next, incubated for 10 min and measured in duplicate on 412 nm wavelength. For blind test, instead of the sample, we used distilled water. The calibration curve was constructed to determine the concentrations of the GSH activity in the samples. It was created by four standards with a known amount of glutathione.

Mentioned parameters were determined using Shimadzu UV 1800 spectrophotometer (Shimadzu corporation, Nishinokyo-Kuwabaracho, Nakagyo-KU, Kyoto, Japan) as previously described [12,48].

4.7. Cardiac Function Monitored In Vivo

Transthoracic echocardiography evaluation was performed in the last week of chronic protocol, after three-week administration of DATS, using a Hewlett-Packard Sonas 5500, Andover, MA, USA sector scanner equipped with a 15.0 MHz phased-array transducer. Rats were anaesthetized with an intraperitoneal injection of a combination of 0.025 mL ketamine (100 mg/mL; Ketalar, Pfizer Pharmaceuticals, Groton, CT, USA) and 0.025 mL xylazine (20 mg/mL; Xyla, Interchemie, Holland). The cursor was positioned perpendicularly, and images were acquired from M-mode. The following structural variables were measured: interventricular septal wall thickness at end-diastole (IVSd) and end-systole (IVSs), left ventricle (LV) internal dimension at end-diastole (LVIDd) and end-systole (LVIDs), LV posterior wall thickness at end-diastole (LVPWd) and ended-systoleVPWs), as well as fractional shortening (FS) percentage. Average values were obtained from no less than five cardiac sets on M-mode tracking. Additionally, Teicholz formula was used for calculation of ejection fraction (EF) values [52]. Furthermore, echocardiographic measurements were performed in all animals before any manipulation before initiation of DATS, STZ injection, or HFd feeding) to ensure that the cardiodynamic parameters of the animals included in the study were within the physiological range.

Blood pressure (BP) and heart rate (HR) were measured a day before sacrificing animals, by a tail-cuff non-invasive technique (Rat Tail Cuff Method Blood Pressure Systems (MRBP-R), IITC Life Science Inc, Los Angeles, CA, USA) [45]. To eliminate potential variations in blood pressure values due to stress all rats were placed for 30 min in a chamber two days before final BP testing. In each round 8–10 determinations are made, based on which mean values are calculated.

4.8. Ex Vivo Experimental Protocol

To examine the heart function in detail, we used the Langendorff apparatus (Experimetria Ltd., Budapest, Hungary) for retrograde heart perfusion and ex vivo-induced I/R injury. Namely, the rats were anaesthetized with an intraperitoneal injection of 0.025 mL ketamine (100 mg/mL; Ketalar, Pfizer, New York, NY, USA) and 0.025 mL xylazine (20 mg/mL; Xyla, Interchemie, Holland) and heart was isolated and perfused with Krebs–Henseleit solution through an aortic cannula on Langendorff apparatus. The left atrium was incised, and mitral valves were separated to provide the placement of the sensor in the LV. After the heart reached a stable steady-state (S), 30 min global ischemia was caused by complete cessation of flow followed by 60 min reperfusion (flow was turned on) [12].

4.8.1. Cardiodynamic and Oxidative Stress Parameters

At the steady-state, as well in the 1st, 3rd, 5th, 10th, 15th, 30th, 45th, and 60th minute of reperfusion cardiodynamic parameters: maximum rate of left ventricular pressure development (marked as dp/dt max, unit: mmHg), a minimum rate of left ventricular pressure development (marked as dp/dt min, unit: mmHg), systolic left ventricular pressure (marked as SLVP, unit: mmHg), diastolic left ventricular pressure (marked as DLVP, unit: mmHg), heart rate (marked as HR, unit: bpm) were monitored. Furthermore, coronary flow (marked as CF unit: mL/min) was followed and coronary venous effluent was collected. All oxidative stress parameters measured in plasma TBARS, NO_2^-, O_2^- and H_2O_2, were also measured in the coronary venous effluent. Based on these parameters in the coronary venous effluent during I/R injury is directly estimated oxidative stress in the endocardium of the left ventricle and endothelium of coronary circulation. The principle of determination is similar to those in plasma; only a few steps differ [12,48].

4.8.2. Pathohistological Analysis of Myocardial Tissue

After ex vivo protocol on Langendorff apparatus, all hearts were fixed in 4% buffered paraformaldehyde solution on room temperature. Tissues were two times dehydrated with 95% ethanol for 30 min, soaked in xylene for 60 min 60–70 °C and put 12 h in paraffin. The stained tissues were cut into 4 μm sections and then stained with hematoxylin/eosin. To visualize collagen deposition, paraffin heart sections were stained with Picrosirius red (Sigma, Direct Red 80, St. Louis, MO, USA) as previously described [53]. Quantification of red-stained collagen in heart sections stained with Picrosirius red was performed using ImageJ software (National Institute of Health, Bethesda, MD, USA), on 10 fields/section, as previously described [54].

For the violation of the specificity and quality of deoxynucleotidyl transfer-mediated dUTP nick end-labelling (TUNEL) staining in this study [55], we used a positive control. Lymph node tissue, which was previously found to have cells with a TUNEL positive nucleus, was used for this purpose (Figure 10). Positive control sections were treated in the same manner and at the same time as the tested tissues of the heart.

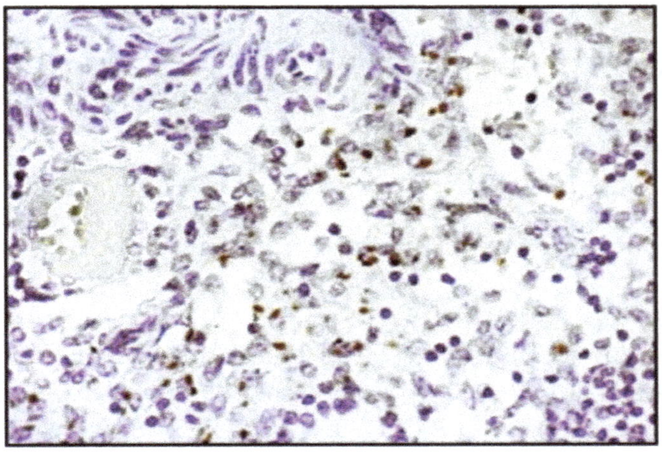

Figure 10. Representative lymph node section (positive external control). Original magnification 40×.

For immunohistochemical staining 5 μm thick heart tissue sections, were dewaxed, rehydrated and treated with citrate buffer (pH 6.0) in the microwave for antigen retrieval. Staining was visualized by using the EXPOSE Rabbit specific HRP/DAB detection IHC Kit (ab80437, Abcam, UK) and sections were counterstained with Mayer's hematoxylin. The slices were incubated with cardiac troponin T (ab209813), vimentin (working dilution 1:100; Novocastra, Burlingame, CA, USA), recombinant anti-Bax (ab32503), Bcl2 (ab32124), anti-cleaved Caspase 3 (ab2302) and anti-HSP70 (ab5439) overnight at room temperature. Sections were photomicrographed with a digital camera mounted on a light microscope (Olympus Corporation, BX51, Shinjuku-ku, Tokyo, Japan), digitized and analyzed. The analysis was performed on 10 fields/section (×40) using ImageJ software (National Institute of Health, Bethesda, MD, USA). Results are presented as mean count of positively stained cells per field or percentage of immunoreactive area.

Microscopic analysis of the hearts longitudinal sections of all rats was performed by a pathology specialist. To avoid bias and maximizing objectivity, the pathologist was blinded to the sample group. The emphasis was on histologic changes of the left ventricle, and primarily on the lateral wall, septum, and apex.

4.8.3. Expression of Antioxidative, (anti)Apoptotic and (anti)Inflammation Genes in the LV of Heart Tissue

The total RNA (μg) from LV tissue samples was isolated using TRIzol reagent (Invitrogen, Carlsbad, CA, USA) according to the manufacturer's protocol. Total RNA (μg) was reverse transcribed using High Capacity cDNA Reverse Transcription Kit (Applied Biosystems, Foster City, CA, USA). Real-time quantitative polymerase chain reaction (RT-PCR) was performed using Thermo Scientific Luminaris Color HiGreen qPCR Master Mix (Applied Biosystems, Foster City, CA, USA) and mRNA specific primer for oxidative stress markers: SOD-1, SOD-2, eNOS; (anti)apoptotic markers: Bax, Bcl-2, caspase-3, caspase-9; (anti)inflammation markers: NFkB, TNFα, IL-6, IL-10, and IL-17A.

β-actin (Invitrogen, Carlsbad, CA, USA) was used as a housekeeping gene (Table 1). PCR reactions were performed in a Mastercycler ep realplex (Eppendorf, Hamburg, Germany). Data were analyzed and relative gene expression was calculated according to Livak and Schmittgen.

Table 1. Primers used for RT-PCR analysis.

	Left Primers	Right Primers
β-actin	GATCAGCAAGCAGGAGTACGAT	GTAACAGTCCGCCTAGAAGCAT
SOD-1	TGAAGAGAGGCATGTTGGAGAC	CACACGATCTTCAATGGACACA
SOD-2	AATCAACAGACCCAAGCTAGGC	CACAATGTCACTCCTCTCCGAA
eNOS	GAGGGAGTCAGCCTAAATCCTG	ATCAAAGCATACGAAGAGGGCA
Bcl-2	GCAAAGCACATCCAATAAAAGCG	GTACTTCATCACGATCTCCCGG
Bax	GCTACAGGGTTTCATCCAGGAT	ATGTTGTTGTCCAGTTCATCGC
Caspase-3	GGAAGATCACAGCAAAAGGAGC	GCAGTAGTCGCCTCTGAAGAAA
Caspase-9	TGTACTCCAGGGAAGATCGAGA	CGTTGTTGATGATGAGGCAGTG
NF-kB	GTTTGGTTTGAGACATCCCTGC	CTGTCTTATGGCTGAGGTCTGG
TNF-α	GAAAGCATGATCCGAGATGTGG	CAGGAATGAGAAGAGGCTGAGG
IL-6	GATACCACCCACAACAGACCAG	GTGCATCATCGCTGTTCATACA
IL-10	CTTACTGGCTGGAGTGAAGACC	CTGGGAAGTGGGTGCAGTTATT
IL-17	GCAAGAGATCCTGGTCCTGAAG	AGGTCTCTGTTTAGGACGCATG

4.9. Statistical Analysis

All presented data are shown as mean ± standard deviation (SD). Figures and tables were made in Microsoft Excel for Mac version 16. Unless otherwise stated, data were assessed by one-way ANOVA followed by Tukey's multiple comparison post hoc test, using IBM-SPSS, version 20. p values less < 0.05 were considered statistically significant.

5. Conclusions

The main advantage of this study is the use of DATS that naturally exists in garlic and is unlikely to cause serious side effects, so it can be a great option for clinical relevance. It is important to note that the efficacy of DATS is impossible to achieve just by eating garlic, but further clinical studies in which the optimized formulations of DATS would be applied are needed. In our experimental study, it seems to be well-tolerated, but since its structure is sensitive to chemical transformations, poor water solubility, and the generation of various by-products after H_2S release [56], larger multi-faceted studies are necessary for a full DATS pharmacodynamic and pharmacokinetic profile. Although it should be kept in mind that not all findings obtained on animals can be directly translated into humans [57], the results of our study are an important cornerstone for future clinical studies in which various formulations of DATS would be examined.

Furthermore, we previously described the positive effects on the cardiovascular system in rats with chemically induced diabetes mellitus type 1; however, the effects of DATS on rats with MetS is barely known. Although we accept the fact that mechanisms through which DATS accomplished its protective effects are similar, used model by itself is completely pathophysiological different. Taken together our results undoubtedly show protective effects of DATS and its potential to control metabolic disorders and prevent their cardiovascular complications. In addition to the previous report which demonstrates antiapoptotic, antioxidative and anti-inflammatory effects of DATS, in this study we also identified its potential to alter levels of homocysteine, H_2S, lipid status, blood pressure and fibrosis. The relationship between DATS and HSP70 is barely known and with this study, we show that it is possible for DATS to achieve cardioprotection by triggering high expression of HSP70. In this way, we attained a deeper insight into the mechanisms of the protective effects of DATS.

Based on our findings, DATS, a phytochemical derived from garlic, has the potential to be used as a herbal-based supplement in the management of MetS and its related manifestations. The mechanism underlying the cardioprotective effects of DATS against ex vivo induced I/R injury in MetS hearts could be mainly attributed to the ability of this compound to ameliorate oxidative stress, apoptosis and inflammation in the heart. These results suggest that diallyl trisulfide is at least partially responsible for the epidemiologically established cardioprotective and anti/MetS effect of garlic.

Author Contributions: Conceptualization, N.S.J. and J.N.J.; methodology, V.I.Z.; validation, I.M.M. and J.V.B.; formal analysis, S.L.M.; investigation, J.N.J. and N.U.J.; writing—original draft preparation, J.N.J. and J.V.B.; writing—review and editing, I.M.S.; visualization, S.B.B. and A.A.S.; supervision, V.L.J. and S.C.T.; project administration, N.S.J. All authors have read and agreed to the published version of the manuscript.

References

1. Heusch, G.; Libby, P.; Gersh, B.; Yellon, D.; Böhm, M.; Lopaschuk, G.; Opie, L. Cardiovascular remodelling in coronary artery disease and heart failure. *Lancet* **2014**, *383*, 1933–1943. [CrossRef]
2. Andreadou, I.; Iliodromitis, E.K.; Rassaf, T.; Schulz, R.; Papapetropoulos, A.; Ferdinandy, P. The role of gasotransmitters NO, H_2S and CO in myocardial ischaemia/reperfusion injury and cardioprotection by preconditioning, postconditioning and remote conditioning. *Br. J. Pharmacol.* **2015**, *172*, 1587–1606. [CrossRef] [PubMed]
3. Hausenloy, D.J.; Yellon, D.M. The therapeutic potential of ischemic conditioning: An update. *Nat. Rev. Cardiol.* **2011**, *8*, 619–629. [CrossRef] [PubMed]
4. Grassi, G.; Dell'oro, R.; Quarti-Trevano, F.; Scopelliti, F.; Seravalle, G.; Paleari, F.; Gamba, P.L.; Mancia, G. Neuroadrenergic and reflex abnormalities in patients with metabolic syndrome. *Diabetologia* **2015**, *48*, 1359–1365. [CrossRef] [PubMed]
5. Heusch, G.; Boengler, K.; Schulz, R. Inhibition of mitochondrial permeability transition pore opening: The Holy Grail of cardioprotection. *Basic Res. Cardiol.* **2010**, *105*, 151–154. [CrossRef] [PubMed]
6. Subramanian, M.S.; Nandagopal MS, G.; Amin Nordin, S.; Thilakavathy, K.; Joseph, N. Prevailing Knowledge on the Bioavailability and Biological Activities of Sulphur Compounds from Alliums: A Potential Drug Candidate. *Molecules* **2020**, *25*, 4111. [CrossRef] [PubMed]
7. Sivarajah, A.; McDonald, M.C.; Thiemermann, C. The production of hydrogen sulfide limits myocardial ischemia and reperfusion injury and contributes to the cardioprotective effects of preconditioning with endotoxin, but not ischemia in the rat. *Shock* **2006**, *26*, 154–161. [CrossRef] [PubMed]

8. Sodha, N.R.; Clements, R.T.; Feng, J.; Liu, Y.; Bianchi, C.; Horvath, E.M.; Szabo, C.; Stahl, G.L.; Sellke, F.W. Hydrogen sulfide therapy attenuates the inflammatory response in a porcine model of myocardial ischemia/reperfusion injury. *J. Thorac. Cardiovasc. Surg.* **2009**, *138*, 977–984. [CrossRef]
9. Kimura, Y.; Goto, Y.; Kimura, H. Hydrogen sulfide increases glutathione production and suppresses oxidative stress in mitochondria. *Antioxid. Redox Sign.* **2010**, *12*, 1–13. [CrossRef]
10. Pluth, M.D.; Bailey, T.S.; Hammers, M.D.; Hartle, M.D.; Henthorn, H.A.; Steiger, A.K. Natural Products Containing Hydrogen Sulfide Releasing Moieties. *Synlett* **2015**, *26*, 2633–2643. [CrossRef]
11. Kuo, W.W.; Wang, W.J.; Tsai, C.Y.; Way, C.L.; Hsu, H.H.; Chen, L.M. Diallyl trisulfide (DATS) suppresses high glucose-induced cardiomyocyte apoptosis by inhibiting JNK/NFκB signaling via attenuating ROS generation. *Int. J. Cardiol.* **2013**, *168*, 270–280. [CrossRef] [PubMed]
12. Jeremic, J.N.; Jakovljevic, V.L.; Zivkovic, V.I.; Srejovic, I.M.; Bradic, J.V.; Bolevich, S.; Nikolic Turnic, T.R.; Mitrovic, S.L.; Jovicic, N.U.; Tyagi, S.C.; et al. The cardioprotective effects of diallyl trisulfide on diabetic rats with ex vivo induced ischemia/reperfusion injury. *Mol. Cell Biochem.* **2019**, *460*, 151–164. [CrossRef]
13. McCracken, E.; Monaghan, M.; Sreenivasan, S. Pathophysiology of the metabolic syndrome. *Clin. Dermatol.* **2018**, *36*, 14–20. [CrossRef] [PubMed]
14. Lenzen, S. The mechanisms of alloxan- and streptozotocin-induced diabetes. *Diabetologia* **2008**, *51*, 216–226. [CrossRef] [PubMed]
15. Skovso, S. Modeling type 2 diabetes in rats using high fat diet and streptozotocin. *J. Diabetes Investig.* **2014**, *5*, 349–358. [CrossRef] [PubMed]
16. Pérez-Torres, I.; Torres-Narváez, J.C.; Pedraza-Chaverri, J.; Rubio-Ruiz, M.E.; Díaz-Díaz, E.; Del Valle-Mondragón, L.; Martínez-Memije, R.; Varela López, E.; Guarner-Lans, V. Effect of the Aged Garlic Extract on Cardiovascular Function in Metabolic Syndrome Rats. *Molecules* **2016**, *21*, 1425. [CrossRef] [PubMed]
17. Ha, A.W.; Ying, T.; Kim, W.K. The effects of black garlic (Allium satvium) extracts on lipid metabolism in rats fed a high fat diet. *Nutr. Res. Pract.* **2015**, *9*, 30–36. [CrossRef]
18. Aouadi, R.; Aouidet, A.; Elkadhi, A.; Ben Rayana, C.M.; Jaafoura, H.; Tritar, B.; Nagati, K. Effect of fresh garlic (allium sativum) on lipid metabolism in male rats. *Nutr. Res.* **2000**, *20*, 273–280. [CrossRef]
19. Thomson, M.; Al-Qattan, K.K.; Bordia, T. Including Garlic in the Diet May Help Lower Blood Glucose, Cholesterol, and Triglycerides. *J. Nutr.* **2006**, *136*, 800–802. [CrossRef]
20. Shrivastava, A.; Chaturvedi, U.; Sonkar, R.; Saxena, J.K.; Khanna, A.K.; Bhatia, G. Antidyslipidemic, antiatherogenic and antioxidant activity of Allium sativum in Charles Foster rats. *Int. J. Curr. Pharm. Rev. Res. IJCPR* **2011**, *2*, 110–119.
21. Sun, L.; Zhang, S.; Yu, C.; Pan, Z.; Liu, Y.; Zhao, J.; Wang, X.; Yun, F.; Zhao, H.; Yan, S.; et al. Hydrogen sulfide reduces serum triglyceride by activating liver autophagy via the AMPK-mTOR pathway. *Am. J. Physiol. Metab.* **2015**, *309*, E925–E935. [CrossRef] [PubMed]
22. Padiya, R.; Banerjee, S.K. Garlic as an Anti-Diabetic Agent: Recent Progress and Patent Reviews. *Recent Pat. Food Nutr. Agric.* **2013**, *5*, 105–127. [CrossRef] [PubMed]
23. Sujithra, K.; Srinivasan, S.; Indumathi, D.; Vinothkumar, V. Allyl methyl sulfide, a garlic active component mitigates hyperglycemia by restoration of circulatory antioxidant status and attenuating glycoprotein components in streptozotocin-induced experimental rats. *Toxicol. Methods* **2019**, *29*, 165–176. [CrossRef] [PubMed]
24. Tripathi, P.; Gupta, P.P.; Lal, V.K. Effect of Co-administration of Allium sativum extract and metformin on blood glucose of Streptozotocin induced diabetic rats. *J. Intercult. Ethnopharmacol.* **2013**, *2*, 81–84. [CrossRef]
25. Belemkar, S.; Dhameliya, K.; Pata, M.K. Comparative study of garlic species (Allium sativum and Allium porrum) on glucose uptake in diabetic rats. *Ind. J. Clin. Biochem.* **2013**, *8*, 80–85. [CrossRef]
26. Ceriello, A. Oxidative stress and diabetes-associated complications. *Endocr. Pract.* **2006**, *12*, 60–62. [CrossRef]
27. Jang, E.K.; Seo, J.H.; Lee, S.P. Physiological activity and antioxidative effects of aged black garlic (*Allium sativum* L.) extract. *Korean J. Food Sci. Technol.* **2008**, *40*, 443–448.
28. Ahmad, M.S.; Pischetsrieder, M.; Ahmed, A. Aged garlic extract and S-allyl cysteine prevent formation of advanced glycation endproducts. *Eur. J. Pharmacol.* **2007**, *561*, 32–38. [CrossRef]
29. Qu, Z.; Mossine, V.V.; Cui, J.; Sun, G.Y.; Gu, Z. Protective effects of AGE and its components on neuroinflammation and neurodegeneration. *Neuromol. Med.* **2016**, *18*, 474–482. [CrossRef]

30. Jeremic, N.; Bradic, J.; Petkovic, A.; Weber, G. Role of Oxidative Stress in Hyperhomocysteinemia-Induced Heart Diseases. In *Modulation of Oxidative Stress in Heart Disease*; Springer: Singapore, 2019; Volume 1, pp. 365–375.
31. Hayden, M.R.; Tyagi, S.C. Homocysteine and Reactive Oxygen Species in Metabolic Syndrome, Type 2 Diabetes Mellitus, and Atheroscleropathy: The Pleiotropic Effects of Folate Supplementation. *Nutr. J.* **2004**, *3*, 4. [CrossRef]
32. Muellner, M.K.; Schreier, S.M.; Laggner, H.; Hermann, M.; Esterbauer, H.; Exner, M.; Gmeiner, B.M.; Kapiotis, S. Hydrogen sulfide destroys lipid hydroperoxides in oxidized LDL. *Biochem. J.* **2009**, *420*, 277–281. [CrossRef] [PubMed]
33. Reinhart, K.M.; Coleman, C.I.; Teevan, C.; Vachhani, P.; White, C.M. Effects of garlic on blood pressure in patients with and without systolic hypertension: A meta-analysis. *Ann. Pharmacother.* **2008**, *42*, 1766–1771. [CrossRef] [PubMed]
34. Brankovic, S.; Radenkovic, M.; Kitic, D.; Veljkovic, S.; Ivetic, V.; Pavlovic, D.; Miladinovic, B. Comparison of the hypotensive and bradycardic activity of ginkgo, garlic, and onion extracts. *Clin. Exp. Hypertens.* **2011**, *33*, 95–99. [CrossRef]
35. Asdaq, S.M.; Inamdar, M.N. Potential of garlic and its active constituent, S-allyl cysteine, as antihypertensive and cardioprotective in presence of captopril. *Phytomedicine* **2010**, *17*, 1016–1026. [CrossRef] [PubMed]
36. Jain, S.K.; Bull, R.; Rains, J.L.; Bass, P.F.; Levine, S.N.; Reddy, S.; McVie, R.; Bocchini, J.A. Low levels of hydrogen sulfide in the blood of diabetes patients and streptozotocin-treated rats causes vascular inflammation? *Antioxid. Redox Signal.* **2010**, *12*, 1333–1337. [CrossRef] [PubMed]
37. Grundy, S.M. Metabolic syndrome update. *Trends Cardiovasc. Med.* **2016**, *26*, 364–373. [CrossRef]
38. Bian, J.S.; Yong, Q.C.; Pan, T.T.; Feng, Z.N.; Ali, M.Y.; Zhou, S.; Moore, P.K. Role of hydrogen sulfide in the cardioprotection caused by ischemic preconditioning in the rat heart and cardiac myocytes. *J. Pharmacol. Exp. Ther.* **2006**, *316*, 670–678. [CrossRef] [PubMed]
39. Eisen, A.; Fisman, E.Z.; Rubenfire, M.; Freimark, D.; McKechnie, R.; Tenenbaum, A.; Motro, M.; Adler, Y. Ischemic preconditioning: Nearly two decades of research. A comprehensive review. *Atherosclerosis* **2004**, *172*, 201–210. [CrossRef]
40. Zhao, W.; Zhang, J.; Lu, Y.; Wang, R. The vasorelaxant effect of H(2)S as a novel endogenous gaseous KATP channel opener. *Eur. Mol. Biol. Organ. J.* **2001**, *20*, 6008–6016. [CrossRef]
41. Geng, B.; Chang, L.; Pan, C.; Qi, Y.; Zhao, J.; Pang, Y.; Du, J.; Tang, C. Endogenous hydrogen sulfide regulation of myocardial injury induced by isoproterenol. *Biochem. Biophys. Res. Commun.* **2004**, *318*, 756–763. [CrossRef]
42. Calvert, J.W.; Jha, S.; Gundewar, S.; Elrod, J.W.; Ramachandran, A.; Pattillo, C.B.; Kevil, C.G.; Lefer, D.J. Hydrogen sulfide mediates cardioprotection through Nrf2 signaling. *Circ. Res.* **2009**, *105*, 365–374. [CrossRef] [PubMed]
43. Ondruschka, B.; Rosinsky, F.; Trauer, H.; Schneider, E.; Dreßler, J.; Franke, H. Drug- and/or trauma-induced hyperthermia? Characterization of HSP70 and myoglobin expression. *PLoS ONE* **2018**, *13*, e0194442. [CrossRef] [PubMed]
44. Kukreja, R.C.; Kontos, M.C.; Loesser, K.E.; Batra, S.K.; Qian, Y.Z.; Gbur Jr, C.J.; Naseem, S.A.; Jesse, R.L.; Hess, M.L. Oxidant stress increases heat shock protein 70 mRNA in isolated perfused rat heart. *Am. J. Physiol. Heart Circ. Physiol.* **1994**, *267*, H2213–H2219. [CrossRef]
45. Tripatara, P.; Patel, N.S.; Collino, M.; Gallicchio, M.; Kieswich, J.; Castiglia, S.; Benetti, E.; Stewart, K.N.; Brown, P.A.; Yaqoob, M.M.; et al. Generation of endogenous hydrogen sulfide by cystathionine gamma-lyase limits renal ischemia/reperfusion injury and dysfunction. *Lab. Investig.* **2008**, *88*, 1038–1048. [CrossRef] [PubMed]
46. Elrod, J.W.; Calvert, J.W.; Morrison, J.; Doeller, J.E.; Kraus, D.W.; Tao, L.; Jiao, X.; Scalia, R.; Kiss, L.; Szabo, C.; et al. Hydrogen sulfide attenuates myocardial ischemia-reperfusion injury by preservation of mitochondrial function. *Proc. Natl. Acad. Sci. USA* **2007**, *104*, 15560–15565. [CrossRef] [PubMed]
47. Zou, C.G.; Banerjee, R. Homocysteine and redox signalling. *Antioxid. Redox Signal.* **2005**, *7*, 547–559. [CrossRef] [PubMed]
48. Jakovljevic, V.; Milic, P.; Bradic, J.; Jeremic, J.; Zivkovic, V.; Srejovic, I.; Nikolic Turnic, T.; Milosavljevic, I.; Jeremic, N.; Bolevich, S.; et al. Standardized Aronia melanocarpa Extract as Novel Supplement against Metabolic Syndrome: A Rat Model. *Int. J. Mol. Sci.* **2019**, *20*, 6. [CrossRef]
49. Liu, C.T.; Hse, H.; Lii, C.K.; Chen, P.S.; Sheen, L.Y. Effects of garlic oil and diallyl trisulfide on glycemic control in diabetic rats. *Eur. J. Pharmacol.* **2005**, *516*, 165–173. [CrossRef]

50. Salloum, F.N.; Chau, V.Q.; Hoke, N.N.; Abbate, A.; Varma, A.; Ockaili, R.A.; Toldo, S.; Kukreja, R.C. Phosphodiesterase-5 inhibitor, tadalafil, protects against myocardial ischemia/reperfusion through protein-kinase g-dependent generation of hydrogen sulfide. *Circulation* **2009**, *120*, S31–S36. [CrossRef]
51. Meng, B.; Gao, W.; Wei, J.; Yang, J.; Wu, J.; Pu, L.; Guo, C. Quercetin reduces serum homocysteine level in rats fed a methionine-enriched diet. *Nutrition* **2013**, *29*, 661–666. [CrossRef]
52. Stypmann, J.; Engelen, M.A.; Troatz, C.; Rothenburger, M.; Eckardt, L.; Tiemann, K. Echocardiographic assessment of global left ventricular function in mice. *Lab. Anim.* **2009**, *43*, 127–137. [CrossRef] [PubMed]
53. Junqueira, L.C.; Bignolas, G.; Brentani, R.R. Picrosirius staining plus polarization microscopy, a specific method for collagen detection in tissue sections. *Histochem. J.* **1979**, *11*, 447–455. [CrossRef] [PubMed]
54. Hadi, A.M.; Mouchaers, K.T.; Schalij, I.; Grunberg, K.; Meijer, G.A.; Vonk-Noordegraaf, A.; van der Laarse, W.J.; Belien, J.A. Rapid quantification of myocardial fibrosis: A new macro-based automated analysis. *Anal. Cell. Pathol.* **2010**, *33*, 257–269. [CrossRef]
55. Fishbein, M.C.; Wang, T.; Matijasevic, M.; Hong, L.; Apple, F.S. Myocardial tissue troponins T and I. An immunohistochemical study in experimental models of myocardial ischemia. *Cardiovasc. Pathol.* **2003**, *12*, 65–71. [CrossRef]
56. Bayan, L.; Koulivand, P.H.; Gorji, A. Garlic: A review of potential therapeutic effects. *Avicenna J. Phytomed.* **2014**, *4*, 1–14.
57. Polhemus, D.; Kondo, K.; Bhushan, S.; Bir, S.C.; Kevil, C.G.; Murohara, T.; Lefer, D.J.; Calvert, J.W. Hydrogen sulfide attenuates cardiac dysfunction following heart failure via induction of angiogenesis. *Circ. Heart Fail.* **2013**, *6*, 1077–1086. [CrossRef]

3

Sex Differences in the Influence of Sleep on Body Mass Index and Risk of Metabolic Syndrome in Middle-Aged Adults

Hyun-E Yeom [1] and Jungmin Lee [2,*]

1 College of Nursing, Chungnam National University, Munhwaro 266, Junggu, Daejeon 35015, Korea; yeom@cnu.ac.kr

2 Youth Independence & Competencies Research Office, National Youth Policy Institute, Social Policy BLDG, Sejong National Research Complex, 370, Sicheong-daero, Sejong-si 30147, Korea

* Correspondence: mhlee77@gmail.com

Abstract: Poor sleep and obesity are intimately related to cardiovascular diseases. We aimed to examine whether the influence of sleep and body mass index (BMI) on the risk of metabolic syndrome (MetS) differed by sex in middle-aged people. It is a cross-sectional study of 458 Korean participants who completed self-administered surveys; the data were analyzed using the PROCESS macro for SPSS. We found that both sleep and BMI were significant predictors of MetS risk in women, particularly by the role of BMI connecting the impact of sleep to MetS risk. However, the association was not found in men, showing that BMI, but not sleep, was a significant predictor of MetS. This sex-related difference was due to different relationships between sleep and BMI, indicating that BMI was more dependent on sleep quality for women than for men. Therefore, a sex-specific approach to decrease the risk of MetS is warranted.

Keywords: body mass index; metabolic syndrome; sex characteristics; sleep disorders

---

1. Introduction

Cardiovascular diseases are one of the leading causes of increasing mortality and reduced quality of life globally. Metabolic syndrome (MetS), a condition clustered with cardiovascular risk factors (hypertension, central obesity, dyslipidemia in lower high-density lipoprotein (HDL), elevated triglycerides, and elevated fasting glucose), is a critical, life-threatening issue [1]. Recent data show that with increases in obesity in Asian countries, the prevalence of cardiovascular diseases and the risk of MetS have also increased. Asian populations are thought to have a relatively low risk of cardiovascular diseases [2]. However, a recent comparative study of Asian and European populations indicated the prevalence was similar to, or higher than, some less developed Asian countries than in Europe [3]. Also, according to recent South Korean national health statistics, the incidence of MetS was 26%, and 73.2% of adults who had received health screening services and had one or more MetS risk factors [4].

The prevalence of MetS is related to lifestyle factors, such as physical activity, diet, smoking, and drinking alcohol [5]. In particular, a large body of literature [6,7] indicates the key role of sleep in increasing the risks of MetS, showing intimate interrelatedness of sleep characteristics, such as duration, regular patterns, and overall quality, to risks of various cardiovascular diseases. Also, an increasing number of studies have provided a scientific mechanism for the link between sleep and obesity. Sleep affects energy balance and appetite-related hormones, such as ghrelin and leptin; these, in turn, are linked to physiological metabolic function. There is strong evidence that sleep deprivation is also associated with overall adiposity [6,7].

In addition, sleep and obesity are key contributors to the risk of MetS [5–7]. However, their interrelatedness and relative impact on MetS varies depending on sex, possibly due to differences in body composition. A comparative study of adolescents has reported sex-related differences in relationships between sleep, body mass index (BMI), and risk of obesity [8]. Some studies have shown that males' body weight tends to be more sensitive to changes in sleep hours [8], while others have reported that females' weight tends to be more sensitive to changes in sleep quality [9]. However, empirical evidence on sex-related differences in the relationship between sleep and BMI is inconclusive.

Midlife is accompanied by multifaceted aging-related declines in physiological and cardiometabolic functions that may cause sleep disturbance and increase BMI, which increases the risk of cardiovascular disorders and MetS [10]. Studies have shown that the risk of MetS increases with age, particularly after midlife in women with dramatic hormone declines with menopause (i.e., estrogen) [10,11]. Global epidemic evidence has shown that the prevalence of MetS is higher in men under 50 years old but higher in women over 60 [11]. Additionally, for women, sleep plays a pivotal role in cardiovascular health with increasing age, particularly after menopause; the relationship is not clear for men [12].

Thus, although numerous studies have shown the interrelationship among sleep, BMI, and risk of MetS, it remains unclear how it differs by sex in middle-aged people. The aims of this study were to examine sex-related differences in the relationship between sleep and BMI and to investigate whether the impacts of sleep and BMI on the risk of MetS differed by sex in middle-aged Korean people.

Figure 1 displays our hypothesized model. We hypothesized that (1) the relationship between sleep and BMI differs by sex, and (2) such a sex-related difference produces different impacts of sleep and body mass index on the risk of MetS in middle-aged men and women.

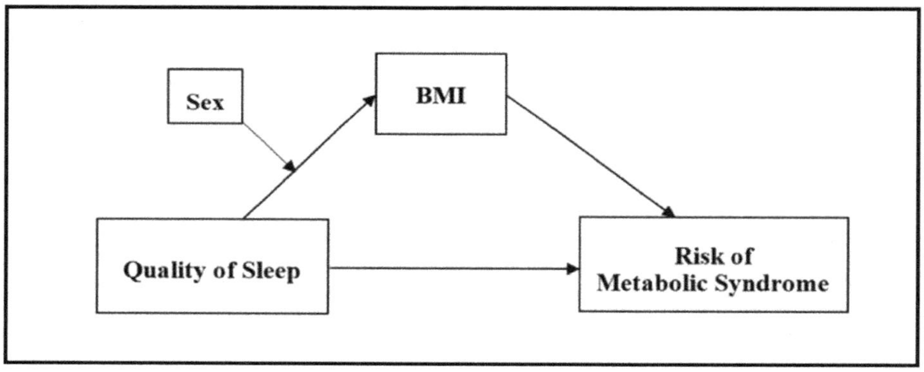

Figure 1. Hypothesized sex-moderated mediation model for the relationship between quality of sleep, body mass index (BMI), and risk of metabolic syndrome (MetS).

2. Materials and Methods

2.1. Participants and Procedures

In this cross-sectional study, we conducted a secondary analysis of data from two primary studies that aimed to investigate the characteristics of physiological and psychosocial experiences in midlife and perceptual and behavioral factors related to MetS risk factors in the Korean population.

Participants were recruited from multiple outpatient sites at two hospitals and two local clinics and community centers in the city of Daegu and the province of Gyeongbuk, South Korea. Data for 458 adults aged 45–64 years were collected through self-administered questionnaires. The exclusion criterion was individuals who had emergent health issues, such as stroke and coronary artery disease.

Ethical considerations: Procedures for the two primary studies were approved by the Institutional Review Board of Chungnam National University (approval numbers: 201711-SB-081-01, 201809-SB-137-01). The study's purposes and procedures, protection of participants' rights, and measures for the physical and psychological well-being of human participants were explained to participants, along with the potential benefits and risks of participation. Participants provided written informed consent.

Sample size adequacy was validated by G * Power 3.1.9.2 [13]. For post-hoc testing under the conditions of type 1 error (alpha = 0.05), medium effective size (0.15) [14] for linear multiple regression analysis with 10 predictors and total sample size of 450, achieved power (1-β error probability) was 0.99.

2.2. Measures

2.2.1. Risk of MetS

People with MetS have multiple risk factors for cardiovascular diseases, including type II diabetes, hypertension, and hyperlipidemia. The assessment of MetS risk was conducted via participant self-reporting on five dichotomous questions evaluating whether or not the participant met any of the five criteria announced by the National Cholesterol Education Program Expert Panel [15]: (1) high systolic (≥130 mm Hg) and/or diastolic (≥85 mm Hg) blood pressure or being treated with antihypertensive agents; (2) hyperglycemia (fasting blood glucose ≥ 100 mg/dL) or taking medication prescribed for diabetes; (3) hypertriglyceridemia (fasting plasma triglyceride ≥ 150 mg/dL) or taking medication prescribed for hyperlipidemia; (4) low high-density lipoprotein cholesterol (men < 40 mg/dL, women < 50 mg/dL) or taking medication prescribed for hyperlipidemia; and (5) central obesity, based on World Health Organization guidelines for Asian populations (abdominal circumference ≥90 cm in men, ≥85 cm in women) [16]. Participants were classified into the MetS risk group if they met two or more of the criteria.

2.2.2. Sleep

Characteristics of sleep were assessed using the Korean version of the Pittsburgh Sleep Quality Index (PSQI), a valid global scale encompassing dimensions of subjective quality of sleep, latency, duration, and disturbances initiating and maintaining sleep; use of medication for sleep; and daytime dysfunction related to sleep [17]. The PSQI consists of 19 items on a 4-point Likert-type scale, ranging from 0 to 3. The quality of sleep score was calculated by an algorithm; higher scores indicate poorer quality of sleep. The reliability in this study was Cronbach's alpha = 0.88.

2.2.3. Socioeconomic and Health-Related Characteristics

As potential covariates, we assessed sociodemographic variables including age, sex, current job status, education, whole-family monthly income, and living status. For general health-related characteristics, an individual's height and weight were self-reported and we calculated BMI using the formula (kg/m^2). We also assessed engagement in healthy behaviors with the Health Behavior scale [18]. The scale is composed of 25 items that ask the frequency of health behaviors along several dimensions, including dietary habits (8 items), physical activities (4 items), stress management (5 items), health responsibility (5 items), and smoking (3 items). Responses are provided on a 4-point Likert scale from 1 (never) to 4 (routinely). The mean score of all items is calculated and a higher overall score means more active engagement in healthy lifestyles. The Health Behavior scale has been validated to assess the characteristics of healthy behavior to prevent cardiovascular diseases [18] and the reliability in this study was Cronbach's alpha = 0.82.

2.3. Statistical Analyses

Data were analyzed using SPSS 26.0 (IBM Corp., Armonk, NY, USA). Sociodemographic and health-related characteristics were analyzed using descriptive statistics (frequency, percentage, mean, standard deviation. Bivariate correlation analysis was conducted to assess the relationship among study variables. For Pearson correlations, all categorical variables (i.e., level of education, living status, employment, level of family income, and MetS risk) were created as binary variables (like dummy variables) to interpret the finding as a point-biserial correlation coefficient. Finally, covariates were determined based on the correlation coefficients.

We hypothesized that the effect of quality of sleep on BMI may differ by sex, and the quality of sleep may affect MetS risk through BMI in a sex-dependent manner. The moderated mediation effects of quality of sleep, sex, and BMI in predicting MetS risk were tested using Hayes' PROCESS macro for SPSS [19]. PROCESS applies a logistic regression when there is a dichotomous dependent variable (i.e., MetS risk), and conducts a series of logistic regressions to estimate direct and indirect effects and the proposed mediator path [19,20]. To test our proposed moderated mediation model (see Figure 1), the PROCESS macro first estimated an effect of sex moderating the relationship between quality of sleep and BMI, which was an interaction effect of sex and quality of sleep in predicting BMI. In the second step, it estimated an effect of BMI mediating the effect of quality of sleep on MetS risk; in other words, an indirect effect of quality of sleep on MetS risk through BMI. In the final step, it tested whether an indirect effect of the quality of sleep on MetS risk through BMI differed by sex, which would indicate a moderated mediation effect. Results of the three steps allowed us to determine whether there was a sex-moderated mediation effect of BMI in the relationship between quality of sleep and MetS risk.

3. Results

3.1. Descriptive Characteristics of Participants

Table 1 presents the sociodemographic information of the participants depending on sex. The number of participants in the MetS risk group was 226 (49.3%). Prevalence of MetS risk did not differ based on sex ($t = 0.08$, $p = 0.780$) and 52.2% of the MetS risk group were women. The average age of participants was 54.57 years (SD = 8.5 years). Approximately 64% were college graduates or beyond and most of the participants lived with family (92.4%) and were currently employed (78.2%). As for health-related characteristics, the average score of healthy behaviors in all participants was 2.57 (SD = 0.05) and did not differ by sex ($t = 1.00$, $p = 0.317$).

Table 1. General characteristics of the participants and sex-related differences ($N = 458$).

Variables	Categories	All	Sex		Differences by Sex
			Women ($n = 236$)	Men ($n = 222$)	
		M ± SD or n (%)	M ± SD or n (%)	M ± SD or n (%)	t or χ^2 (p)
Age		54.57 ± 8.5	55.81 ± 9.1	53.24 ± 7.7	3.27 (0.001)
High education (≥College)	Yes	291 (63.5)	113 (47.9)	178 (80.2)	51.51 (0.000)
	No	167 (36.5)	123 (52.1)	44(19.8)	
Living alone	Yes	35 (7.6)	23 (9.7)	12 (5.4)	3.05 (0.081)
	No	423(92.4)	213 (90.3)	210 (94.6)	
Currently employed	Yes	358 (78.2)	153 (64.8)	205 (92.3)	52.54 (0.000)
	No	96 (20.9)	81 (34.3)	15 (6.8)	
	Missing	4 (0.9)	2 (0.9)	2 (0.9)	
High family income(≥4,000,000 won/mon)	Yes	239 (52.2)	89 (37.7)	120 (54.1)	12.02 (0.001)
	No	209 (45.6)	141 (59.8)	98 (44.1)	
	Missing	10 (2.2)	6 (2.5)	4 (1.8)	
Health behaviors		2.57 ± 0.5	2.6 ± 0.5	2.5 ± 0.5	1.00 (0.317)
Body mass index		24.25 ± 3.2	23.4 ± 2.8	25.2 ± 3.3	−6.34 (0.000)
Quality of sleep		6.16 ± 3.3	6.5 ± 3.4	5.8 ± 3.0	2.61 (0.009)
Risk of Metabolic Syndrome	Yes	226 (49.3)	118 (50.0)	108 (48.6)	0.08 (0.780)
	No	232 (50.7)	118 (50.0)	114 (51.4)	

The mean levels of the main study variables were 6.16 (SD = 3.3) for quality of sleep and 24.25 (SD = 3.2) for BMI. The number (percent) of participants who were classified as overweight (BMI = 23–24.9 kg/m^2), obese (BMI = 25–29.9 kg/m^2), and severely obese (BMI ≥ 30 kg/m^2) was 123 (26.9%), 151 (33.0%), and 20 (4.4%), respectively. Both quality of sleep ($t = 2.61$, $p = 0.009$) and BMI ($t = -6.34$, $p < 0.001$) did differ significantly by sex. Additional characteristics are presented in Table 1.

3.2. Correlations between the Main Study Variables and Sex-Related Differences

Bivariate correlation analysis showed that the risk of MetS was related to quality of sleep ($r = 0.161$, $p < 0.001$), BMI ($r = 0.296$, $p < 0.001$), age ($r = 0.387$, $p < 0.001$), level of education ($r = -0.386$, $p < 0.001$), living status ($r = 0.094$, $p < 0.05$), employment ($r = -0.179$, $p < 0.001$), and family income ($r = -0.293$, $p < -0.001$). Thus, these were included as covariates to assess the effect of sleep quality on BMI and MetS risk.

Table 2 shows different correlational relationships among the main variables between men and women. For women, quality of sleep was significantly correlated with BMI ($r = 0.165$, $p < 0.05$) and MetS risk ($r = 0.234$, $p < 0.001$). Also, there was a significant correlation between BMI and MetS risk ($r = 0.321$, $p < 0.001$). For men, quality of sleep was not significantly related to BMI ($r = -0.040$, $p = 0.552$) or MetS risk ($r = 0.069$, $p = 0.307$). A significant correlation was found only for BMI and MetS risk ($r = 0.305$, $p < 0.001$).

Table 2. Correlations between demographic and main variables by sex ($N = 458$).

		Men (n = 222)								
Variables		Age	Education §1	Living Status §2	Employment §3	Family Income §4	Health Behaviors	Quality of Sleep	BMI	Mets Risk §5
Women (n = 236)	Age	-	−0.046 **	−0.060	−0.438 **	−0.186 **	0.256 **	0.125	−0.223 **	0.220 **
	Education §1	−0.534 **	-	−0.231 **	0.367 **	0.438 **	0.091	−0.186 **	0.018	−0.375 **
	Living status §2	0.335 **	−0.201 **	-	−0.253 **	−0.146 *	−0.044	0.154 *	−0.039	0.006
	Employment §3	−0.295 **	0.272 **	−0.152 **	-	0.242 **	0.001	−0.196 **	0.024	−0.242 **
	Family income §4	−0.525 **	0.487 **	−0.228 **	0.239 **	-	0.048	−0.043	−0.059	−0.226 **
	Health behaviors	0.169 **	−0.103	−0.057	−0.104	0.093	-	−0.245 **	−0.046	−0.026
	Quality of sleep	0.205 **	−0.228 **	0.059	−0.024	−0.156 *	−0.149 *	-	−0.040	0.069
	BMI	0.163 *	−0.207 **	0.072	−0.074	−0.084	−0.111	0.165 *	-	0.305 **
	Mets risk §5	0.527 **	−0.433 **	0.157 **	−0.171 **	−0.363 **	0.053	0.234 **	0.321 **	-

Note. § Dummy variable; Reference groups: [1] = high education (≥College); [2] = living alone; [3] = currently employed; [4] = high family income (≥4,000,000 won/mon); [5] = MetS risk group. * $p < 0.05$, ** $p < 0.001$.

3.3. Sex Difference in Effects of Quality of Sleep on BMI and MetS Risk

The PROCESS macro model 7 results for the effect of sex on the relationship between quality of sleep, BMI, and risk of MetS are as follows (see Table 3). First, a significant interaction between quality of sleep and sex (B = −0.21, t = −2.24, $p < 0.05$) was found in predicting BMI. It indicates that the relationship between quality of sleep and BMI differed by sex and sex moderated the effect of quality of sleep on BMI. Figure 2 displays the relationship between sleep quality and BMI by sex; for women, worse sleep quality predicted higher BMI, and for men, the reverse.

Table 3. Sex-related different effects of quality of sleep on BMI and MetS risk (n = 439).

Predictor	BMI			
	B	**SE**	***t/z***	***p***
Quality of sleep	0.12	0.06	1.98	0.05
Sex §,1	3.40	0.66	5.16	0.00
Quality of sleep × sex §,1	−0.21	0.09	−2.24	0.03
Covariates				
Constant	26.26	1.53	17.18	0.00
Age	−0.04	0.02	−1.80	0.07
Education §,2	−0.87	0.41	−2.09	0.04
Living alone §,3	0.03	0.58	0.06	0.95
Employment §,4	−0.26	0.42	−0.61	0.54
Family income §,5	−0.14	0.34	−0.40	0.69
Health behaviors	−0.34	0.32	−1.06	0.29
R^2 = 11.29%, F (9, 429) = 6.07, $p < 0.000$				
Predictor	**MetS risk**			
	B	**SE**	***t/z***	***p***
BMI	0.31	0.04	7.00	0.00
Quality of sleep	0.03	0.04	0.73	0.46
Covariates				
Constant	−12.07	1.80	−6.72	0.00
Age	0.10	0.02	5.19	0.00
Education §,2	−0.94	0.31	−3.06	0.00
Living alone §,3	−0.32	0.49	−0.65	0.51
Employment §,4	−0.01	0.34	−0.02	0.98
Family income §,5	−0.65	0.26	−2.49	0.01
Health behaviors	−0.05	0.26	−0.19	0.85
Logistic regression summary				
McFadden's R^2= 26.83, CoxSnell's R^2=31.03, Nagelkrk's R^2 = 41.40; F (8, 430) = 163.11, $p < 0.000$				
Sex difference in indirect effects of quality of sleep on MetS risk BMI				
Sex §,1	Boot indirect effect	Boot SE	LL 95% CI	UL 95% CI
Men	−0.03	0.02	−0.076	0.019
Women	0.04	0.02	0.001	0.083
Index of sex-moderated mediation effect for the relationship between quality of sleep, BMI, and MetS risk				
	Index	Boot SE	LL 95% CI	UL 95% CI
BMI	−0.07	0.03	−0.13	−0.01

Note. MetS = metabolic syndrome. § Dummy variable; Reference groups: 1 = Men; 2 = high education (≥College); 3 = living alone; 4 = currently employed; 5 = high family income (≥4,000,000 won/mon).

Second, the indirect effect of quality of sleep on the risk of MetS through BMI was significant in women (indirect effect = 0.04, 95% CI = 0.001, 0.083) but not in men (indirect effect = −0.03, 95% CI = −0.076, 0.019). It indicates a difference in indirect effects of quality of sleep on MetS risk through BMI between women and men.

Finally, the result for the whole model 7 indicated that sex moderated the effect of BMI, mediating the relationship between quality of sleep and risk of MetS, confirming a moderated mediation effect (Index = −0.07, 95% CI = −0.13, −0.01).

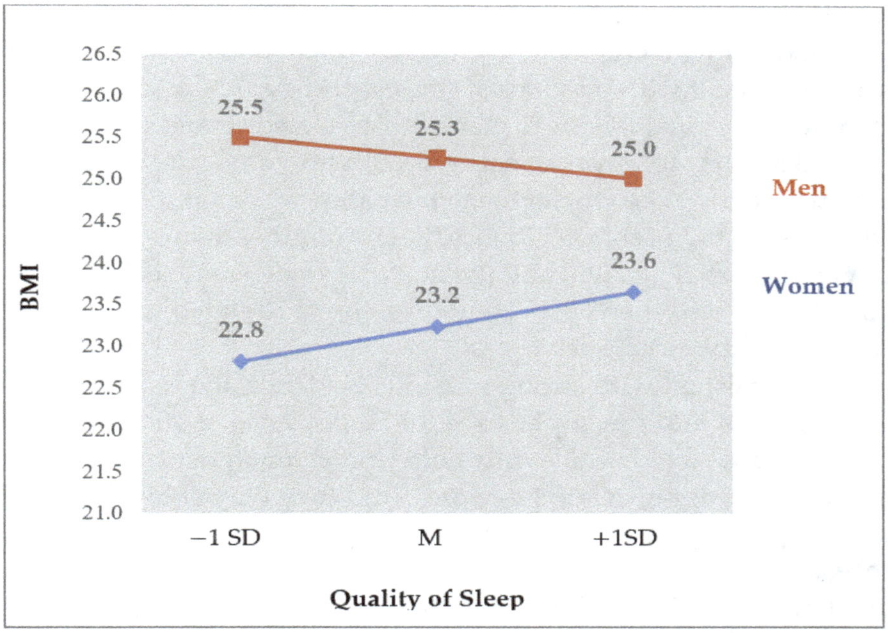

Figure 2. Sex differences in the relationship between worsening of quality of sleep and BMI.

4. Discussion

Despite extensive evidence of interrelatedness among sleep, obesity, and MetS, the information about sex differences in the impacts of sleep and obesity on the risk of MetS is inconsistent. The findings of the current study describe the sophisticated mechanism by which sex changes the ways sleep and BMI contribute to increased risks for MetS. The sex-related differences in the relationship between sleep and BMI account for variances in how sex impacts increased risk of MetS in middle-aged people.

A key finding is that quality of sleep is a primary factor affecting the risk of MetS through the joint impact with BMI, but with a difference by sex. The women in midlife who have poorer quality of sleep tended to have higher BMI, leading to an increase in the risk of MetS. Notably, BMI played a role as a mediator for the relationship between sleep and the risk of MetS. However, such an association was not found in midlife men. The findings indicate that deterioration of quality of sleep and an increase of BMI need to be considered relevant predictors for the risk of MetS in women. Comparably, sleep in men was a relatively less influential factor for BMI; therefore, BMI rather than sleep needs to be considered a relatively more meaningful factor related to the risk of MetS.

It is noteworthy that the sex-dependent distinguished impacts of sleep and BMI on MetS risk were associated with the different connections of sleep to BMI, comparable by sex. Women's BMI tended to be intimately related to the quality of sleep; this tendency was not detected in men. This finding conflicts with prior evidence that sleep was closely related to BMI in both men and women [3]. Some studies have addressed that sex-related physiological distinctiveness may cause such a difference [9]. A recent study [21] reported a significant relationship between sleep disorders and obesity in postmenopausal women, and another study [22] addressed the changes in women's sleep with regard to sex hormone-related changes beginning from the perimenopausal period. Participants in this study were middle-aged, and it is known that women tend to experience more turbulent physiological changes during the menopause period. Therefore, further study is necessary to include physiological characteristics for a more concrete understanding of the sex-related differences in the relationship between sleep and BMI. It is also notable that the current study added empirical evidence that the impacts of sleep and BMI on MetS risk differed by sex, distinguishing the relationship between sleep and BMI depending on sex. This study found that despite strong evidence for the impact of sleep on MetS, its contribution to increasing the risk of MetS differed according to sex when considering its interrelatedness with BMI, since BMI was associated with sleep only in women.

Another interesting finding included confirmation of additional sex-related differences in BMI changes by age. BMI tended to increase with age for women, whereas this tendency was reversed for men. The findings are consistent with previous studies reporting that women have a high tendency to gain weight with increasing age, mainly due to menopause-related changes including body composition and cardiometabolic risks [10]. Moreover, consistent with previous studies [23,24] we found that the quality of sleep in women tends to be worse as age increases, while this tendency was not observed in men. This finding does conflict with some evidence that men rather than women tended to suffer worse sleep deterioration with increased age [25] and the quality of sleep tended to decrease as age increased in middle-aged (46–60 years old) men [24]. Therefore, the sex-related difference in the relationship between sleep and aging is still inconclusive.

On the other hand, consistent with strong previous evidence, the risk of MetS increases with age in both men and women. The finding emphasizes the importance of efforts to prevent various MetS risks at a younger age. Middle-aged adults' physiological characteristics are unstable and turbulent, depending on individualized aging-related declines, and they may show substantial variation even within this sexual homogeneity. Therefore, further study is warranted to confirm and clarify the sex-related differences.

The other considerable finding is the interrelatedness between sleep and lifestyles in men and women. We found that individuals of both sexes who more actively engage in healthy lifestyle practices, such as physical exercise and diet, tended to report better quality of sleep. This finding is congruent with existing evidence on the benefits of health behavior for better sleep [26]. However, a noticeable relationship between healthy lifestyle practices and BMI was not found, despite considerable evidence supporting these links [27]. Prior research has indicated the necessity of healthcare behavioral strategies targeting specific health outcomes [28]. Therefore, future studies focusing on the link between the risk of MetS and healthy behavior by type are suggested.

Strengths and Limitations

A major contribution of the current study is that it clearly indicated that for women, but not men, quality of sleep has a substantial impact on risk of MetS with increased BMI, due to the intimate connection between sleep quality and BMI. Therefore, the present study provides a sex-differentiated concrete association among sleep, BMI, and the risk of MetS; in particular, a different role of BMI by sex in the relationship between sleep and the risk of MetS.

Several limitations of this study need to be addressed. First is its cross-sectional design, which aimed to confirm the causal effect of sleep and BMI on MetS. Further longitudinal studies are necessary for more convincing, predictive evidence of this relationship. Additionally, the population of this study was ethnically homogeneous. Empirical studies have shown that the prevalence of MetS varies by ethnicity. A recent study [3] that compared Asian and European populations reported differences in the prevalence of MetS and risk factors by sex and ethnicity; its prevalence was higher in women than in men among the Asian population, while the tendency was reversed in the European population. In addition, factors contributing to MetS were inconsistent, although hypertension was the most common risk factor for MetS in both populations. Furthermore, a global report [29] has shown a considerable variation in the prevalence of risk factors of MetS even within Asia-Pacific countries, with a much higher rate in low-middle- and low-income countries compared to developed countries. Therefore, further cross-cultural studies are necessary for an integrated understanding of the behavioral and bio-social factors related to the risk of MetS. Also, the current study employed BMI rather than abdominal obesity. Some prior studies have indicated a need to distinguish overall obesity and abdominal obesity based on differences in their relationships with MetS [3]. For both Asian (Indonesian) and European (Dutch) populations, the prevalence of MetS had a stronger relationship with abdominal circumference than with BMI (and thus with abdominal adiposity than overall adiposity) [3]. Thus, a further study focusing on abdominal obesity's contribution to the risk of MetS, with consideration of sex-related differences, is suggested.

5. Conclusions

The current study highlights the need to consider sex-related differences to reduce the risk of metabolic syndrome by demonstrating that, for women, both sleep quality and BMI are influential predictive factors for the risk of MetS, whereas for men, BMI but not the quality of sleep is a critical issue. The differences in the roles of BMI were based on different relationships between sleep and BMI by sex. Sex-specific strategies that target the prevention of MetS and effective management of its risk factors are highly warranted.

Author Contributions: Conceptualization, H.-E.Y. and J.L.; Methodology, H.-E.Y. and J.L.; Project administration: H.-E.Y.; Investigation, H.-E.Y.; Formal analysis: J.L.; Validation, H.-E.Y. and J.L.; Writing—Original draft preparation, H.-E.Y. and J.L.; Writing—Review and editing, H.-E.Y. and J.L. Both authors have read and agreed to the published version of the manuscript.

References

1. Alberti, K.G.; Eckel, R.H.; Grundy, S.M.; Zimmet, P.Z.; Cleeman, J.I.; Donato, K.A.; Fruchart, J.C.; James, W.P.; Loria, C.M.; Smith, S.C., Jr.; et al. Harmonizing the metabolic syndrome: A joint interim statement of the International Diabetes Federation Task Force on Epidemiology and Prevention; National Heart, Lung, and Blood Institute; American Heart Association; World Heart Federation; International Atherosclerosis Society; and International Association for the Study of Obesity. *Circulation* **2009**, *120*, 1640–1645. [CrossRef] [PubMed]
2. Peters, S.A.; Wang, X.; Lam, T.H.; Kim, H.C.; Ho, S.; Ninomiya, T.; Knuiman, M.; Vaartjes, I.; Bots, M.L.; Woodward, M. Clustering of risk factors and the risk of incident cardiovascular disease in Asian and Caucasian populations: Results from the Asia Pacific Cohort Studies Collaboration. *BMJ Open* **2018**, *8*, e019335. [CrossRef] [PubMed]
3. Sigit, F.S.; Tahapary, D.L.; Trompet, S.; Sartono, E.; Willems van Dijk, K.; Rosendaal, F.R.; De Mutsert, R. The prevalence of metabolic syndrome and its association with body fat distribution in middle-aged individuals from Indonesia and the Netherlands: A cross-sectional analysis of two population-based studies. *Diabetol. Metab. Syndr.* **2020**, *12*, 2. [CrossRef] [PubMed]
4. 2017 National Health Screening Statistical Yearbook by National Health Insurance Service. Available online: https://www.nhis.or.kr/nhis/together/wbhaec07000m01.do?mode=view&articleNo=127944&article.offset=0&articleLimit=10 (accessed on 13 December 2020).
5. Barbaresko, J.; Rienks, J.; Nöthlings, U. Lifestyle Indices and Cardiovascular Disease Risk: A Meta-analysis. *Am. J. Prev. Med.* **2018**, *55*, 555–564. [CrossRef] [PubMed]
6. Kwok, C.S.; Kontopantelis, E.; Kuligowski, G.; Gray, M.; Muhyaldeen, A.; Gale, C.P.; Peat, G.M.; Cleator, J.; Chew-Graham, C.; Loke, Y.K.; et al. Self-Reported Sleep Duration and Quality and Cardiovascular Disease and Mortality: A Dose-Response Meta-Analysis. *J. Am. Heart Assoc.* **2018**, *7*, e008552. [CrossRef]
7. Lin, J.; Jiang, Y.; Wang, G.; Meng, M.; Zhu, Q.; Mei, H.; Liu, S.; Jiang, F. Associations of short sleep duration with appetite-regulating hormones and adipokines: A systematic review and meta-analysis. *Obes. Rev.* **2020**, *21*, e13051. [CrossRef]
8. Knutson, K.L. Sex differences in the association between sleep and body mass index in adolescents. *J. Pediatr.* **2005**, *147*, 830–834. [CrossRef]
9. St-Onge, M.P.; Perumean-Chaney, S.; Desmond, R.; Lewis, C.E.; Yan, L.L.; Person, S.D.; Allison, D.B. Gender Differences in the Association between Sleep Duration and Body Composition: The Cardia Study. *Int. J. Endocrinol.* **2010**, *2010*, 726071. [CrossRef]
10. Karvonen-Gutierrez, C.; Kim, C. Association of Mid-Life Changes in Body Size, Body Composition and Obesity Status with the Menopausal Transition. *Healthcare* **2016**, *4*, 42. [CrossRef]
11. Jiang, B.; Zheng, Y.; Chen, Y.; Chen, Y.; Li, Q.; Zhu, C.; Wang, N.; Han, B.; Zhai, H.; Lin, D.; et al. Age and gender-specific distribution of metabolic syndrome components in East China: Role of hypertriglyceridemia in the SPECT-China study. *Lipids Health Dis.* **2018**, *17*, 92. [CrossRef]

12. Chair, S.Y.; Wang, Q.; Cheng, H.Y.; Lo, S.W.; Li, X.M.; Wong, E.M.; Sit, J.W. Relationship between sleep quality and cardiovascular disease risk in Chinese post-menopausal women. *BMC Womens Health* **2017**, *17*, 79. [CrossRef] [PubMed]
13. Faul, F.; Erdfelder, E.; Lang, A.-G.; Buchner, A. G*Power 3: A flexible statistical power analysis program for the social, behavioral, and biomedical sciences. *Behav. Res. Methods* **2007**, *39*, 175–191. [CrossRef] [PubMed]
14. National Cholesterol Education Program (US). Expert Panel on Detection, Evaluation, and Treatment of High Blood Cholesterol in Adults. Executive summary of the third report of the National Cholesterol Education Program (NCEP) Expert panel on detection, evaluation, and treatment of high blood cholesterol in adults (Adult Treatment Panel III). *JAMA* **2001**, *285*, 2486–2497. [CrossRef] [PubMed]
15. Cohen, J. *Statistical Power Analysis for the Behavioral Sciences*, 2nd ed.; Lawrence Erlbaum Associates: Hillsdale, NJ, USA, 1988.
16. WHO Expert Consultation. Appropriate body-mass index for Asian populations and its implications for policy and intervention strategies. *Lancet* **2004**, *363*, 157–163. [CrossRef]
17. Buysse, D.J.; Reynolds, C.F.; Monk, T.H.; Berman, S.R.; Kupfer, D.J. The Pittsburgh Sleep Quality Index: A new instrument for psychiatric practice and research. *Psychiatry Res.* **1989**, *28*, 193–213. [CrossRef]
18. Song, R.; June, K.J.; Kim, C.G.; Jeon, M.Y. Comparisons of motivation, health behaviors, and functional status among elders in residential homes in Korea. *Public Health Nurs.* **2004**, *21*, 361–371. [CrossRef]
19. Hayes, A.F. *Introduction to Mediation, Moderation, and Conditional Process Analysis: A regression-Based Approach*, 2nd ed.; The Guilford Press: New York, NY, USA, 2018.
20. Hayes, A.F.; Matthes, J. Computational procedures for probing interactions in OLS and logistic regression: SPSS and SAS implementations. *Behav. Res. Methods* **2009**, *41*, 924–936. [CrossRef]
21. Naufel, M.F.; Frange, C.; Andersen, M.L.; Girão, M.J.B.C.; Tufik, S.; Beraldi Ribeiro, E.; Hachul, H. Association between obesity and sleep disorders in postmenopausal women. *Menopause* **2018**, *25*, 139–144. [CrossRef]
22. Pengo, M.F.; Won, C.H.; Bourjeily, G. Sleep in Women across the Life Span. *Chest* **2018**, *154*, 196–206. [CrossRef]
23. Zhang, B.; Wing, Y.K. Sex differences in insomnia: A meta-analysis. *Sleep* **2006**, *29*, 85–93. [CrossRef]
24. Madrid-Valero, J.J.; Martínez-Selva, J.M.; Ribeiro do Couto, B.; Sánchez-Romera, J.F.; Ordoñana, J.R. Age and gender effects on the prevalence of poor sleep quality in the adult population. *Gac. Sanit.* **2017**, *31*, 18–22. [CrossRef] [PubMed]
25. Mander, B.A.; Winer, J.R.; Walker, M.P. Sleep and Human Aging. *Neuron* **2017**, *94*, 19–36. [CrossRef] [PubMed]
26. Murawski, B.; Wade, L.; Plotnikoff, R.C.; Lubans, D.R.; Duncan, M.J. A systematic review and meta-analysis of cognitive and behavioral interventions to improve sleep health in adults without sleep disorders. *Sleep Med. Rev.* **2018**, *40*, 160–169. [CrossRef] [PubMed]
27. Min, D.; Cho, E. Associations among health behaviors, body mass index, hypertension, and diabetes mellitus: A path analysis. *Medicine* **2018**, *97*, e10981. [CrossRef] [PubMed]
28. Kesavachandran, C.; Bihari, V.; Mathur, N. Can physical activity maintain normal grades of body mass index and body fat percentage? *Int. J. Yoga* **2009**, *2*, 26–29. [CrossRef] [PubMed]
29. OECD/World Health Organization. Mortality from cardiovascular disease. In *Health at a Glance: Asia/Pacific 2018: Measuring Progress Towards Universal Health Coverage*; OECD Publishing: Paris, France, 2018. [CrossRef]

4

Assessment of Sodium Knowledge and Urinary Sodium Excretion among Regions of the United Arab Emirates

Amjad H. Jarrar [1], Lily Stojanovska [1,2], Vasso Apostolopoulos [2], Leila Cheikh Ismail [3,4], Jack Feehan [2,5], Eric O. Ohuma [6,7], Ala Z. Ahmad [1], Asma A. Alnoaimi [1], Latifa S. Al Khaili [1], Najah H. Allowch [1], Fatima T. Al Meqbaali [1], Usama Souka [1] and Ayesha S. Al Dhaheri [1,*]

1 Food, Nutrition and Health Department, College of Food and Agriculture, United Arab Emirates University, Al Ain 15551, UAE; AmjadJ@uaeu.ac.ae (A.H.J.); lily.stojanovska@uaeu.ac.ae (L.S.); 201050547@uaeu.ac.ae (A.Z.A.); 201050511@uaeu.ac.ae (A.A.A.); 201005105@uaeu.ac.ae (L.S.A.K.); 201050006@uaeu.ac.ae (N.H.A.); fatmadiab@uaeu.ac.ae (F.T.A.M.); usamasouka@uaeu.ac.ae (U.S.)

2 Institute for Health and Sport, Victoria University, Melbourne 14428, Australia; vasso.apostolopoulos@vu.edu.au (V.A.); jfeehan@student.unimelb.edu.au (J.F.)

3 Clinical Nutrition and Dietetics Department, College of Health Sciences, University of Sharjah, Sharjah 27272, UAE; lcheikhismail@sharjah.ac.ae

4 Nuffield Department of Women's & Reproductive Health, University of Oxford, Oxford OX1 2JD, UK

5 Department of Medicine—Western Health, The University of Melbourne, Melbourne 3021, Australia

6 Maternal, Adolescent, Reproductive & Child Health (MARCH) Centre, London School of Hygiene &Tropical Medicine (LSHTM), London WC1E 7HT, UK; eric.ohuma@ndm.ox.ac.uk

7 Centre for Tropical Medicine and Global Health, Nuffield Department of Medicine, University of Oxford, Oxford OX3 7LG, UK

* Correspondence: ayesha_aldhaheri@uaeu.ac.ae

Abstract: Non-communicable diseases (NCDs) such as cardiovascular disease, cancer and diabetes, are increasing worldwide and cause 65% to 78% of deaths in the Gulf Cooperation Council (GCC). A random sample of 477 healthy adults were recruited in the United Arab Emirates (UAE) in the period March–June 2015. Demographic, lifestyle, medical, anthropometric and sodium excretion data were collected. A questionnaire was used to measure knowledge, attitude and practice regarding salt. Mean sodium and potassium excretion were 2713.4 ± 713 mg/day and 1803 ± 618 mg/day, respectively, significantly higher than the World Health Organization (WHO) recommendations for sodium (2300 mg/day) and lower for potassium (3150 mg/day). Two-thirds (67.4%) exceeded sodium guidelines, with males 2.6 times more likely to consume excessively. The majority of the participants add salt during cooking (82.5%) and whilst eating (66%), and 75% identified processed food as high source of salt. Most (69.1%) were aware that excessive salt could cause disease. Most of the UAE population consumes excess sodium and insufficient potassium, likely increasing the risk of NCDs. Despite most participants being aware that high salt intake is associated with adverse health outcomes, this did not translate into salt reduction action. Low-sodium, high-potassium dietary interventions such as the Mediterranean diet are vital in reducing the impact of NCDs in the UAE.

Keywords: urinary sodium excretion; urinary potassium excretion; salt; sodium; non-communicable diseases; United Arab Emirates

---

1. Introduction

Chronic diseases are long-lasting conditions with continuous effects, and include cardiovascular disease (CVD), chronic respiratory disease (CRD), cancer and type 2 diabetes (T2D). Globally, their incidence is increasing becoming a growing burden to global economies and people's quality of life. Collectively, these non-communicable diseases (NCDs) are the leading cause of death globally [1], making it a significant priority in healthcare systems. In some countries, up to 40% of those dying from NCDs are younger than 60 years of age [1].

The rapid improvement in the socio-economic status of the countries making up the Gulf Cooperation Council (GCC) (Bahrain, Kuwait, Oman, Qatar, Saudi Arabia and the United Arab Emirates (UAE) has contributed to changing food consumption patterns, lifestyle habits and health status over the last four decades, with diet quality decreasing through the addition of more processed Westernized food. These changes have resulted in an increasingly sedentary lifestyle, high blood pressure and obesity, known to be major risk factors of NCDs [2,3]. Thus, it is not surprising that CVD is the major cause of morbidity and mortality in the Gulf region [4]. It is estimated that NCDs cause between 65% and 78% of deaths in the GCC member countries [5].

In particular, the lifestyle of the Emirati population has changed considerably in the last 40 years due to rapid improvement in socio-economic indicators in the UAE. This transition has led to less physical activity and altered eating habits, including increased intake of processed foods. These changes, in addition to the adoption of a Western lifestyle and diet, have led to the rise in prevalence of overweight, obesity and the risk of metabolic syndrome in the UAE. In the UAE, CVD accounts for more than 25% of all deaths countrywide, however, this has increased in the major metropolitan center, accounting for 29% of all deaths in the Emirate of Abu Dhabi [6].

Diet, environmental factors, lifestyle, physical inactivity and genetics have been shown to contribute to the risk of NCDs [1]. Control of these primary risk factors could reduce the incidence of some NCDs by up to 80% and cancers by 40% [1]. As such, in recent years, there has been a significant effort to improve diet and increase physical activity to control the prevalence of NCDs. Hypertension is the most common outcome of excessive sodium intake independent of age and is a key risk factor for many NCDs [7]. Globally, over 7.5 million people die from hypertension-related complications per year, which surpasses deaths from tobacco smoking (5 million), obesity (2.8 million) and cholesterol (2.6 million) [8]. Hypertension, secondary to excessive salt consumption, is a major risk factor for CVD, responsible for 62% of strokes and 49% of coronary heart disease (CHD) [7]. In the UAE, approximately 30% of the population is hypertensive, [9] and the disease is thought to be widely underdiagnosed [10]. High salt intake is considered one of the major contributors to premature adult death in developed and developing countries [11]. A systematic review and meta-analysis of 5508 participants across 61 studies showed that higher salt intake was associated with significantly increased risk of stroke, stroke mortality and coronary heart disease [11]. Unfavorably high sodium intake remains prevalent worldwide and varies widely, ranging from 4–17 g/day, with mainland China having the greatest intake, and some less developed island nations the lowest [12], but for many countries it remains well above the World Health Organization (WHO) recommendation of less than 5 g of salt intake per day [13]. The UK Food Standards Agency highlighted in 2012 that 75% of salt intake comes from processed foods and proposed that a reduction in the sodium content of processed food and drink would be required to achieve the recommended daily intake in the community [14,15].

Alongside appropriate sodium consumption, ensuring adequate intake of potassium is vital to ensuring normal mineral homeostasis and healthy blood pressure. Potassium is the paired ion for sodium in a range of different physiologies—from nerve transmission to renal function. Having adequate potassium in the diet ensures that the kidney is able to remove sodium from the plasma, and hence allows more effective regulation of blood pressure. While frank potassium deficiency (hypokalemia) is well understood and monitored, chronic, insufficient dietary intake is not, despite being associated with an increase in systolic blood pressure, and in the face of declining diet quality, insufficient intake is becoming more common [16]. Despite its important role in health, potassium intake has not been investigated in the UAE, however, globally, it has been reported that there is widespread dietary insufficiency, and this is likely to be mirrored in the Gulf region.

The impact of diet on NCDs is critical, and dietary approaches such as the Mediterranean diet have been suggested to have a role in improving health outcomes globally. The Mediterranean diet, with its high fruit and vegetable and low meat and processed food content, is an effective way to reduce salt and sodium intake, leading to a subsequent improvement in health outcomes [17]. Its high vegetable content also lends itself to improving potassium intake—making it an effective intervention to reduce hypertension [17].

There are numerous methods used for assessing salt intake, including estimation by weighing ingested food, dietary recall questionnaires, estimating the salt content of food before ingestion and taking measurements of 24-h (hr) sodium excretion [18]. Measurement of 24-h urinary sodium excretion is considered to be the golden standard for estimating daily sodium intake on the premise that the majority (90–95%) of sodium ingested is excreted via the urine [18].

The aim of this study was to assess sodium intake using 24-h urinary sodium excretion from a sample of the healthy UAE population and to assess their knowledge, attitudes and practices (KAP) surrounding salt intake.

2. Materials and Methods

2.1. Study Design and Participants

A cross-sectional study with an anonymized self-reported questionnaire and the collection of 24-h urine for the assessment of sodium, potassium and creatinine excretion was conducted between March 2015 and June 2015 in the UAE. The questionnaire consisted of items to assess participants' attitudes, behavior and knowledge (KAP) regarding salt consumption and knowledge. The sample size was calculated based on the following formula to be representative of the UAE, with a confidence interval level of 95%.

Sample size of an unknown population was calculated by Cochrane's formula ($n = z^2 \times p \times (1 - p)/e2$), with z = level of confidence (for a level of confidence of 95%, z = 1.96); *p* = the estimated proportion of the population that presents the characteristic of having high knowledge *p* = 0.5; e = margin of error accepted, e = 0.05; N (sample size) = 385 participants, plus 20% estimated dropouts = approximately 461 participants. Hence, a sample of 530 healthy individuals were recruited to participate in the study from the seven Emirates (Abu Dhabi, Dubai, Sharjah, Ajman, Ras Al Khaimah, Fujairah and Umm Al Quwain) aged between 20 and 65 years. Two methods were used for recruitment: face to face recruitment at community, school or university events and posters displayed in shopping malls, health centers, schools and university hostels. The WHO/PAHO (2010) protocol for 24-h urine collection and analysis was used. Four age groups were considered for recruitment in the current study; 20–30, 31–40, 41–50 and 51–65 years old with a ratio of 1:1 male to female. This demographic was used to ensure a sample of the 'healthy' population—participants older than 65 are likely to have comorbid disease which may have affected the urine analysis. All participants provided written informed consent to participate in the study.

A screening questionnaire was designed to collect data regarding demographic information, lifestyle habits, past medical history, medication and current health status. Questionnaires were administered by the research team. Exclusion criteria at screening were those with self-reported chronic diseases (i.e., heart disease, using medication for hypertension, renal failure, liver disease), pregnant and lactating women, those on diuretics and women who had their menstrual period during the time of urine collection. Inclusion and exclusion criteria are summarized in Table 1. Inclusion criteria at screening were participants aged 20 to 65 years for both genders, non-pregnant and non-lactating, no known chronic kidney disease, renal failure, hypertension with medications and liver diseases, no medical condition(s) or medication(s) known to affect urination and able to collect 24-h (hr) urine. Exclusion criteria following urine collection included those that were unable to collect adequate urine within the 24-h time period (i.e., volume < 500 mL), and creatinine levels below 500 or above 2000 mg/day, which is equivalent to <9 or >26 mg/kg of body mass for female participants and <13 or >29 mg/kg of body mass for male participants [19]. Forty-one participants were excluded due to limited urine sample collection (<500 mL urine) or being unable to effectively urinate into the collection bottle, and 12 participants due to creatinine levels below 500 mg. The creatinine cutoffs were used to screen for renal abnormalities that may have skewed the results [19]. One urine sample was also excluded during testing due to abnormalities, leaving 476 urine samples for the final urine analysis, alongside 477 questionnaire responses. The enrolment process of the study participants is shown in Figure 1.

Table 1. Summary of inclusion and exclusion criteria.

Inclusion	Exclusion
Age 20–65	Renal or urinary pathology
Non-pregnant	Chronic disease
Non-lactating	Current menstrual period
No chronic kidney disease	24-h urine volume <500 mL
No medical conditions	Urine creatinine <500 mg or >2000 mg
Not currently taking prescribed medications known to affect urine	

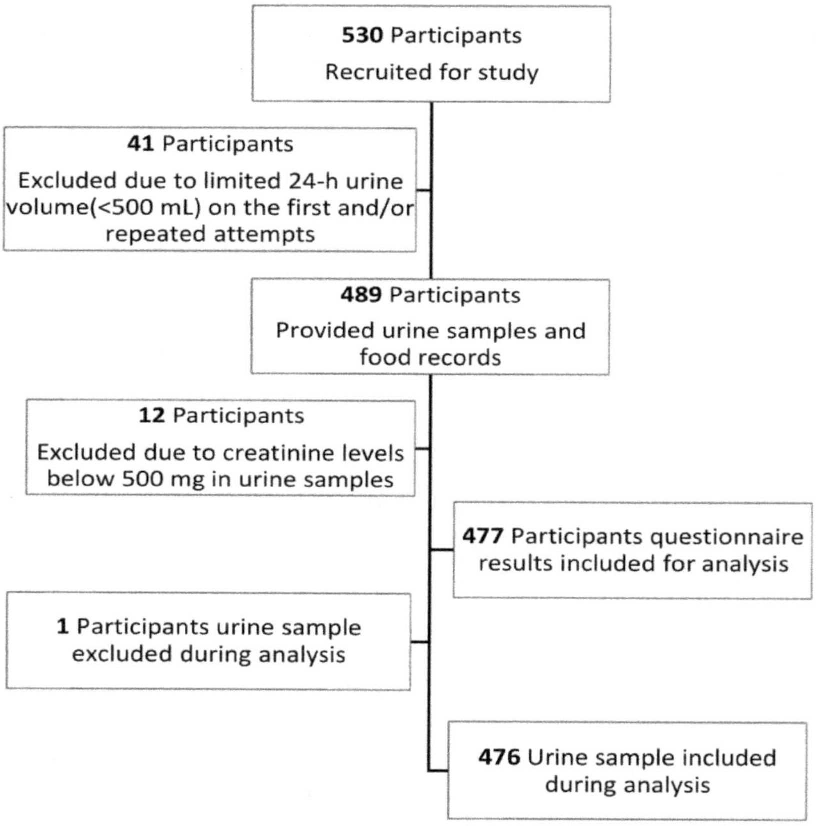

Figure 1. Flow diagram of the study design.

Participants were given full details of the study protocol with the opportunity to ask questions after which written informed consent to participate was sought. Each participant was allocated a personal identification number to provide anonymity and data confidentiality. Ethical approval for the study protocol was obtained from the UAE University (UAEU) Scientific Research Ethics Committee (Reference number: DVCRGS/36/2015).

2.2. *Anthropometric Measurements*

Body weight and height were measured for each participant and their body mass index (BMI) was calculated as weight (kg) divided by height (m) squared (kg/m^2). Height was recorded to the nearest 1 cm using a stadiometer (Seca Stadiometer, Seca Ltd., Birmingham, UK) and weight was recorded using a balance (Biospace Co., Seoul, Korea) to the nearest 0.1 kg having removed their shoes and heaviest clothing. An appropriately trained member of the research team took all the measurements [20].

2.3. *Knowledge, Attitude and Practice (KAP) Questionnaire*

Participants were asked to complete a self-reported questionnaire. The questionnaire assessed knowledge relating to salt and health outcomes, frequency of consumption and their perceived salt consumption, and was developed according to the WHO/PAHO recommendations for the assessment of population sodium intake and behaviors. The development and performance of the specific questionnaire has been described elsewhere [21].

2.4. *24-h Urine Collections and Analysis*

A single timed 24-h urine collection was obtained for the estimation of sodium excretion. Participants were given written and verbal instructions for the 24-h urine collection procedure. A 3-L coded plastic bottle was given to each participant for urine collection. Participants were asked to discard the first urine of the day and to collect all urine in the plastic bottle provided over the following 24-h. Participants were also asked to write on a separate sheet the time and date at the start and end of the urine collection, indicating occasions they missed urination. Urine samples with less than 500 mL or those who missed urine collection were rejected and participants were asked to repeat the process on another day.

Urine analysis for sodium, potassium and creatinine were conducted in the College of Food and Agriculture laboratories at UAEU. For the measurement of sodium and potassium levels in the urine, 50 mL of the urine sample was mixed with 200 μL of 1% nitric acid. Analytical solutions were introduced to a Varian ICP-OES model 710-ES spectrometer for sodium and potassium measurements [18]. Urinary creatinine was measured using a Cary 50 MPR Micro plate Reader-Varian and the concentration determined using a standard curve [22].

2.5. *Statistical Analysis*

Continuous variables were summarized by means and standard deviations or medians and inter-quartile ranges (25th–75th percentile) as appropriate. Continuous variables were checked visually for any departure from normality using histograms and quantile-quantile plots (Q–Q plots). All continuous data were reasonably normally distributed and therefore no transformations were applied. Categorical variables from the KAP questionnaire were reported as the percentage of responses per category. The Student's *t*-test was used to compare the mean difference in sodium and potassium excretion in urine against the recommended dietary allowance. Measures of association for categorical variables were evaluated using a chi-square or Fisher's exact test as appropriate. All analyses were conducted using the Statistical Package for the Social Sciences (SPSS) version 21. All statistical significance was determined at 5%.

3. Results

3.1. *Characteristics of the Study Population*

A total of 530 participants provided urine specimens, out of which 41 participants were excluded due to limited urine sample collection (<500 mL urine), and 12 participants due to creatinine levels below 500 mg in the urine, to give a final sample size of 477. One urine sample was excluded from the sample during analysis, due to excessive creatinine levels, leading to one less participant in the urine analysis (n = 476). The mean age was 37.31 years (standard deviation (SD) = 12.5 years, range 20–65 years), of which 55% were female (Table 2). The mean weight, height and BMI for participants were 73.37 ± 15.4 kg, 165.8 ± 8.95 cm and 26.7 ± 5.15 kg/m^2, respectively (Table 2). The prevalence of underweight, normal weight, overweight and obese individuals was 3.14%, 37.11%, 36.06% and 23.69%, respectively.

Table 2. Summary of study population demographics (N = 477).

Variable	Mean ± SD
Age (years)	37.31 ± 12.5
Weight (kg)	73.37 ± 15.4
Height (cm)	165.8 ± 8.95
Body Mass Index (BMI)	26.7 ± 5.15
	N (%)
Emirates [1]	
Abu Dhabi (West)	137 (28.72)
Al-Ain (East)	150 (31.45)
Northern Emirates [2]	190 (39.83)
Age Category (years)	
20–30	156 (32.70)
31–40	113 (23.69)
41–50	123 (25.78)
51–65	85 (17.82)
BMI Classifications (WHO definition)	
Underweight (<18.5 kg/m^2)	15 (3.14)
Normal-weight (18.5–24.9 kg/m^2)	177 (37.11)
Overweight (25.0–29.9 kg/m^2)	172 (36.06)
Obese (30.0–34.9 kg/m^2)	113 (23.69)
Gender Distribution, N (%)	
Males	214 (44.86)
Females	263 (55.14)

[1] Geographic divisions of United Arab Emirates; [2] Dubai, Sharjah, Ajman, Umm Al Quwain and Fujairah.

3.2. Major Findings of the Knowledge, Attitude and Practice (KAP) Questionnaire

The knowledge, attitude and practice (KAP) questionnaire (Table 3) indicated that the majority of the participants added salt during cooking (N = 393; 82.4%) and while eating (N = 315; 66%). Most participants reported that they always or sometimes use stock cubes during cooking (N = 346; 72.6%), and 69.1% reported that they were aware that high salt intake could cause serious health problems. However, a large proportion (62.1%) thought that their salt consumption was within the recommended amounts, with 60% claiming to have tried to control their salt or sodium intake. Most of the participants (45.2%) reported that high salt intake was associated with high blood pressure, followed by kidney stones (18.7%) and obesity (17.8%), but only 11.7% associated it with heart disease, and 6.5% with T2D. More than 75% of the participants reported that they considered processed foods as a high source of salt.

Table 3. Knowledge, attitude and practice (KAP) of salt intake and participants' knowledge on health consequences (N = 477). * This question is multiple choice with more than one selection allowed.

	Gender				Age Category (Year)				
Do you Add Salt during Cooking (Missing Answers = 0)	**Male N = 214 (%)**	**Female N = 263 (%)**	**Total N = 477 (%)**	**Chi-Square (*p*-Value)**	**20–30 N = 156 (%)**	**31–40 N = 113 (%)**	**41–50 N = 123 (%)**	**51–65 N = 85 (%)**	**Chi-Square (*p*-Value)**
Never	46 (21.6)	38 (14.1)	84 (17.5)		28 (18.0)	26 (23.0)	13 (10.6)	17 (19.0)	
Sometimes	80 (37.6)	96 (36.6)	176 (37.1)	5.60 (0.061)	65 (41.7)	42 (37.2)	46 (37.4)	23 (27.4)	20.01 (0.01)
Always	88 (40.8)	129 (49.2)	217 (45.5)		63 (40.4)	45 (39.8)	64 (52.0)	45 (54.2)	
Do you Add Salt to Food at the Table (Missing Answers = 1)	**Male N (%)**	**Female N (%)**	**Total N = 476 N (%)**	**Chi-Square (*p*-Value)**	**20–30 N (%)**	**31–40 N (%)**	**41–50 N (%)**	**51–65 N (%)**	**Chi-Square (*p*-Value)**
Never	71 (33.3)	90 (34.4)	161 (33.8)		54 (34.6)	31 (27.4)	40 (32.8)	36 (42.8)	
Sometimes	93 (43.7)	122 (46.60	215 (45.2)	2.12 (0.548)	75 (48.1)	53 (46.9)	51 (41.8)	36 (42.8)	12.71 (0.391)
Always	49 (23.0)	51 (19.0)	100 (21.0)		27 (17.3)	29 (25.7)	31 (25.4)	13 (14.3)	
Do you Use Stock Cubes during Cooking (Missing Answers = 0)	**Male N (%)**	**Female N (%)**	**Total N = 477 N (%)**	**Chi-Square (*p*-Value)**	**20–30 N (%)**	**31–40 N (%)**	**41–50 N (%)**	**51–65 N (%)**	**Chi-Square (*p*-Value)**
Never	55 (25.8)	76 (28.6)	131 (27.4)		39 (25.0)	30 (26.6)	33 (26.8)	29 (34.1)	
Sometimes	61 (28.6)	74 (28.2)	135 (28.4)	0.50 (0.779)	42 (26.9)	35 (31.0)	36 (29.2)	22 (25.9)	4.65 (0.794)
Always	98 (45.5)	113 (43.1)	211 (44.2)		75 (48.1)	48 (42.5)	54 (44.0)	34 (40.0)	
How Much Salt do you Think you Consume (Missing Answers = 0)	**Male N (%)**	**Female N (%)**	**Total N = 477 N (%)**	**Chi-Square (*p*-Value)**	**20–30 N (%)**	**31–40 N (%)**	**41–50 N (%)**	**51–65 N (%)**	**Chi-Square (*p*-Value)**
Too much	49 (23.0)	47 (17.6)	96 (20.0)		32 (20.5)	26 (23.0)	22 (18.0)	16 (19.1)	
Just the right amount	125 (58.2)	171 (65.3)	296 (62.1)	2.85 (0.240)	96 (61.5)	70 (62.0)	80 (65.0)	50 (59.5)	3.101 (0.928)
Far too little	40 (18.8)	45 (17.2)	85 (17.9)		28 (17.9)	17 (15.0)	21 (17.0)	19 (21.4)	
Do you Think that High Salt Diet could Cause Serious Health Problems? (Missing Answers = 0)	**Male N (%)**	**Female N (%)**	**Total N = 477 N (%)**	**Chi-Square (*p*-Value)**	**20–30 N (%)**	**31–40 N (%)**	**41–50 N (%)**	**51–65 N (%)**	**Chi-Square (*p*-Value)**
Yes	149 (69.6)	181 (68.8)	330 (69.1)		113 (72.4)	73 (64.6)	84 (68.4)	60 (70.0)	
No	45 (21.0)	68 (25.8)	113 (23.7)	3.682 (0.158)	32 (20.6)	32 (28.3)	31 (25.2)	18 (23.7)	4.782 (0.780)
Don't know	20 (9.3)	14 (5.4)	34 (7.2)		11 (7.1)	8 (7.1)	8 (6.56)	7 (8.4)	
What are the Health Problems Associated with High Salt Intake *	**Male N (%)**	**Female N (%)**	**Total N = 477N (%)**	**Chi-Square (*p*-Value)**	**20–30 N (%)**	**31–40 N (%)**	**41–50 N (%)**	**51–65 N (%)**	**Chi-Square (*p*-Value)**
High blood pressure	90 (42.1)	126 (47.9)	216 (45.2)		73 (46.8)	47 (41.6)	59 (48.0)	37 (43.5)	
Kidney stones	43 (20.1)	46 (17.5)	89 (18.7)		31 (19.9)	22 (19.5)	21 (17.1)	15 (17.6)	
Obesity	38 (17.8)	47 (17.9)	85 (17.8)	3.43 (0.414)	25 (16.0)	23 (20.3)	18 (14.6)	19 (22.3)	4.23 (0.624)
Diabetes	18 (8.4)	13 (4.9)	31 (6.5)		8 (5.1)	9 (8.0)	8 (6.5)	6 (7.1)	
Heart disease	25 (11.7)	31 (11.8)	56 (11.7)		19 (12.2)	12 (10.6)	17 (13.8)	8 (9.4)	
Do you Think Processed Foods are High in Sodium? (Missing Answers = 0)	**Male N (%)**	**Female N (%)**	**Total N = 477 (%)**	**Chi-Square (*p*-Value)**	**20–30 N (%)**	**31–40 N (%)**	**41–50 N (%)**	**51–65 N (%)**	**Chi-Square (*p*-Value)**
Yes	159 (74.2)	207 (78.6)	366 (76.7)	1.620 (0.444)	123 (78.9)	88 (77.9)	88 (71.5)	68 (80.0)	6.578 (0.574)
No	55 (25.8)	56 (21.4)	111 (23.3)		33 (21.1)	25 (22.1)	35 (28.5)	17 (20.0)	
Do you do Anything on a Regular Basis to Control your Salt or Sodium Intake? (Missing Answers = 0)	**Male N (%)**	**Female N (%)**	**Total N = 477 (%)**	**Chi-Square (*p*-Value)**	**20–30 N (%)**	**31–40 N (%)**	**41–50 N (%)**	**51–65 N (%)**	**Chi-Square (*p*-Value)**
Yes	131 (61.2)	158 (60.1)	289 (60.6)	0.935 (0.626)	88 (56.4)	69 (61.1)	76 (61.8)	56 (65.9)	4.823 (0.764)
No	83 (38.8)	105 (39.9)	188 (39.4)		68 (43.6)	44 (38.9)	47 (38.2)	29 (34.1)	

3.3. High Levels of Sodium Secretion in the UAE Population within 24-h Urine Collection

The mean 24-h urine volume was 1338.3 ± 553 mL, with a range of 550–4000 mL. The mean sodium excretion in urine was 2713.4 ± 713 mg. The average values for sodium excretion in urine exceeded the WHO recommendations of sodium intake of less than 2300 mg (Table 4) [23]. Of the 476 participants, 320 (67.4%) had a sodium excretion above the WHO recommended level of 2300 mg. Males were more likely (51.6%) to exceed the WHO recommendation compared to females (odds ratio (OR): 2.60; 95% confidence interval (CI): 1.71 to 3.96; $p < 0.001$). However, there were no significant differences by age of those surpassing the recommendation (OR: 0.99; 95% CI: 0.98 to 1.02; $p = 0.98$).

Table 4. Mean sodium, potassium and creatinine urinary excretion and ratio of sodium to potassium (n = 476).

Nutrients	Mean ± SD	Recommendation	*p*-Value
Mean 24-h sodium excretion in urine (mg)	2713.40 ± 713	<2300 mg	<0.001
Mean 24-h potassium excretion in urine (mg)	1803.30 ± 618.03	>3510 mg	<0.001
Mean 24-h creatinine excretion in urine (mg)	1284.81 ± 607.0		
Mean 24-h creatinine (mg/kg body mass)	16.83 ± 4.84		
Mean 24-h creatinine (mg/kg body mass)—female	13.42 ± 1.95		
Mean 24-h creatinine (mg/kg body mass)—male	21.81 ± 3.80		
Mean 24-h urinary Na/K ratio	1.64 ± 0.55		

Mean urinary excretion for potassium and creatinine and the sodium to potassium ratio were 1803.30 ± 618.03 mg, 1284.81 ± 607.0 mg and 1.64 ± 0.55 mg, respectively (Table 4). While it is challenging to use potassium excretion to estimate intake, it is likely that it is well below the WHO recommendations of 3500 mg/day [24]. Moreover, mean urinary excretion for creatinine for female participants was 13.42 ± 1.95 mg/kg body mass, with a minimum to maximum reading of 10.23 to 19.87 mg/kg body mass, while for male participants it was 21.81 ± 3.80 mg/kg body mass, with a minimum to maximum reading of 13.60 to 28.63 mg/kg body mass (Table 4). Mean urinary excretions for sodium, potassium and creatinine for male and female participants according to the different age groups are shown in Figure 2.

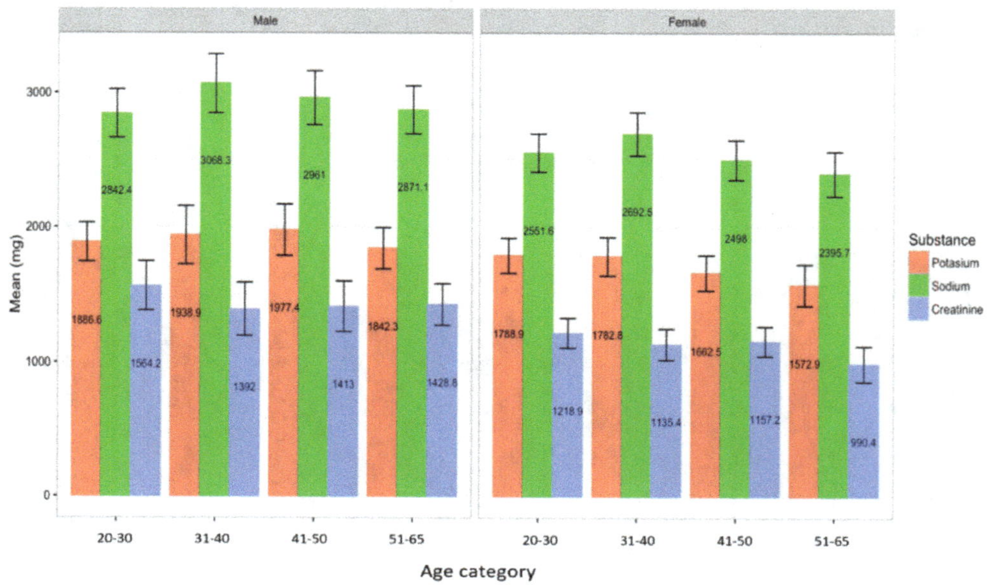

Figure 2. Mean creatinine, sodium and potassium levels for male (left panel) and female (right panel) participants according to age groups. The capped bars represent the 95% confidence intervals of the means.

4. Discussion

This study showed that sodium intake of the participants exceeds WHO recommendations with concurrent low intakes of potassium. Moreover, most of the participants were unaware that their consumption was beyond the recommended levels of the WHO, however, most were able to identify some common sources of sodium, such as stock cubes and processed foods, as well as its deleterious effect on health. To our knowledge, this is the first study in the UAE reporting 24-h urinary sodium excretion. A 24-h collection period is necessary to capture the marked diurnal variation in sodium, chloride and water excretion. Electrolyte excretion in healthy individuals normally reaches the maximum at or before midday, and the minimum at night towards the end of sleep [25]. This study is also the first to report on potassium excretion in the UAE, another critical indicator of dietary hypertension risk.

The results from the current study were similar to the results in a study conducted in Eastern Saudi Arabia that showed the mean intake of sodium assessed by 24-h sodium excretion to be 3200 ± 1100 mg/day and 2700 ± 850 mg/day for men and women, respectively [26]. Similar findings were noted in a Jordan study using 24-h urinary sodium excretion, which showed that the average sodium intake was 4100 mg/day (10.4 g/day salt) and sodium intake was higher in males, 4300 mg, compared with 4000 mg by females. It was clear that the Jordanian participants consumed at least double the current WHO recommended daily sodium amount of 2000 mg (5 g salt) [27]. Likewise, a study conducted in Oman using the National Nutrition Survey based on a 24-h dietary recall noted the average intake of salt to be 11–12 g/day [28], again significantly higher than the WHO recommendation. Two further studies analyzing food consumption in Kuwait [29,30] reported the average salt intake to be within 8–10 g/day. These results, and our own, are strong indicators that consumption of sodium exceeds the WHO recommendations in the GCC countries. It is well known high sodium intake is associated with hypertension and stroke, as well as contributes to myocardial infarction and heart and kidney failure [31,32]. Consequently, this prevalent increase in sodium consumption is likely to contribute to the incidence of NCDs in the UAE. Globally, the mean intake of sodium is high in East Asia, Central Asia, Eastern Europe, Central Europe and the Middle East/North Africa, in the range of 3900–4200 mg/day, which is equivalent to 9.75–10.5 g/day of salt [33], far exceeding the WHO recommendations, and is similar to our findings. While higher than the recommendations, the results of our study would suggest that the UAE was at the lower end of the scale of sodium intake in these geographic areas, however, comparisons between urinary excretion and sodium intake must be drawn with care. This may reflect the relatively high levels of education and other key socio-economic indicators when compared to these countries, which may manifest in more health-promoting behaviors. Urinary excretion of sodium as a function of intake has also been assessed in other nations, with generally higher socio-economic and health indicators. For example, in Japan and the United Kingdom (UK), sodium intake was 4470 ± 1600 mg/day and 3289 mg/day, respectively, and was attributed to a high intake of canned and processed foods [34,35].

High dietary sodium and low dietary potassium intakes are associated with hypertension and increased risk of cardiovascular disease (CVD) [36]. In the current study, the sodium to potassium ratio was 1.64 ± 0.55, suggesting that not only did sodium intake exceed WHO recommendations but insufficient dietary potassium was also prevalent. The amount of potassium excreted in 24-h urine is well correlated with dietary potassium intake [37]. A high urinary sodium–potassium ratio is an indicator of a need to reduce sodium and increase potassium intake [1,3]. The WHO has suggested that achieving guidelines for sodium and potassium intake would yield a sodium–potassium ratio close to 1.00 [23,24].

In our study, 67.4% of the participants exceeded the WHO recommendations for salt intake, with more males (51.6%) than females exceeding the recommendations. This finding is consistent with previous studies conducted in Kuwait, where males (74.7%) and females (50.9%) exceeded recommendations [29]. Similarly, a study conducted in Eastern Saudi Arabia also found that males tend to consume more sodium compared to females [26]. This finding is also consistent outside the GCC countries. In Brazil, 90% of the of study population exceeded WHO recommendations for salt intake with excess consumption again more common in males [38]. Another study aimed to estimate sodium intake in New York City, noting the mean sodium intake to be 3239 mg/day, with 81% of participants exceeding recommendations [39]. Brown et al. (2013), reported that sodium intake tends to be higher in men than women, based on 5693 participants recruited in 1984–1987 aged 20–59 years from 29 North American and European samples [31]; the findings again echoed those in our study. The sex differences in sodium excretion could have a number of causes, however, it is likely that increased appetite and calorie consumption is a major driver behind the variance. It is also possible that socio-cultural norms lead men to make more salt-heavy diet choices in both social and home situations, both in the UAE and globally. This is particularly relevant when viewed against the increased risk profile of a number of NCDs in men, and also makes it more challenging for males to meet sodium guidelines, as they are required to reduce their intake considerably compared to women.

The data on urinary potassium excretion is also of significant importance to the health of the population of the UAE. It is well known that potassium is a key part of effective blood pressure regulation, because of its role in effective sodium clearance. The mean potassium intake shown in this study was well below the WHO guidelines, providing opportunities for improvement of the health of the UAE. Encouraging a varied diet, high in fruit and leafy vegetables, would provide a ready means of improving health outcomes. Potassium is not amenable to fortification, due to the negative consequences of excessive intake and a flavor-masking effect of common chemical formats of the mineral, which means improving diet quality is the major means of increasing intake in the community.

It was also found that 82.5% of the participants in this study added salt sometimes or always during cooking, which is similar to that noted in Lebanon, where 100% of the participants have been found to add salt during cooking [40]. In the current study, the majority of participants reported that they added stock cubes and additional table salt while eating, sometimes or always. These findings are similar to the Lebanon study which showed that 60% of the participants used table salt [40]. Likewise, 61% of university students in the UAE reported adding salt while cooking, and 14% of the participants often added salt to food even before tasting it [21].

Despite the fact that 67.4% of the participants exceeded the WHO recommended salt intake in the current study, only 20.0% reported that their consumption was beyond the recommended threshold (Table 3). In light of our data showing widespread sodium excess, this suggests that many people are unaware of how much they are consuming. In this regard, education and public awareness programs are required so that the general population is more aware of salt portion sizes and the sodium content of processed foods, drinks and other foods in general.

Interestingly, about 60% of the participants claimed to be taking measures to control their salt intake, again similar to reports from Lebanon (65.8%) [40]. These findings are also similar to a study conducted in five sentinel countries of the Americas (Argentina, Canada, Chile, Costa Rica and Ecuador), where almost 90% of the participants reported excess intake of salt is associated with adverse health conditions, and over 60% of the participants indicated they were conscious of their salt intake and taking measures to reduce it. They also found that more than 30% of their participants believed that reducing dietary salt intake was highly important [41]. Most of these studies reported that the majority of the participants were aware that high salt intake was associated with adverse health outcomes, however, this awareness does not translate into effective behavioral change in salt reduction. These interesting findings have some important implications for strategies to reduce sodium intake. One of the mainstays of sodium reduction is public education, however, these results would indicate that the general knowledge is adequate. However, education campaigns on effective ways to reduce intake, while increasing potassium and hydration, would play a role in the general reduction in sodium across the UAE, alongside effective regulations and sodium targets.

The results of the current study indicate that there is prevalent high sodium and low potassium intake within the general population of the UAE, which consequently may increase the risk of hypertension, CVD and other NCDs. This emphasizes the need for coordinated salt reduction programs to aid in the reduction of NCDs in the UAE. Strategies such as educational campaigns, regulation of sodium content of widely consumed food items and setting targets for sodium intake will allow for a more cohesive approach to improving the health of the UAE in this regard. In the last two decades, a number of countries have put sodium reduction strategies in place, and they have generally been somewhat successful, however, there are still significant strides to be made [42]. The most effective population interventions are likely to be salt reduction targets in common food stuffs, specific to the geographical areas and the local cuisines. In the metropolitan centers of the UAE, this will likely need to target processed and fast foods, which are becoming more of a staple in the Emirati diet, however, future research to identify significant sources of sodium in the UAE is needed to guide policy makers. Other nations with successful sodium reduction strategies have used salt targets, typically between 5–8 g/day [42], to help guide these regulations and interventions. Decreasing the sodium consumption of the UAE will also require regulation of industry to offer more low-salt options, as well as improve standards on labeling and nutritional declaration on packaged foodstuffs.

The Mediterranean diet could play a role in combatting the widespread salt imbalance in the UAE. The Mediterranean diet is inherently low in sodium and high in potassium due to its high vegetable and low meat and processed food content. The Mediterranean diet is also accessible to the local region, as it contains a number of similarities to traditional food practices in the Arab nations, such as an emphasis on vegetables, dairy, grains and spices, however, the Emirati cuisine traditionally features meat products more strongly [43]. The Mediterranean diet has been shown to reduce hypertension [44], however, there is some debate surrounding the role of sodium in this. Some authors have found that the Mediterranean diet does not readily offer reductions in sodium [45], however, this may be due to variations in adherence and specific components of the diet, as well as the amount of other minerals, such as potassium, which are abundant in plant-rich diets.

Despite the significant findings, a limitation of this study was that urinary sodium was assessed by a single 24-h urine collection and this may not represent the average sodium intake in a person due to daily individual variability. However, a single urine measurement is considered a more accurate measure of sodium intake at a population level [18], though it may possibly be less accurate for individuals. There is also a potential that the recruited population may have been broadly healthier, as they were likely more health conscious, better educated and possibly of a higher socio-economic status. Future studies should account for key socio-economic indicators, such as years of education and household income in both their recruitment and analysis to ensure a representative sample of the population. This may have led to an underestimation of the UAE's sodium intake found in this study. Additionally, while the KAP questionnaire used in this study captures some important facets of the participants' knowledge and behavior surrounding salt, there is further room for additional information, particularly surrounding important sources of sodium in the modern diet. An expanded questionnaire, and other measures such as food diaries, would provide more reliable information on the true intake of sodium, and how that compares to the participants' knowledge. Despite these limitations, the study described was statistically sound and powered to reliably identify the sodium practices in the UAE. The large sample, with demographically representative participants, and the validated analytical methods, are also strengths of the research presented here.

5. Conclusions

In this cross-sectional sample of the UAE population, the majority consumed salt well above the international WHO recommendations with a concurrent low intake of potassium, suggesting significant room for improvement in the intake of these minerals. There are significant differences by gender, with males more likely to exceed the WHO recommendations for salt and sodium intake.

It is imperative for communities, as well as local and national governments, to play a leading role in the development and implementation of salt reduction strategies, such as increasing adherence to the Mediterranean diet, as well as setting standards for industry. Future research should aim to validate these findings with larger studies, as well as to identify important sources of sodium in the diet of the UAE. Awareness programs should be established to educate the population about the risk factors for excess salt consumption. A nationwide assessment should be conducted to evaluate the level of the problem, and to enable identification of appropriate priorities for the implementation of population-based diet-related interventions to reduce the prevalence of NCDs and their associated rates of morbidity and mortality.

Author Contributions: Conceptualization, A.S.A.D.; Formal analysis, E.O.O., F.T.A.M. and U.S.; Investigation, A.H.J., A.Z.A., A.A.A., L.S.A.K. and N.H.A.; Methodology, A.S.A.D.; Resources, A.S.A.D.; Supervision, A.H.J. and A.S.A.D.; Writing—original draft, A.H.J. and A.S.A.D.; Writing—review and editing, A.H.J., L.S., V.A., L.C.I., J.F., E.O.O. and A.S.A.D. All authors have read and agreed to the published version of the manuscript.

Acknowledgments: Authors would like to express their sincere gratitude to everyone who participated in the study.

References

1. World Health Organization. *Plan of Action for the Prevention and Control of Noncommunicable Diseases in the Eastern Mediterranean Region*; World Health Organization: Geneva, Switzerland, 2011.
2. Stamler, J.; Rose, G.; Stamler, R.; Elliott, P.; Dyer, A.; Marmot, M. Intersalt study findings. Public health and medical care implications. *Hypertension* **1989**, *14*, 570–577. [CrossRef] [PubMed]
3. He, F.J.; MacGregor, G.A. Effect of modest salt reduction on blood pressure: A meta-analysis of randomized trials. Implications for public health. *J. Hum. Hypertens.* **2002**, *16*, 761–770. [CrossRef] [PubMed]
4. Morrison, A.C.; Ness, R.B. Sodium intake and cardiovascular disease. *Ann. Rev. Public Health* **2011**, *32*, 71–90. [CrossRef]
5. World Health Organization. *Noncommunicable Diseases Country Profiles 2018*; World Health Organization: Geneva, Switzerland, 2018.
6. Loney, T.; Aw, T.-C.; Handysides, D.G.; Ali, R.; Blair, I.; Grivna, M.; Shah, S.M.; Sheek-Hussein, M.; El-Sadig, M.; Sharif, A.A. An analysis of the health status of the United Arab Emirates: The 'Big 4'public health issues. *Glob. Health Action* **2013**, *6*, 20100. [CrossRef] [PubMed]
7. He, F.J.; Burnier, M.; MacGregor, G.A. Nutrition in cardiovascular disease: Salt in hypertension and heart failure. *Eur. Heart J.* **2011**, *32*, 3073–3080. [CrossRef]
8. World Health Organization. Global Status Report on Noncommunicable Diseases 2010, Geneva. 2011. Available online: http://www.who.int/nmh/publications/ncd_report_full_en.pdf (accessed on 28 August 2020).
9. Shah, S.M.; Loney, T.; Sheek-Hussein, M.; El Sadig, M.; Al Dhaheri, S.; El Barazi, I.; Al Marzouqi, L.; Aw, T.-C.; Ali, R. Hypertension prevalence, awareness, treatment, and control, in male South Asian immigrants in the United Arab Emirates: A cross-sectional study. *BMC Cardiovasc. Disord.* **2015**, *15*, 30. [CrossRef]
10. Abdulle, A.M.; Nagelkerke, N.J.; Abouchacra, S.; Pathan, J.Y.; Adem, A.; Obineche, E.N. Under-treatment and under diagnosis of hypertension: A serious problem in the United Arab Emirates. *BMC Cardiovasc. Disorders* **2006**, *6*, 24. [CrossRef]
11. Aburto, N.J.; Ziolkovska, A.; Hooper, L.; Elliott, P.; Cappuccio, F.P.; Meerpohl, J.J. Effect of lower sodium intake on health: Systematic review and meta-analyses. *BMJ* **2013**, *346*, f1326. [CrossRef]
12. Brown, I.J.; Tzoulaki, I.; Candeias, V.; Elliott, P. Salt intakes around the world: Implications for public health. *Int. J. Epidemiol.* **2009**, *38*, 791–813. [CrossRef]
13. World Health Organization. *Diet, Nutrition, and the Prevention of Chronic Diseases: Report of a Joint WHO/FAO Expert Consultation*; World Health Organization: Geneva, Switzerland, 2003; Volume 916, p. 5.
14. Chobanian, A.V.; Bakris, G.L.; Black, H.R.; Cushman, W.C.; Green, L.A.; Izzo, J.L., Jr.; Jones, D.W.; Materson, B.J.; Oparil, S.; Wright, J.T., Jr. The seventh report of the joint national committee on prevention, detection, evaluation, and treatment of high blood pressure: The JNC 7 report. *JAMA* **2003**, *289*, 2560–2571. [CrossRef]
15. Wyness, L.A.; Butriss, J.L.; Stanner, S.A. Reducing the population's sodium intake: The UK Food Standards Agency's salt reduction programme. *Public Health Nutr.* **2012**, *15*, 254–261. [CrossRef] [PubMed]

16. Newberry, S.J.; Chung, M.; Anderson, C.A.; Chen, C.; Fu, Z.; Tang, A.; Zhao, N.; Booth, M.; Marks, J.; Hollands, S.; et al. *Sodium and Potassium Intake: Effects on Chronic Disease Outcomes and Risks*; Agency for Healthcare Research and Quality: Rockville, MD, USA, 2018.
17. Kokkinos, P.; Panagiotakos, D.B.; Polychronopoulos, E. Dietary influences on blood pressure: The effect of the Mediterranean diet on the prevalence of hypertension. *J. Clin. Hypertens.* **2005**, *7*, 165–172. [CrossRef] [PubMed]
18. Wielgosz, A.; Robinson, C.; Mao, Y.; Jiang, Y.; Campbell, N.R.; Muthuri, S.; Morrison, H. The impact of using different methods to assess completeness of 24-hour urine collection on estimating dietary sodium. *J. Clin. Hypertens.* **2016**, *18*, 581–584. [CrossRef] [PubMed]
19. Johnson, R.J.; Feehally, J.; Floege, J. *Comprehensive Clinical Nephrology E-Book*; Elsevier Health Sciences: Amsterdam, The Netherlands, 2014.
20. Lee, R.; Nieman, D. *Nutritional Assessment*; McGraw-Hill Education: New York, NY, USA, 2012.
21. Ismail, L.C.; Hashim, M.; Jarrar, A.H.; Mohamad, M.N.; Saleh, S.T.; Jawish, N.; Bekdache, M.; Albaghli, H.; Kdsi, D.; Aldarweesh, D. Knowledge, Attitude, and Practice on Salt and Assessment of Dietary Salt and Fat Intake among University of Sharjah Students. *Nutrients* **2019**, *11*, 941. [CrossRef] [PubMed]
22. Bowers, L.D.; Wong, E.T. Kinetic serum creatinine assays. II. A critical evaluation and review. *Clin. Chem.* **1980**, *26*, 555–561. [CrossRef]
23. World Health Organization. *Guideline: Sodium Intake for Adults and Children*; 9241504838; World Health Organization (WHO): Geneva, Switzerland, 2012.
24. World Health Organization. *Guideline: Potassium Intake for Adults and Children*; World Health Organization: Geneva, Switzerland, 2012.
25. Wesson, L.G. Electrolyte excretion in relation to diurnal cycles of renal function: Plasma electrolyte concentrations and aldosterone secretion before and during salt and water balance changes in normotensive subjects. *Medicine* **1964**, *43*, 547–592. [CrossRef]
26. Alkhunaizi, A.; Al Jishi, H.; Al Sadah, Z. Salt intake in Eastern Saudi Arabia. *East Mediterr. Health J.* **2013**, *19*, 915–918. [CrossRef]
27. Alawwa, I.; Dagash, R.; Saleh, A.; Ahmad, A. Dietary salt consumption and the knowledge, attitudes and behavior of healthy adults: A cross-sectional study from Jordan. *Libyan J. Med.* **2018**, *13*, 1479602. [CrossRef]
28. Al-Ghannami, S.; Library of Ministry of Health; Ministry of Health; Sultanate of Oman. National Nutrition Survey. 2004. Available online: https://www.moh.gov.om/en/web/statistics/ (accessed on 1 August 2020).
29. Zaghloul, S.; Al-Hooti, S.N.; Al-Hamad, N.; Al-Zenki, S.; Alomirah, H.; Alayan, I.; Al-Attar, H.; Al-Othman, A.; Al-Shami, E.; Al-Somaie, M. Evidence for nutrition transition in Kuwait: Over-consumption of macronutrients and obesity. *Public Health Nutr.* **2013**, *16*, 596–607. [CrossRef]
30. Alomirah, H.; Al-Zenki, S.; Husain, A. *Assessment of Acrylamide Levels in Heat-Processed Foodstuffs Consumed by Kuwaitis*; KISR No. 9316; Library of the Kuwait Institute of Scientific Research: Safat, Kuwait, 2008.
31. Brown, I.J.; Dyer, A.R.; Chan, Q.; Cogswell, M.E.; Ueshima, H.; Stamler, J.; Elliott, P.; Group ICOR. Estimating 24-hour urinary sodium excretion from casual urinary sodium concentrations in Western populations: The INTERSALT study. *Am. J. Epidemiol.* **2013**, *177*, 1180–1192. [CrossRef]
32. Lichtenstein, A.H.; Appel, L.J.; Brands, M.; Carnethon, M.; Daniels, S.; Franch, H.A.; Franklin, B.; Kris-Etherton, P.; Harris, W.S.; Howard, B. Diet and lifestyle recommendations revision 2006: A scientific statement from the American Heart Association Nutrition Committee. *Circulation* **2006**, *114*, 82–96. [CrossRef] [PubMed]
33. Micha, R.; Khatibzadeh, S.; Shi, P.; Fahimi, S.; Lim, S.; Andrews, K.G.; Engell, R.E.; Powles, J.; Ezzati, M.; Mozaffarian, D. Global, regional, and national consumption levels of dietary fats and oils in 1990 and 2010: A systematic analysis including 266 country-specific nutrition surveys. *BMJ* **2014**, *348*, g2272. [CrossRef] [PubMed]
34. Anderson, C.A.; Appel, L.J.; Okuda, N.; Brown, I.J.; Chan, Q.; Zhao, L.; Ueshima, H.; Kesteloot, H.; Miura, K.; Curb, J.D. Dietary sources of sodium in China, Japan, the United Kingdom, and the United States, women and men aged 40 to 59 years: The INTERMAP study. *J. Am. Diet. Assoc.* **2010**, *110*, 736–745. [CrossRef]
35. Ashford, R.; Jones, K.; Collins, D.; Earl, K.; Moore, S.; Koulman, A.; Yarde, J.; Polly, B.; Swan, G. *Assessment of Salt Intake from Urinary Sodium in Adults (Aged 19 to 64 Years) in England, 2018 to 2019. National Diet and Nutrition Survey*; Public Health England: London, UK, 2020.

36. Geleijnse, J.M.; Witteman, J.C.; Stijnen, T.; Kloos, M.W.; Hofman, A.; Grobbee, D.E. Sodium and potassium intake and risk of cardiovascular events and all-cause mortality: The Rotterdam Study. *Eur. J. Epidemiol.* **2007**, *22*, 763–770. [CrossRef] [PubMed]
37. Taylor, E.N.; Stampfer, M.J.; Mount, D.B.; Curhan, G.C. DASH-style diet and 24-hour urine composition. *Clin. J. Am. Soc. Nephrol.* **2010**, *5*, 2315–2322. [CrossRef]
38. Nilson, E.A. The strides to reduce salt intake in Brazil: Have we done enough? *Cardiovasc. Diagn. Ther.* **2015**, *5*, 243.
39. Angell, S.Y.; Yi, S.; Eisenhower, D.; Kerker, B.D.; Curtis, C.J.; Bartley, K.; Silver, L.D.; Farley, T.A. Sodium intake in a cross-sectional, representative sample of New York City adults. *Am. J. Public Health* **2014**, *104*, 2409–2416. [CrossRef]
40. Nasreddine, L.; Akl, C.; Al-Shaar, L.; Almedawar, M.M.; Isma'eel, H. Consumer knowledge, attitudes and salt-related behavior in the Middle-East: The case of Lebanon. *Nutrients* **2014**, *6*, 5079–5102. [CrossRef]
41. Claro, R.M.; Linders, H.; Ricardo, C.Z.; Legetic, B.; Campbell, N.R. Consumer attitudes, knowledge, and behavior related to salt consumption in sentinel countries of the Americas. *Rev. Panam. Salud. Publica* **2012**, *32*, 265–273. [CrossRef]
42. World Health Organization. *Mapping Salt Reduction Initiatives in the WHO European Region*; WHO Regional Office for Europe: Copenhagen, Denmark, 2013.
43. Berry, E.M.; Arnoni, Y.; Aviram, M. The Middle Eastern and biblical origins of the Mediterranean diet. *Public Health Nutr.* **2011**, *14*, 2288–2295. [CrossRef]
44. La Verde, M.; Mulè, S.; Zappalà, G.; Privitera, G.; Maugeri, G.; Pecora, F.; Marranzano, M. Higher adherence to the Mediterranean diet is inversely associated with having hypertension: Is low salt intake a mediating factor? *Int. J. Food Sci. Nutr.* **2018**, *69*, 235–244. [CrossRef] [PubMed]
45. Magriplis, E.; Farajian, P.; Pounis, G.D.; Risvas, G.; Panagiotakos, D.B.; Zampelas, A. High sodium intake of children through 'hidden' food sources and its association with the Mediterranean diet: The GRECO study. *J. Hypertens.* **2011**, *29*, 1069–1076. [CrossRef] [PubMed]

5

Diet Quality, Saturated Fat and Metabolic Syndrome

Stéphanie Harrison [1,2], Patrick Couture [1,3] and Benoît Lamarche [1,2,*]

1 Centre Nutrition, santé et société (NUTRISS), Institut sur la nutrition et les aliments fonctionnels (INAF), Université Laval, Québec, QC G1V 0A6, Canada; stephanie.harrison.1@ulaval.ca (S.H.); patrick.couture@fmed.ulaval.ca (P.C.)
2 School of Nutrition, Université Laval, Québec, QC G1V 0A6, Canada
3 CHU Research Center, Québec, QC G1V 0A6, Canada
* Correspondence: benoit.lamarche@fsaa.ulaval.ca

Abstract: Indices reflecting overall diet quality are used globally in research to predict the risk of various diseases and metabolic disorders such as metabolic syndrome (MetS). Such indices are built to measure adherence to current dietary guidelines or to best assess the diet–disease relationship. Although mostly food-based, dietary guidelines often include recommendations to limit saturated fatty acid (SFA) intake in order to prevent cardiovascular diseases. However, not all diet quality indices consider SFA in their definition of diet quality. Additionally, the relationship between SFA consumption and the development of MetS remains unclear. The purpose of this short review was to explore the association between MetS and various diet quality indices and dietary patterns, with a focus on how SFA contributes to these associations.

Keywords: saturated fatty acids; metabolic syndrome; diet quality; dietary guidelines; cardiovascular disease

---

1. Introduction

Various scores and indices are available to assess overall diet quality in population-based or interventional studies. These scores measure either adherence to certain dietary patterns, such as the Mediterranean diet (MedDiet) or the Dietary Approach to Stop Hypertension (DASH), or to country-specific dietary guidelines, such as Healthy Eating Indices (HEI). As discussed below, dietary patterns and diet quality indices have been associated with the risk of various diseases, including the metabolic syndrome (MetS), a collection of metabolic disorders that increase the risk of cardiovascular diseases (CVD), stroke or type 2 diabetes [1]. The typical features of MetS are central obesity, insulin resistance, dyslipidemia, hypertension, dysglycemia, and a pro-inflammatory/pro-thrombotic state [1]. The dyslipidemic features of the MetS are hypertriglyceridemia (fasting and postprandial) and low high-density lipoprotein cholesterol (HDL-C). While an elevated low-density lipoprotein cholesterol concentration (LDL-C) is not considered a typical feature of MetS, other features of LDL are. Specifically, patients with MetS generally have smaller and denser LDL particles, which are more prone to oxidative stress and are cleared less rapidly from the circulation than larger LDL particles [2].

Dietary patterns are a multidimensional representation of eating and, by definition, do not focus on singled out nutrients or foods. This is also the case for dietary guidelines, which have shifted from mostly nutrient-based to mostly food-based recommendations in recent years [3]. Nevertheless, most dietary guidelines around the globe still include a recommendation to limit intakes of specific nutrients of public health concern, including saturated fatty acids (SFAs). The recommendation to limit the consumption of SFAs is based largely on their well-established cholesterol-raising effects [4,5]. Data from a number of randomized controlled trials (RCTs) have shown that replacing dietary SFA with unsaturated fats reduces the risk of combined CVD events and are also at the basis of the recommendation to limit SFA intakes [5,6]. Replacing dietary SFA with carbohydrates from whole grains foods may also yield cardiovascular benefits, unlike carbohydrates from refined grains [7–9].

Although SFAs have been considered a major nutritional risk factor of CVD for more than 50 years, recent data have provided new challenging evidence suggesting that the SFA–CVD relationship may not be as straightforward as originally thought [10]. For example, the meta-analysis that showed a significant impact of SFA reduction on combined CVD events and showed no significant effect of SFAs on the risk of fatal myocardial infarction (MI) or coronary heart disease (CHD) mortality [5]. The authors of this meta-analysis emphasized the lack of robust, high-quality data to reach definitive conclusions on many of these associations. Others suggest that the recommendations on healthy dietary patterns capture the inherent risk attributed to variations in SFA intake, implying that specific recommendations on SFA intake are, in that context, redundant [11]. The fact that the increase in LDL-C concentrations seen with higher intakes of SFA intake is generally paralleled by an increase in the size of the LDL is another factor complexifying the association between dietary SFA and CVD risk [11]. Finally, the heterogeneity in the health effects of individual types of SFAs (e.g., myristic, lauric, etc.) [7,12] and the important interindividual variation in response to SFA reduction [13] are additional considerations put forward by those against the specific recommendations on SFA [11].

Beyond its well-known LDL-raising effects, the impact of SFA consumption on cardiometabolic health remains controversial. While data from a recent systematic review suggest that increased intake of SFA is associated with an increased risk of MetS, this association appeared to be dependent on the concurrent variations of other nutrients [9]. The purpose of this short review was therefore to explore the association between MetS and various diet quality indices and dietary patterns, with a focus on how SFA may contribute to these associations.

2. Diet Quality and Metabolic Syndrome

2.1. *The HEI and MetS*

The first HEI was developed in 1995 by the United States Department of Agriculture (USDA) in order to measure adherence to the Dietary Guidelines for Americans (DGA) as well as the Food Guide Pyramid. The HEI's main goal was to serve as a "report card" of Americans' diet, i.e., a measure of overall diet quality. This first HEI had 10 components related to recommendations found in the Food Guide Pyramid (Grains, Vegetables, Fruits, Milk, Meat, and "Other Foods") and in the DGA (Total fat, SFA, Cholesterol, Sodium, and Variety). The HEI-2015 is the most recent healthy eating index in the USA and reflects adherence to the 2015–2020 DGA. It has 13 components, including both adequacy and moderation components (Table 1). The moderation components of the HEI-2015 include a fatty acids sub-score calculated as the ratio of unsaturated fat to SFAs, as well as an SFA sub-score. According to the 2015–2020 DGA, SFA intake should not exceed 10%E per day (the SFA sub-score of the HEI-2015) and should be replaced by unsaturated fats (the fatty acids sub-score of the HEI-2015). As indicated above, those recommendations are based on many studies having shown that replacing SFA with unsaturated fat (notably PUFA) reduces serum levels of total and LDL-cholesterol [4], as well as the risk of CVD events [5]. The rationale for the SFA recommendation (<10% E) in the 2015–2020 DGA is not based on the upper limit instated by the Institute of Medicine. It is based on the notion that in most instances, people with an SFA intake > 10% E cannot meet the recommended intake of all food groups while maintaining an energy balance [3]. SFA intake in the calculation of the HEI-2015 is also partially accounted for in the total protein foods adequacy component, higher fat protein foods receiving fewer points than lower fat protein foods [14]. Finally, the adequacy dairy component of the HEI-2015, which rewards a higher consumption of dairy products irrespective of fat content, as well as the SFA moderation component, which sanctions higher SFA intakes, reflects the 2015–2020 DGA recommendations to favor lower-fat or fat-free dairy products [3].

Surprisingly, very few studies have documented the association between HEIs (2010 or 2015 versions) and the risk of MetS. In a cross-sectional analysis of 1036 Iranian women, participants in the highest quartile of HEI-2010 had a 28% lower risk of MetS compared with those in the first quartile (95% CI 0.50–0.96). Abdominal obesity, high blood pressure, high serum triacylglycerol and low serum HDL-C also decreased across HEI-2010 quartiles [15]. Structural equation modeling analyses of data from a sample of 188 healthy obese adults revealed that the HEI-2015 mediated the association between age and several cardio-metabolic risk factors associated with MetS, including fat mass, fat free mass, systolic blood pressure (SBP) and HDL-C. HEI-2015 scores also mediated the association between gender and waist circumference, SBP, triglyceride and HDL-C [16].

Table 1. Components of different healthy eating indices.

HEI-2015	aHEI	PNNS-GS2
Adequacy		*Adequacy*
1. Total fruits 2. Whole fruits	1. Fruits	1. Vegetables/Fruits
3. Total vegetables	2. Vegetables	
4. Greens and Beans	3. Nuts/Legumes	2. Nuts
		3. Legumes
5. Whole grains	4. Whole grains	4. Whole grain foods
6. Dairy products		5. Milk and dairy products
7. Total protein foods		
8. Seafood and Plant protein		6. Fish and sea foods
9. Fatty acids (UFA/SFA ratio)	5. Trans fat	7. Added fat (prefer vegetable sources)
	6. Long chain n3 fatty acids	
	7. PUFA	
Moderation		*Moderation*
	8. Red/Processed meat	8. Red meat
		9. Processed meat
10. Refined grains		
11. Sodium	9. Sodium	10. Sodium
12. Added sugars	10. SSBs	11. Sweet tasting beverages
		12. Sugary foods
13. SFA		
	11. Alcohol	13. Alcohol

HEI: Healthy Eating Index, PNNS-GS2: Programme National Nutrition Santé-Guideline Score updated to reflect the 2017 French dietary guidelines, UFA: Unsaturated fatty acids, SFA: Saturated fatty acids, PUFA: Polyunsaturated fatty acids, SSBs: Sugar-sweetened beverages. Note: The aHEI does not use the adequacy/moderation classification of its components.

The extent to which each of the HEI-2015 sub-scores, including those related to SFA intake, contribute to modifying individual features of the MetS is a complex question. To the extent that high LDL-C concentrations are not a typical feature of the MetS, adequacy or moderation components of the HEI-2015 having an impact on LDL-C concentrations would not predict changes in the incidence of MetS. However, replacing SFA with PUFA or MUFA slightly reduces HDL-C, total cholesterol, and TG concentrations in healthy adults [4]. Furthermore, replacing SFA by PUFA from different oils or foods reduced HDL-C concentrations in a recently published cross-over randomized controlled trial (RCT) of 36 men and women at risk of CVD, while having no effect on serum TG and glucose levels [17]. The substitution of SFA by PUFA, particularly PUFAs from walnuts, had a small but significant lowering effect on blood pressure but no effect on arterial stiffness in the same RCT [17]. These results suggest that dietary SFA, because of opposing effects on many of the typical features of MetS, cannot explain in and of themselves the favorable association between diet quality, as measured by the HEI-2015, and MetS. On the other hand, consumption of other foods and nutrients accounted for in the HEI-2015 has been more consistently associated with specific features of the MetS. For example, high vs. low dairy consumption has been associated with a lower risk of abdominal obesity and of being overweight [18]. The blood pressure lowering effect of a low sodium diet is well established [19].

Data from observational studies indicate that consumption of fruits and vegetables is associated with a lower risk of MetS [20]. Fruit consumption, independent of vegetable consumption, has also been inversely associated with the incidence of hypertriglyceridemia [21]. Higher consumption of sugar-sweetened beverages (SSBs), one of the main sources of added sugar in the North American diet, has been associated with an increased risk of MetS [22]. Taken together, these results suggest that the SFA component of the HEI-2015 per se cannot explain the favorable association between the HEI-2015 and the risk of MetS.

2.2. *The aHEI and MetS*

Unlike the HEI-2015, which is meant to measure adherence to dietary guidelines, the Alternate HEI (aHEI) was developed not only as a measure of diet quality but also to entail the diet–disease association. It was first developed in 2002 and included 9 components, including vegetables, fruits, and cereal fiber [23]. While the first version of the aHEI included an SFA component, the updated 2010 version of the aHEI does not (Table 1) [24], reflecting to some extent the inconsistent association between SFA consumption and CVD [11]. This is not to say that SFA is not indirectly accounted for in the aHEI. Indeed, a high score resulting from a high consumption of vegetables and fruits, whole grains, nuts and legumes, and PUFA, combined with a low consumption of SSBs, sodium, and red/processed meat, reflects a healthy food pattern that is very likely to be low in SFA.

In a cross-sectional analysis of 12,406 US Hispanics and Latinos from the multicenter, population-based Hispanic Community Health Study/Study of Latinos cohort, a higher aHEI was associated with lower odds of MetS [25]. Interestingly, the association of the aHEI and cardiometabolic factors varied by ethnic background. Specifically, the aHEI was inversely associated with waist circumference, blood pressure, and glucose among Mexicans and Puerto Ricans and with TG among Mexicans only, and was positively associated with HDL-C among Puerto Ricans and Central Americans [25]. We have also shown a similar inverse association between the aHEI and the prevalence of MetS in a cross-sectional analysis of 998 men and women from the province of Québec, in Canada [26]. In a cross-sectional analysis of 775 healthy women from the Nurses' Health Study, the aHEI was inversely associated with leptin and insulin concentrations but showed no association with other cardiometabolic risk factors traditionally associated with MetS [27]. These associations were, however, no longer present after adjusting for body mass index (BMI). Similar to the HEI-2015, this inverse association between the aHEI and the MetS is unlikely to be explained by variations in dietary SFA intake per se.

2.3. *The Programme National Nutrition Santé Guideline Score (PNNSG-GS2) and MetS*

The PNNS-GS2 is a score that reflects adherence to the 2017 French nutritional guidelines (Table 1) [28]. Briefly, it includes 13 components, of which seven are considered as adequacy recommendations and six refer to moderation recommendations. Similar to the aHEI, the PNNS-GS2 has no specific sub-score for SFA, but SFA intake is captured by the recommendation on added fat (to favor vegetable sources of fat vs. animal sources of fat) and indirectly by the recommendation on processed meats. Hence, individuals with a higher PNNS-GS2 consumed less SFA than individuals with a lower score [28]. Cross-sectional data from the Nutrinet-Santé Study have shown that a higher PNNS-GS2 was associated with a lower BMI, lower TG and glucose concentrations, lower systolic and diastolic blood pressures, and with higher concentrations of HDL-C in both men and women [28]. Recent data also suggest that higher adherence to the French dietary guidelines is prospectively associated with a lower risk of being overweight or obese [29]. These observations suggest that the PNNS-GS2 is likely to be inversely associated with the risk of incident MetS, but this needs to be formally confirmed with prospective data. The extent to which each of the components of the PNNS-GS2 are associated with individual features of the MetS is also unknown.

2.4. The Dietary Approaches to Stop Hypertension (DASH) Score and MetS

The Dietary Approaches to Stop Hypertension (DASH) score was created to measure adherence to the DASH diet, a healthy eating pattern that has been repeatedly associated with lower blood pressure and reduced CVD risk [30–35]. It was developed in the 1990s for the DASH trial, a randomized controlled trial in which more than 400 participants were randomized to either the control "American" diet, an "American" diet rich in fruits and vegetables or a DASH diet [36]. Most studies available at the time of the trial had shown no clear association between dietary fat (including SFA) and blood pressure [37]. However, it was argued that strict vegetarian diets (i.e., excluding dairy products) that were low in fat and SFA were associated with lower blood pressure. The DASH eating plan as we know it today promotes the consumption of fruits and vegetables, low-fat dairy products, whole grains, legumes, fish, poultry, and nuts and recommends limited intakes of sweets, SSBs, and red meats. Furthermore, individuals wanting to follow a DASH eating plan should choose foods that are low in sodium, SFA and trans-fat and rich in potassium, calcium, magnesium, fiber, and protein [34]. To that extent, the typical DASH diet is also a healthy eating pattern that is low in SFA [34].

Multiple versions of the DASH diet score are available in the literature [35,38–40]. Most scores include some of or all 8 food groups of the DASH eating plan, namely grains, meat/poultry/fish, vegetables, fruits, low-fat dairy products, fats and oils, nuts/legumes, and sweets. Additionally, most versions of the score include a component related to sodium intake. However, even if the recommendation to choose foods low in SFA and to limit consumption of SFA is included in the typical DASH eating plan, not all versions of the DASH score include a component directly related to SFA intake. For example, the DASH score created by Fung et al. does not include a component pertaining to SFA consumption based on the argument that it is already captured, at least partly, by the inclusion of red and processed meat components of the score [35].

In general, a greater adherence to a DASH score is associated with a lower prevalence of MetS [41,42]. Similar to the aHEI, the DASH score showed variable associations with the MetS and its key features among diverse Hispanic/Latino populations [43]. In a cross-sectional analysis among US women, higher adherence to the DASH eating plan was associated with lower TG concentrations, independent of BMI [27]. In a meta-analysis of available RCTs, consumption of the DASH diet over periods ranging from 2 to 24 weeks reduced systolic and diastolic blood pressure as well as LDL-C concentrations, but had no significant effect on TG, HDL-C, and glucose concentrations [44]. Interestingly, the reduction in blood pressure with the DASH diet has been shown to be similar among individuals with and without MetS [45]. Thus, when applied rigorously, the DASH diet is likely to have an impact on MetS, primarily through its important blood pressure lowering effect. Considering that the DASH diet is low in SFA by definition, it is unsurprising to find that adherence to this healthy dietary pattern also reduces serum LDL-C concentration, but this cannot explain the association between the DASH score and MetS.

2.5. The Mediterranean Diet and MetS

The concept of the MedDiet emerged from the Seven Countries Study in the 1950s, which unraveled particularly low CVD mortality rates in countries around the Mediterranean Sea [46]. Such low CVD rates were attributed, at least partly, to the intrinsically low SFA content of the diet of inhabitants around the Mediterranean (<7% E) compared with inhabitants from northern countries such as Finland [47]. It is now recognized that a MedDiet such as the one recommended in dietary guidelines is not just about SFA, although constitutively, a MedDiet is low in SFA. Typically, a MedDiet is characterized by very high intakes of plant-based foods, such as fruits, vegetables, cereals, beans, nuts and seeds, low to moderate intakes of fish and poultry and occasional consumption of eggs and red meat [48]. Olive oil is often considered the main source of fat in the MedDiet. A low to moderate wine consumption is also included in the MedDiet pattern, mostly consumed with meals [48]. The MedDiet is the most documented and researched healthy eating pattern. It has been repeatedly and consistently associated with lower risks of CVD, type 2 diabetes, and some types of cancer as well as cognitive-related diseases [49–52].

Several MedDiet scores have been created to measure adherence to a MedDiet. According to D'Alessandro and De Pergola, there is a certain degree of variability in the different MedDiet scores currently existing [53]. However, Galbete et al. found little differences in disease risk associations when comparing different MedDiet scores [54]. This is not entirely surprising considering that several core foods (fruit, vegetables, legumes, cereals, meat, dairy, fish, alcohol, and healthy fats) are found in most MedDiet scores [53,54]. It must also be stressed that the MedDiet emphasizes consumption of whole foods, with little if no focus on nutrients. Even if SFA is not part of most of the MedDiet scores per se, this healthy eating pattern is intrinsically low in SFA, in part due to the fact that this pattern focuses on fresh foods and because the recommendation to consume almost exclusively olive oil as a source of fat restricts in and of itself SFA consumption.

The PREDIMED study has shown in subjects without MetS at baseline that consumption of a MedDiet supplemented with either nuts or olive oil for five years had no impact on MetS incidence compared with a control diet. However, reversion occurred in almost 3 out of 10 of participants who had MetS at baseline in both groups consuming the MedDiet [55]. MedDiet participants supplemented with olive oil showed significant reductions in abdominal obesity and in fasting glucose while MedDiet participants supplemented with nuts showed a significant reduction in abdominal obesity only. Interestingly, increases in the biomarkers of foods supplied to the Mediterranean diet groups, namely oleic and α-linolenic acids, have been associated with the incidence, reversion, and prevalence of MetS [56]. Similar to the DASH eating plan, higher adherence to the MedDiet has been associated with lower TG concentrations among US women, independent of BMI [27]. Consumption of the MedDiet has also been associated with improvements in several features of the MetS, including blood lipids, blood pressure, glucose-insulin homeostasis, endothelial function, and inflammation markers [57]. Being nutrient-dense and having a low energy density, the MedDiet has often led to weight loss in intervention studies [58], thus potentially amplifying the cardiometabolic changes seen with the MedDiet [59]. Of note, the weight loss achieved with the MedDiet may be more important than with low-fat diets, but similar to low-carbohydrate diets [60]. Others have suggested that consumption of a MedDiet may also reduce central obesity, which in turn may contribute to reduced obesity-related and MetS-related disease risk [61]. To that extent, the contribution of the low SFA content of the MedDiet to its cardiometabolic benefits may be limited to LDL-C and not to features of the MetS.

3. Conclusions

Deciphering the impact of individual foods and nutrients on cardiometabolic risk factors such as those associated with MetS is very challenging because of the numerous food–nutrient interactions found within complex food patterns. This is certainly the case with SFA. In this short narrative review, we have shown that diet quality indices reflecting adherence to dietary guidelines (HEIs) or healthy dietary patterns (DASH, MedDiet) are quite consistently associated with a reduced risk of MetS. Data reviewed here provide indirect evidence that SFA in and of itself may play a rather limited role in the development of MetS. Indeed, while increased SFA intake in place of PUFA is unarguably associated with raised LDL-C concentrations, high LDL-C is not a typical feature of MetS. Moreover, the extent to which variations in SFA intake contribute to the cardiometabolic benefits associated with healthy eating patterns is likely to be diluted within the effects of numerous other nutrients and foods that constitute these patterns and which have been quite consistently associated with features of MetS. However, this may be of little concern since healthy eating scores that do not account for SFA intake per se inevitably capture this component through other components of the scores.

Author Contributions: S.H. and B.L. wrote the paper together. P.C. revised the paper. All authors agreed to the published version of the manuscript.

References

1. Desroches, S.; Lamarche, B. The evolving definitions and increasing prevalence of the metabolic syndrome. *Appl. Physiol. Nutr. Metab.* **2007**, *32*, 23–32. [CrossRef] [PubMed]
2. Lamarche, B.; Lemieux, I.; Després, J.P. The small, dense LDL phenotype and the risk of coronary heart disease: Epidemiology, patho-physiology and therapeutic aspects. *Diabetes Metab.* **1999**, *25*, 199–211. [PubMed]
3. Department of Health and Human Services. *Dietary Guidelines for Americans 2015–2020*; Department of Health and Human Services: Washington, DC, USA, 2015; p. 122.
4. Mensink, R. *Effects of Saturated Fatty Acids on Serum Lipids and lipo90proteins: A Systematic Review and Regression Analysis*; WHO: Geneva, Switzerland, 2016.
5. Hooper, L.; Martin, N.; Jimoh, O.F.; Kirk, C.; Foster, E.; Abdelhamid, A.S. Reduction in saturated fat intake for cardiovascular disease. *Cochrane Database Syst. Rev.* **2020**. [CrossRef] [PubMed]
6. Mozaffarian, D.; Micha, R.; Wallace, S. Effects on coronary heart disease of increasing polyunsaturated fat in place of saturated fat: A systematic review and meta-analysis of randomized controlled trials. *PLoS Med.* **2010**, *7*, e1000252. [CrossRef]
7. Briggs, M.A.; Petersen, K.S.; Kris-Etherton, P.M. Saturated Fatty Acids and Cardiovascular Disease: Replacements for Saturated Fat to Reduce Cardiovascular Risk. *Healthcare* **2017**, *5*, 29. [CrossRef]
8. Li, Y.; Hruby, A.; Bernstein, A.M.; Ley, S.H.; Wang, D.D.; Chiuve, S.E.; Sampson, L.; Rexrode, K.M.; Rimm, E.B.; Willett, W.C.; et al. Saturated Fats Compared With Unsaturated Fats and Sources of Carbohydrates in Relation to Risk of Coronary Heart Disease: A Prospective Cohort Study. *J. Am. Coll. Cardiol.* **2015**, *66*, 1538–1548. [CrossRef]
9. Julibert, A.; Bibiloni, M.d.M.; Tur, J.A. Dietary fat intake and metabolic syndrome in adults: A systematic review. *Nutr. Metab. Cardiovasc. Dis.* **2019**, *29*, 887–905. [CrossRef]
10. Lamarche, B.; Couture, P. It is time to revisit current dietary recommendations for saturated fat. *Appl. Physiol. Nutr. Metab.* **2014**, *39*, 1409–1411. [CrossRef]
11. Krauss, R.M.; Kris-Etherton, P.M. Public health guidelines should recommend reducing saturated fat consumption as much as possible: NO. *Am. J. Clin. Nutr.* **2020**, *112*, 19–24. [CrossRef]
12. German, J.B.; Dillard, C.J. Saturated fats: What dietary intake? *Am. J. Clin. Nutr.* **2004**, *80*, 550–559. [CrossRef]
13. Lopez-Miranda, J.; Ordovas, J.M.; Mata, P.; Lichtenstein, A.H.; Clevidence, B.; Judd, J.T.; Schaefer, E.J. Effect of apolipoprotein E phenotype on diet-induced lowering of plasma low density lipoprotein cholesterol. *J. Lipid Res.* **1994**, *35*, 1965–1975. [PubMed]
14. Krebs-Smith, S.M.; Pannucci, T.E.; Subar, A.F.; Kirkpatrick, S.I.; Lerman, J.L.; Tooze, J.A.; Wilson, M.M.; Reedy, J. Update of the Healthy Eating Index: HEI-2015. *J. Acad. Nutr. Diet* **2018**, *118*, 1591–1602. [CrossRef] [PubMed]
15. Saraf-Bank, S.; Haghighatdoost, F.; Esmaillzadeh, A.; Larijani, B.; Azadbakht, L. Adherence to Healthy Eating Index-2010 is inversely associated with metabolic syndrome and its features among Iranian adult women. *Eur. J. Clin. Nutr.* **2017**, *71*, 425–430. [CrossRef] [PubMed]
16. Khodarahmi, M.; Asghari-Jafarabadi, M.; Abbasalizad, M.F. A structural equation modeling approach for the association of a healthy eating index with metabolic syndrome and cardio-metabolic risk factors among obese individuals. *PLoS ONE* **2019**, *14*, e0219193. [CrossRef] [PubMed]
17. Tindall, A.M.; Petersen, K.S.; Skulas-Ray, A.C.; Richter, C.K.; Proctor, D.N.; Kris-Etherton, P.M. Replacing Saturated Fat With Walnuts or Vegetable Oils Improves Central Blood Pressure and Serum Lipids in Adults at Risk for Cardiovascular Disease: A Randomized Controlled-Feeding Trial. *J. Am. Heart Assoc.* **2019**, *8*, e011512. [CrossRef] [PubMed]
18. Schwingshackl, L.; Hoffmann, G.; Schwedhelm, C.; Kalle-Uhlmann, T.; Missbach, B.; Knüppel, S.; Boeing, H. Consumption of Dairy Products in Relation to Changes in Anthropometric Variables in Adult Populations: A Systematic Review and Meta-Analysis of Cohort Studies. *PLoS ONE* **2016**, *11*, e0157461. [CrossRef] [PubMed]
19. Huang, L.; Trieu, K.; Yoshimura, S.; Neal, B.; Woodward, M.; Campbell, N.R.C.; Li, Q.; Lackland, D.T.; Leung, A.A.; Anderson, C.A.M.; et al. Effect of dose and duration of reduction in dietary sodium on blood pressure levels: Systematic review and meta-analysis of randomised trials. *BMJ* **2020**, *368*, m315. [CrossRef]
20. Zhang, Y.; Zhang, D.Z. Associations of vegetable and fruit consumption with metabolic syndrome. A meta-analysis of observational studies. *Public Health Nutr.* **2018**, *21*, 1693–1703. [CrossRef]

21. Kodama, S.; Horikawa, C.; Fujihara, K.; Ishii, D.; Hatta, M.; Takeda, Y.; Kitazawa, M.; Matsubayashi, Y.; Shimano, H.; Kato, K.; et al. Relationship between intake of fruit separately from vegetables and triglycerides—A meta-analysis. *Clin. Nutr. ESPEN* **2018**, *27*, 53–58. [CrossRef]
22. Malik, V.S.; Popkin, B.M.; Bray, G.A.; Després, J.P.; Willett, W.C.; Hu, F.B. Sugar-sweetened beverages and risk of metabolic syndrome and type 2 diabetes: A meta-analysis. *Diabetes Care* **2010**, *33*, 2477–2483. [CrossRef]
23. McCullough, M.L.; Feskanich, D.; Stampfer, M.J.; Giovannucci, E.L.; Rimm, E.B.; Hu, F.B.; Spiegelman, D.; Hunter, D.J.; Colditz, G.A.; Willett, W.C. Diet quality and major chronic disease risk in men and women: Moving toward improved dietary guidance. *Am. J. Clin. Nutr.* **2002**, *76*, 1261–1271. [CrossRef]
24. Chiuve, S.E.; Fung, T.T.; Rimm, E.B.; Hu, F.B.; McCullough, M.L.; Wang, M.; Stampfer, M.J.; Willett, W.C. Alternative dietary indices both strongly predict risk of chronic disease. *J Nutr.* **2012**, *142*, 1009–1018. [CrossRef]
25. Mattei, J.; Sotres-Alvarez, D.; Daviglus, M.L.; Gallo, L.C.; Gellman, M.; Hu, F.B.; Tucker, K.L.; Willett, W.C.; Siega-Riz, A.M.; Van Horn, L.; et al. Diet Quality and Its Association with Cardiometabolic Risk Factors Vary by Hispanic and Latino Ethnic Background in the Hispanic Community Health Study/Study of Latinos. *J. Nutr.* **2016**, *146*, 2035–2044. [CrossRef] [PubMed]
26. Lafrenière, J.; Carbonneau, É.; Laramée, C.; Corneau, L.; Robitaille, J.; Labonté, M.; Lamarche, B.; Lemieux, S. Is the Canadian Healthy Eating Index 2007 an Appropriate Diet Indicator of Metabolic Health? Insights from Dietary Pattern Analysis in the PREDISE Study. *Nutrients* **2019**, *11*, 1597. [CrossRef] [PubMed]
27. AlEssa, H.B.; Malik, V.S.; Yuan, C.; Willett, W.C.; Huang, T.; Hu, F.B.; Tobias, D.K. Dietary patterns and cardiometabolic and endocrine plasma biomarkers in US women. *Am. J. Clin. Nutr.* **2016**, *105*, 432–441. [CrossRef] [PubMed]
28. Chaltiel, D.; Adjibade, M.; Deschamps, V.; Touvier, M.; Hercberg, S.; Julia, C.; Kesse-Guyot, E. Programme National Nutrition Santé—Guidelines score 2 (PNNS-GS2): Development and validation of a diet quality score reflecting the 2017 French dietary guidelines. *Br. J. Nutr.* **2019**, *122*, 331–342. [CrossRef] [PubMed]
29. Chaltiel, D.; Julia, C.; Adjibade, M.; Touvier, M.; Hercberg, S.; Kesse-Guyot, E. Adherence to the 2017 French dietary guidelines and adult weight gain: A cohort study. *PLoS Med.* **2019**, *16*, e1003007. [CrossRef] [PubMed]
30. Sacks, F.M.; Svetkey, L.P.; Vollmer, W.M.; Appel, L.J.; Bray, G.A.; Harsha, D.; Obarzanek, E.; Conlin, P.R.; Miller, E.R.; Simons-Morton, D.G., 3rd; et al. Effects on blood pressure of reduced dietary sodium and the Dietary Approaches to Stop Hypertension (DASH) diet. DASH-Sodium Collaborative Research Group. *N. Engl. J. Med.* **2001**, *344*, 3–10. [CrossRef]
31. Hu, E.A.; Steffen, L.M.; Coresh, J.; Appel, L.J.; Rebholz, C.M. Adherence to the Healthy Eating Index-2015 and Other Dietary Patterns May Reduce Risk of Cardiovascular Disease, Cardiovascular Mortality, and All-Cause Mortality. *J. Nutr.* **2020**, *150*, 312–321. [CrossRef]
32. Saneei, P.; Salehi-Abargouei, A.; Esmaillzadeh, A.; Azadbakht, L. Influence of Dietary Approaches to Stop Hypertension (DASH) diet on blood pressure: A systematic review and meta-analysis on randomized controlled trials. *Nutr. Metab. Cardiovasc. Dis.* **2014**, *24*, 1253–1261. [CrossRef]
33. Appel, L.J.; Champagne, C.M.; Harsha, D.W.; Cooper, L.S.; Obarzanek, E.; Elmer, P.J.; Stevens, V.J.; Vollmer, W.M.; Lin, P.H.; Svetkey, L.P.; et al. Effects of comprehensive lifestyle modification on blood pressure control: Main results of the PREMIER clinical trial. *JAMA* **2003**, *289*, 2083–2093. [CrossRef] [PubMed]
34. National Heart Lung and Blood Institute. *DASH Eating Plan*; National Heart Lung and Blood Institute: Bethesda, MD, USA, 2020.
35. Fung, T.T.; Chiuve, S.E.; McCullough, M.L.; Rexrode, K.M.; Logroscino, G.; Hu, F.B. Adherence to a DASH-Style Diet and Risk of Coronary Heart Disease and Stroke in Women. *Arch. Intern. Med.* **2008**, *168*, 713–720. [CrossRef] [PubMed]
36. Appel, L.J.; Moore, T.J.; Obarzanek, E.; Vollmer, W.M.; Svetkey, L.P.; Sacks, F.M.; Bray, G.A.; Vogt, T.M.; Cutler, J.A.; Windhauser, M.M.; et al. A Clinical Trial of the Effects of Dietary Patterns on Blood Pressure. *N. Engl. J. Med.* **1997**, *336*, 1117–1124. [CrossRef] [PubMed]
37. Sacks, F.M.; Obarzanek, E.; Windhauser, M.M.; Svetkey, L.P.; Vollmer, W.M.; McCullough, M.; Karanja, N.; Lin, P.-H.; Steele, P.; Proschan, M.A.; et al. Rationale and design of the Dietary Approaches to Stop Hypertension trial (DASH): A multicenter controlled-feeding study of dietary patterns to lower blood pressure. *Ann. Epidemiol.* **1995**, *5*, 108–118. [CrossRef]

38. Dixon, L.B.; Subar, A.F.; Peters, U.; Weissfeld, J.L.; Bresalier, R.S.; Risch, A.; Schatzkin, A.; Hayes, R.B. Adherence to the USDA Food Guide, DASH Eating Plan, and Mediterranean dietary pattern reduces risk of colorectal adenoma. *J. Nutr.* **2007**, *137*, 2443–2450. [CrossRef]
39. Günther, A.L.; Liese, A.D.; Bell, R.A.; Dabelea, D.; Lawrence, J.M.; Rodriguez, B.L.; Standiford, D.A.; Mayer-Davis, E.J. Association between the dietary approaches to hypertension diet and hypertension in youth with diabetes mellitus. *Hypertension* **2009**, *53*, 6–12. [CrossRef]
40. Mellen, P.B.; Gao, S.K.; Vitolins, M.Z.; Goff, D.C., Jr. Deteriorating dietary habits among adults with hypertension: DASH dietary accordance, NHANES 1988-1994 and 1999-2004. *Arch. Intern. Med.* **2008**, *168*, 308–314. [CrossRef] [PubMed]
41. Kang, S.H.; Cho, K.H.; Do, J.Y. Association Between the Modified Dietary Approaches to Stop Hypertension and Metabolic Syndrome in Postmenopausal Women Without Diabetes. *Metab. Syndr. Relat. Disord.* **2018**, *16*, 282–289. [CrossRef]
42. Saneei, P.; Fallahi, E.; Barak, F.; Ghasemifard, N.; Keshteli, A.H.; Yazdannik, A.R.; Esmaillzadeh, A. Adherence to the DASH diet and prevalence of the metabolic syndrome among Iranian women. *Eur. J. Nutr.* **2015**, *54*, 421–428. [CrossRef]
43. Joyce, B.T.; Wu, D.; Hou, L.; Dai, Q.; Castaneda, S.F.; Gallo, L.C.; Talavera, G.A.; Sotres-Alvarez, D.; Van Horn, L.; Beasley, J.M.; et al. DASH diet and prevalent metabolic syndrome in the Hispanic Community Health Study/Study of Latinos. *Prev. Med. Rep.* **2019**, *15*, 100950. [CrossRef]
44. Siervo, M.; Lara, J.; Chowdhury, S.; Ashor, A.; Oggioni, C.; Mathers, J.C. Effects of the Dietary Approach to Stop Hypertension (DASH) diet on cardiovascular risk factors: A systematic review and meta-analysis. *Br. J. Nutr.* **2015**, *113*, 1–15. [CrossRef] [PubMed]
45. Hikmat, F.; Appel, L.J. Effects of the DASH diet on blood pressure in patients with and without metabolic syndrome: Results from the DASH trial. *J. Hum. Hypertens.* **2014**, *28*, 170–175. [CrossRef] [PubMed]
46. Toshima, H.; Keys, A.; Koga, Y.; Blackburn, H. *Lessons for Science from the Seven Countries Study: A 35-Year Collaborative Experience in Cardiovascular Disease Epidemiology*; Springer: Tokyo, Japan, 2012.
47. Keys, A.; Menotti, A.; Karvonen, M.J.; Aravanis, C.; Blackburn, H.; Buzina, R.; Djordjevic, B.S.; Dontas, A.S.; Fidanza, F.; Keys, M.H.; et al. The Diet and 15-Year Death Rate in the Seven Countries Study. *Am. J. Epidemiol.* **2017**, *185*, 1130–1142. [CrossRef] [PubMed]
48. Willett, W.C.; Sacks, F.; Trichopoulou, A.; Drescher, G.; Ferro-Luzzi, A.; Helsing, E.; Trichopoulos, D. Mediterranean diet pyramid: A cultural model for healthy eating. *Am. J. Clin. Nutr.* **1995**, *61* (Suppl. 6), 1402s–1406s. [CrossRef] [PubMed]
49. Singh, B.; Parsaik, A.; Mielke, M.M.; Erwin, P.; Knopman, D.; Petersen, R.C.; Roberts, R. Association of Mediterranean Diet with Mild Cognitive Impairment and Alzheimer's Disease: A Systematic Review and Meta-Analysis. *J. Alzheimers Dis.* **2014**, *39*, 271–282. [CrossRef] [PubMed]
50. Schwingshackl, L.; Schwedhelm, C.; Galbete, C.; Hoffmann, G. Adherence to Mediterranean Diet and Risk of Cancer: An Updated Systematic Review and Meta-Analysis. *Nutrients* **2017**, *9*, 63. [CrossRef]
51. Schwingshackl, L.; Missbach, B.; König, J.; Hoffmann, G. Adherence to a Mediterranean diet and risk of diabetes: A systematic review and meta-analysis. *Public Health Nutr.* **2015**, *18*, 1292–1299. [CrossRef]
52. Rosato, V.; Temple, N.J.; La Vecchia, C.; Castellan, G.; Tavani, A.; Guercio, V. Mediterranean diet and cardiovascular disease: A systematic review and meta-analysis of observational studies. *Eur. J. Nutr.* **2019**, *58*, 173–191. [CrossRef]
53. D'Alessandro, A.; De Pergola, G. The Mediterranean Diet: Its definition and evaluation of a priori dietary indexes in primary cardiovascular prevention. *Int. J. Food Sci. Nutr.* **2018**, *69*, 647–659. [CrossRef]
54. Galbete, C.; Schwingshackl, L.; Schwedhelm, C.; Boeing, H.; Schulze, M.B. Evaluating Mediterranean diet and risk of chronic disease in cohort studies: An umbrella review of meta-analyses. *Eur. J. Epidemiol.* **2018**, *33*, 909–931. [CrossRef]
55. Babio, N.; Toledo, E.; Estruch, R.; Ros, E.; Martínez-González, M.A.; Castañer, O.; Bulló, M.; Corella, D.; Arós, F.; Gómez-Gracia, E.; et al. Mediterranean diets and metabolic syndrome status in the PREDIMED randomized trial. *CMAJ* **2014**, *186*, E649–E657. [CrossRef]
56. Mayneris-Perxachs, J.; Sala-Vila, A.; Chisaguano, M.; Castellote, A.I.; Estruch, R.; Covas, M.I.; Fitó, M.; Salas-Salvadó, J.; Martínez-González, M.A.; Lamuela-Raventós, R.; et al. Effects of 1-year intervention with a Mediterranean diet on plasma fatty acid composition and metabolic syndrome in a population at high cardiovascular risk. *PLoS ONE* **2014**, *9*, e85202. [CrossRef]

57. Kastorini, C.-M.; Milionis, H.J.; Esposito, K.; Giugliano, D.; Goudevenos, J.A.; Panagiotakos, D.B. The Effect of Mediterranean Diet on Metabolic Syndrome and its Components: A Meta-Analysis of 50 Studies and 534,906 Individuals. *J. Am. Coll. Cardiol.* **2011**, *57*, 1299–1313. [CrossRef]
58. Esposito, K.; Kastorini, C.M.; Panagiotakos, D.B.; Giugliano, D. Mediterranean diet and weight loss: Meta-analysis of randomized controlled trials. *Metab. Syndr. Relat. Disord.* **2011**, *9*, 1–12. [CrossRef]
59. Richard, C.; Couture, P.; Desroches, S.; Charest, A.; Lamarche, B. Effect of the Mediterranean diet with and without weight loss on cardiovascular risk factors in men with the metabolic syndrome. *Nutr. Metab. Cardiovasc. Dis.* **2011**, *21*, 628–635. [CrossRef]
60. Mancini, J.G.; Filion, K.B.; Atallah, R.; Eisenberg, M.J. Systematic Review of the Mediterranean Diet for Long-Term Weight Loss. *Am. J. Med.* **2016**, *129*, 407–415.e4. [CrossRef]
61. Bendall, C.L.; Mayr, H.L.; Opie, R.S.; Bes-Rastrollo, M.; Itsiopoulos, C.; Thomas, C.J. Central obesity and the Mediterranean diet: A systematic review of intervention trials. *Crit. Rev. Food Sci. Nutr.* **2018**, *58*, 3070–3084. [CrossRef]

6

Waist Circumference and Abdominal Volume Index Can Predict Metabolic Syndrome in Adolescents, but only When the Criteria of the International Diabetes Federation are Employed for the Diagnosis

Javier S. Perona [1], Jacqueline Schmidt-RioValle [2,*], Ángel Fernández-Aparicio [2], María Correa-Rodríguez [2], Robinson Ramírez-Vélez [3] and Emilio González-Jiménez [2]

1 Instituto de la Grasa-CSIC, Campus Universidad Pablo de Olavide, Edificio 46, 41013 Seville, Spain; perona@ig.csic.es

2 Department of Nursing, University of Granada, Av. Ilustración, 60, 18016 Granada, Spain; anfeapa@ugr.es (Á.F.-A.); macoro@ugr.es (M.C.-R.); emigoji@ugr.es (E.G.-J.)

3 Department of Health Sciences, Public University of Navarra, Navarrabiomed- IdiSNA, Pamplona, 31006 Navarra, Spain; robin640@hotmail.com

* Correspondence: jschmidt@ugr.es

Abstract: We previously reported, using the diagnostic criteria of the International Diabetes Federation (IDF), that waist circumference (WC) and abdominal volume index (AVI) were capable of predicting metabolic syndrome (MetS) in adolescents. This study was aimed at confirming this finding when other diagnostic criteria are used. A cross-sectional study was performed on 981 Spanish adolescents (13.2 ± 1.2 years). MetS was diagnosed by eight different criteria. Ten anthropometric indexes were calculated and receiver-operator curves (ROC) were created to determine their discriminatory capacity for MetS. Of all diagnostic criteria, the ones proposed by the IDF showed the highest mean values for weight, WC and systolic blood pressure in boys and girls with MetS, and the lowest for glucose and triglycerides in boys. ROC analysis showed that only WC, AVI and body roundness index (BRI) achieved area under the curve (AUC) values above 0.8 in boys, and that fat content, body mass index (BMI), WC, AVI, BRI and pediatric body adiposity index (BAIp) showed AUC values above 0.8 in girls. Importantly, this occurred only when diagnosis was carried out using the IDF criteria. We confirm that WC and AVI can predict MetS in adolescents but only when the IDF's diagnostic criteria are employed.

Keywords: anthropometric indexes; diagnosis criteria; metabolic syndrome; adolescents; obesity

---

1. Introduction

Metabolic syndrome (MetS) is defined as the clustering of risk factors for cardiovascular disease (CVD) and type 2 diabetes mellitus, such as hypertension, central obesity, atherogenic dyslipidemia, and insulin resistance [1]. It is now recognized that MetS is not only a problem of adulthood. Children that suffer changes in their metabolic profile present a higher risk of developing this condition in early stages of their lives, like adolescence [2,3], with the resulting risk of developing type 2 diabetes mellitus and cardiovascular disease [4].

For this reason, it is necessary to identify early changes in the metabolic profile for the diagnosis of this condition in children and adolescents [5]. In addition, scientific evidence shows that the use of anthropometric indexes is a simple and innocuous method that can discriminate regional fat to predict disorders as MetS in adolescents. In a previous study with 981 Spanish adolescents, we concluded that waist circumference (WC) and abdominal volume index (AVI) are the anthropometric indexes that best predict MetS in this population Perona et al. [6]. In that study, however, only the criteria of the International Diabetes Federation (IDF) for the diagnosis of MetS [7] were considered.

There is currently no consensus over the most effective criterion for the diagnosis of MetS in the adolescent population [8,9], in all likelihood because of the different sets of components used in the different diagnostic criteria [10]. In recent years, adaptations of the criteria established for the diagnosis of MetS in adults, such as the National Cholesterol Education Program—Adult Treatment Panel III (NCEP–ATP III) [11], modified by Cook et al. [12], Weiss et al. [13], Duncan et al. [14], and de Ferranti et al. [15], have been used. Unlike others, the criteria established by the IDF [7] consider the presence of abdominal obesity as a pre-requisite for the diagnosis of MetS. In contrast, Cook et al. [12], Cruz and Goran [16], de Ferranti et al. [15], and Rodríguez et al. [17] consider the presence of three or more impaired components for the diagnosis, even if adolescents do not have abdominal obesity. Viner et al. [18], following modified WHO criteria adapted for children (Alberti and Zimmet [19]), considered the presence of at least four impaired components as necessary for the diagnosis of MetS.

This variability in the criteria leads to striking differences in the diagnosis of MetS and might affect the results of our previous study. Therefore, the present study is aimed at verifying whether WC and AVI still maintain their predictive capacity for MetS in adolescents when other criteria, such as those aforementioned, are used together with the ones proposed by the IDF.

2. Materials and Methods

2.1. Study Design and Participants

This cross-sectional study included 981 adolescents (456 boys and 525 girls) with a mean age of 13.2 ± 1.2 years (11–16 years old). All of the participants had been born in Spain and also resided there. They came from families of a similar socio-economic level and attended 18 educational centers in the provinces of Granada and Almeria (southeastern Spain). Ten of these schools were public, and eight were private. The principals were sent a letter inviting their schools to participate in the study. In all cases, the invitation was accepted. In each school, two classes of a total of three per grade were randomly selected for participation. The flow diagram in Figure 1 shows the recruiting process. The Education Boards of Granada and Almeria gave their approval to the research study before it was carried out. The study also received the authorization of the principals of the participating school.

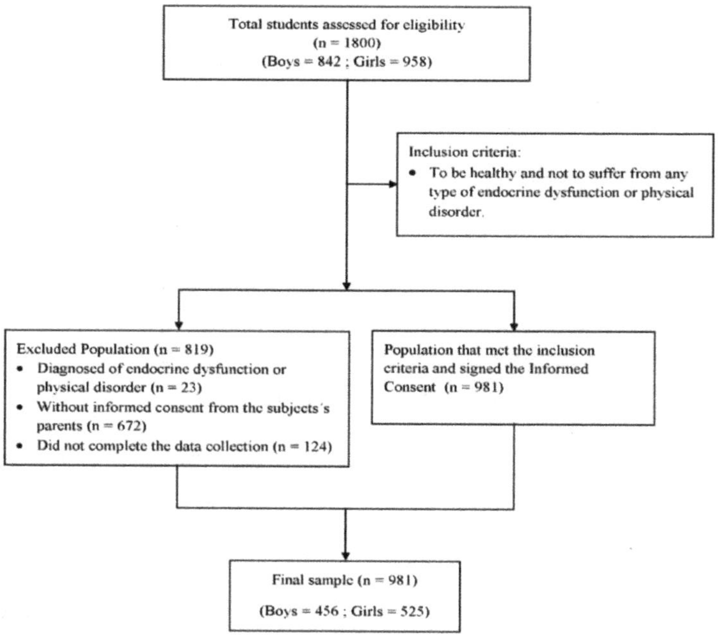

Figure 1. Flow diagram of the recruitment progress.

The Ethics Committee of the University of Granada approved both the study and the model of informed consent used. The parents and legal guardians of the participants gave their written informed consent at the beginning of the study. In addition, the study complied with the International Code of Medical Ethics of the World Medical Association and the Helsinki Declaration. To be included in the study, students had to be healthy and not suffer from any endocrine or physical disorder.

2.2. *Anthropometric Measurements*

All participants underwent an anthropometric evaluation, which was performed by a member of the research team, trained for that purpose. The evaluation was carried out according to the criteria established by the International Society for the Advancement of Kinanthropometry (ISAK) [20]. All body measurements were taken in the morning after a 12-h fasting period and 24-h without any physical exercise. The body weight of each participant was measured twice on a self-calibrating SECA 861 class (III) digital floor scale (Saint Paul, MI, USA) with a precision of up to 100 g. All participants were asked to wear light clothes and to remove their shoes beforehand.

Height measurements were taken with a SECA anthropometer (Model 214). Participants without shoes were measured in an upright position with their back and heels in permanent contact with the vertical height rod of the anthropometer and their head oriented in the Frankfurt plane. The horizontal headpiece was then placed on top of their heads. In all cases, the participants' height and weight were measured twice. The final value was the average of the two measurements.

In addition, the BMI was calculated as the participant's weight divided by the square of his/her height (kg/m^2). The WC and hip circumference were measured with a SECA flexible, inextensible measuring tape with an accuracy of 1mm. The WC was measured on a horizontal plane at a point that was equidistant from the lowest floating rib and the upper border of the iliac crest. In all cases, this measurement was taken after exhalation.

Hip circumference was also measured on the horizontal plane and at the maximum protuberance of the buttocks, which coincides in the front with the ischiopubic symphysis. The waist-to-hip ratio (WHR) was calculated by dividing the waist perimeter by the hip perimeter. Also measured were the triceps, biceps, subscapular, and suprailiac skinfolds. The instrument used for this purpose was a Holtain skinfold caliper (Holtain Ltd., Crymych, UK), with an accuracy of 0.1–0.2 mm. The percentage of body fat was based on these skinfold measurements.

Previously, the Brook equation was used to calculate body density [21]. Once the body density value had been obtained, the body fat percentage was determined with the Siri equation [22]. In each educational center, all anthropometric measurements were taken in a classroom that had been especially prepared for this purpose. The privacy of the students was thus guaranteed.

The rest of the anthropometric indexes, abdominal volume index (AVI), body roundness index (BRI), body adiposity index (BAI), body adiposity index for pediatrics (BAIp), conicity index (C-Index), and body shape index (ABSI), were calculated using the following Equations [23–28]:

$$\text{AVI} = (2\text{Waist Circumference}^2\ (\text{cm}) + 0.7(\text{Waist Circumference} - \text{Hip Circumference})^2\ (\text{cm}))/1000$$

$$\text{BRI} = 364.2 - 365.5\ [1 - \pi^{-2}\ \text{Waist Circumference}^2\ (\text{m})\ \text{Height}^{-2}\ (\text{m})]^{1/2}$$

$$\text{BAI} = [\text{Hip circumference (m)}/\text{Height}^{2/3}\ (\text{m})] - 18$$

$$\text{BAIp} = \text{Hip circumference (cm)}/\text{Height (m)}^{0.8} - 38$$

$$\text{C-Index} = 0.109^{-1}\ \text{Waist Circumference (m)}\ [\text{Weight (kg)}/\text{Height (m)}]^{-1/2}$$

$$\text{ABSI} = \text{WC (m)}/(\text{BMI}^{2/3}(\text{kg/m2})\text{Height}^{1/2}\ (\text{m}))$$

2.3. Serum Biochemical Examination

Blood collection was performed after a 12-h fast. At 8:00 a.m., a nurse member of the research team extracted 10 mL of blood from the median cubital vein of the right arm. For this purpose, a vacutainer system was used with a vacuum blood collection tube. Once the blood had been collected, the glucose concentration was measured with an enzymatic colorimetric method (glucose oxidase-phenol aminophenazone (GOD-PAP); Human Diagnostics, Germany). Also measured were concentrations of HDL-C, total cholesterol, and triglycerides by means of enzymatic colorimetric methods. This was done with an Olympus analyzer.

Four hours after the blood extraction, the samples were centrifuged at 1300 g for 15 minutes (Z400 K, Hermle, Wehingen, Germany). This process separated the red blood cells from the serum, which was then frozen at −80 °C for subsequent analysis. The estimation of low-density-lipoprotein cholesterol (LDL-C) was obtained with the Friedewald equation:

$$\text{LDL-C} = \text{Total Cholesterol} - \text{HDL-C} - (\text{TG}/5)$$

where TG = concentration of triglycerides. Serum insulin was determined by radioimmunoanalysis (Insulin Kit; DPC, Los Angeles, EEUU). Insulin resistance was quantified by Homeostatic Model Assessment (HOMA) [29] with the following equation: fasting glucose (mmol/L) × fasting insulin (mU/L)/22.5.

2.4. Blood Pressure Determination

Blood pressure levels were measured by a calibrated aneroid sphygmomanometer and a Littmann® stethoscope (Saint Paul, MI, USA), according to most widely accepted international recommendations [30]. Systolic blood pressure (SBP) ≥130 and/or diastolic blood pressure (DBP) ≥85 mm Hg were considered to be a risk factor of MetS.

2.5. Diagnostic Criteria of Metabolic Syndrome

Eight different criteria were used to diagnose MetS in the adolescent sample studied: Cook et al. [12], Weiss et al. [13], Duncan et al. [14], de Ferranti et al. [15], Cruz and Goran [16], Rodríguez-Moran et al. [17], and Viner et al. [18], as well as the IDF criteria as published by Zimmet et al. [7]. The details of the criteria employed may be consulted in Table 1.

2.6. Statistical Analysis

The normality of the distribution was assessed using the Kolmogorov-Smirnov test. Results were reported as mean ± SD, except for the number of girls and boys with or without MetS, which was expressed as a number. Student's t-test was used to assess mean differences between boys and girls. The area under receiver operating characteristic (ROC) curves was calculated to evaluate the abilities of the anthropometric indices to predict MetS. Cutoff points were proposed after calculation of the Youden's Index (sensitivity+specificity-1). The areas under the ROC curves were compared using DeLong et al.'s [31] non-parametric approach. Based on the assumption that abdominal obesity is a component of MetS, we conducted a multicollinearity test for the anthropometric indexes that included WC (AVI, BRI and ABSI), and the variance inflation factor (VIF) was calculated. Comparisons of means were assessed by ANOVA, followed by Tukey's test. SPSS v24.0 (IBM, Armonk, NY, USA) was used to perform statistical analyses. Statistical significance was defined as $p < 0.05$.

Table 1. Diagnostic criteria for the MetS in adolescents.

	IDF	Cook	De Ferranti	Weiss	Viner	Duncan	Rodríguez-Moran	Cruz & Goran
Age (years)	10–16	12–19	≥12	4–20	2–18	12–19	10–18	8–13
Number of components	Obesity + 2 components	≥3	≥3	≥3	≥4	≥3	≥3	≥3
Obesity	WC > 90 percentile	WC > 90 percentile	WC > 75 percentile	BMI z-score ≥ 2	BMI ≥ 95 percentile	WC ≥ 90 percentile	WC ≥ 90 percentile	WC ≥ 90 percentile
Glucose (mg/dL)	≥100	≥110	≥110	≥140	≥110	≥110	≥110	<100
TG (mg/dL)	≥150	≥110	≥100	>95 percentile	≥150	≥110	≥90 percentile	≥90 percentile
HDL-cholesterol (mg/dL)	≤40	≤40	<50 girls <45 boys	<5 percentile	≤35	<40	-	<10 percentile
SBP (mmHg)	≥130	>90 percentile	>90 percentile	>95 percentile	>95 percentile	≥90 percentile	≥90 percentile	≥90 percentile
DBP (mmHg)	≥85	-	-	-	-	-	-	-

Notes: IDF, International Diabetes Federation; TG, triglycerides; HDL, high-density lipoprotein; SBP, systolic blood pressure, DBP, diastolic blood pressure, WC, waist circumference; BMI, body mass index.

3. Results

3.1. Baseline Characteristics of the Participants

Table 2 shows the characteristics of the participants, including anthropometric and biochemical measures, including HOMA-IR. On average, variables were within normal limits, and for most of them, no differences were observed between boys and girls. However, girls showed significantly lower body weight, WC and SBP and higher fat content.

Table 2. Baseline characteristics of participants.

Variables	Boys (n = 456)		Girls (n = 525)	
	Mean	SD	Mean	SD
Age (years)	13.2	1.2	13.3	1.2
Weight (kg)	57.1	14.1	53.1	11.0 ***
Fat (%)	27.3	8.3	29.6	7.8 ***
BMI (kg/m^2)	21.5	4.0	21.1	3.6
WC (cm)	73.7	11.8	71.3	9.6 ***
Glucose (mg/dL)	86.2	31.2	85.2	28.7
TG (mg/dL)	129.2	59.3	125.0	46.2
Cholesterol (mg/dL)	81.8	17.3	81.4	15.7
LDL-c (mg/dL)	93.4	23.6	92.9	22.5
HDL-c (mg/dL)	40.1	2.8	40.0	3.1
SBP (mmHg)	119.6	15.7	116.9	15.1 **
DBP (mmHg)	64.5	9.2	63.9	8.8
Insulin (mU/mL)	21.0	10.2	20.2	9.0
HOMA-IR	4.5	2.9	4.3	3.1

Notes: Fat (%), body fat percentage; BMI, body mass index; WC, waist circumference; TG, triglycerides; LDL-c, low-density lipoprotein cholesterol; HDL-c, high-density lipoprotein cholesterol; SBP, systolic blood pressure, DBP, diastolic blood pressure, HOMA-IR, homeostatic model assessment of insulin resistance. Differences between means were assessed by an unpaired Student's t-test. **, $p < 0.05$; ***, $p < 0.001$.

Tables 3 and 4 show the characteristics of boys and girls, respectively, diagnosed of MetS according to the different diagnostic criteria studied. The number of diagnosed participants varied with the criteria from 25 to 68 boys. In these subjects, the criteria proposed by Viner et al. [18] resulted in 25 individuals with MetS, while those proposed by Duncan et al. [14], Rodriguez-Moran et al. [17] and Cruz and Goran [16] resulted in 68 individuals. Since these latter subjects were actually the same, the mean values of all variables studied (weight, fat %, BMI, WC, fasting glucose, triglycerides, cholesterol, LDL-cholesterol, HDL-cholesterol, SBP, DBP, insulin and HOMA-IR) were also the same. The criteria proposed by the IDF consistently showed the highest mean values for weight, WC, HDL-cholesterol, SBP, DBP and insulin and the lowest for glucose, triglycerides, cholesterol and LDL-cholesterol. In contrast, using the criteria proposed by Viner et al. [18], resulted in the highest mean levels of glucose, triglycerides, cholesterol, LDL-cholesterol and HOMA-IR. Among the components of the MetS, the highest mean values for WC, HDL-cholesterol and SBP were 86.0 cm, 35.7 mg/dL and 137.2 mmHg, respectively, (IDF) and for glucose and triglycerides, 193.7 mg/dL and 338.9 mg/dL, respectively [18]. The lowest mean values for WC, HDL-cholesterol and SBP were 74.6 cm (Cook et al. [12]), 32.4 mg/dL (Viner et al. [18]) and 121.6 mmHg (Cook et al. [12]), respectively. No significant differences were observed in age, fat content and BMI among adolescent boys with MetS, regardless of the criteria used.

Table 3. Characteristics of boys diagnosed of MetS according to the different diagnostic criteria.

Variables	IDF		Cook		De Ferranti		Weiss		Viner		Duncan		Rodríguez-Moran		Cruz & Goran	
	Mean	SD	Mean	SD	Mean	SD	Mean	SD	Mean	SD	Mean	SD	Mean	SD	Mean	SD
MetS (number)	41		39		63		32		25		68		68		68	
Age (y)	13.6 ^{a}	1.0	12.9 ^{a}	1.2	13.0 ^{a}	1.0	13.2 ^{a}	1.2	13.0 ^{a}	1.2	13.1 ^{a}	1.1	13.1 ^{a}	1.1	13.1 ^{a}	1.1
Weight (kg)	69.3 ^{a}	13.6	54.9 ^{b}	14.3	59.8 ^{b}	15.6	59.3 ^{ab}	17.4	59.1 ^{ab}	17.0	60.3 ^{ab}	15.3	60.3 ^{ab}	15.3	60.3 ^{ab}	15.3
Fat (%)	34.1 ^{a}	6.5	29.3 ^{a}	7.8	32.1 ^{a}	7.7	29.4 ^{a}	8.4	30.3 ^{a}	8.1	31.3 ^{a}	7.8	31.3 ^{a}	7.8	31.3 ^{a}	7.8
BMI (kg/m^2)	25.2 ^{a}	4.3	21.8 ^{a}	4.2	23.6 ^{a}	4.7	22.4 ^{a}	5.5	22.4 ^{a}	5.0	23.4 ^{a}	4.5	23.4 ^{a}	4.5	23.4 ^{a}	4.5
WC (cm)	86.0 ^{a}	9.9	74.6 ^{b}	11.7	80.2 ^{ab}	12.7	76.9 ^{b}	14.0	77.8 ^{ab}	13.5	79.5 ^{ab}	12.4	79.5 ^{ab}	12.4	79.5 ^{ab}	12.4
Glucose (mg/dL)	128.4 ^{a}	53.5	172.9 ^{b}	47.4	139.5 ^{a}	56.9	191.4 ^{b}	27.8	193.7 ^{b}	24.4	136.0 ^{a}	56.2	136.0 ^{a}	56.2	136.0 ^{a}	56.2
TG (mg/dL)	193.0 ^{a}	120.1	257.9 ^{a}	146.4	210.1 ^{ac}	133.9	295.0 ^{bc}	143.9	338.9 ^{b}	132.5	204.0 ^{a}	130.6	204.0 ^{a}	130.6	204.0 ^{a}	130.6
Chol (mg/dL)	129.6 ^{a}	35.6	151.6 ^{ab}	27.1	134.6 ^{a}	35.7	163.0 ^{b}	7.3	163.2 ^{b}	8.1	133.4 ^{a}	35.4	133.4 ^{a}	35.4	133.4 ^{a}	35.4
LDL-c (mg/dL)	101.9 ^{a}	23.8	119.7 ^{b}	24.9	107.2 ^{ab}	26.7	126.3 ^{c}	19.8	126.0 ^{c}	21.3	107.2 ^{ab}	25.3	107.2 ^{ab}	25.3	107.2 ^{ab}	25.3
HDL-c (mg/dL)	35.7 ^{a}	3.4	33.1 ^{bc}	2.2	35.0 ^{a}	3.4	32.3 ^{c}	1.6	32.4 ^{c}	1.8	34.9 ^{ab}	3.2	34.9 ^{ab}	3.2	34.9 ^{ab}	3.2
SBP (mmHg)	137.2 ^{a}	14.7	121.6 ^{b}	17.0	123.5 ^{b}	17.3	122.9 ^{b}	17.9	123.4 ^{b}	18.8	124.0 ^{b}	16.6	124.0 ^{b}	16.6	124.0 ^{b}	16.6
DBP mmHg)	74.1 ^{a}	11.4	64.6 ^{b}	8.6	65.5 ^{b}	9.0	65.1 ^{b} ,	9.0	63.9 ^{b}	9.2	66.3 ^{b}	8.7	66.3 ^{b}	8.7	66.3 ^{b}	8.7
Insulin (mU/mL)	28.7 ^{a}	15.1	20.9 ^{a}	10.4	25.5 ^{a}	13.6	23.7 ^{a}	14.2	24.0 ^{a}	14.3	24.9 ^{a}	13.3	24.9 ^{a}	13.3	24.9 ^{a}	13.3
HOMA-IR	8.8 ^{a}	6.0	9.1 ^{a}	5.7	8.3 ^{a}	5.1	10.7 ^{a}	5.6	11.1 ^{a}	6.2	8.0 ^{a}	5.0	8.0 ^{a}	5.0	8.0 ^{a}	5.0

Notes: Fat (%), body fat percentage; BMI, body mass index; WC, waist circumference; TG, triglycerides; Chol, cholesterol; LDL-c, low-density lipoprotein cholesterol; HDL-c, high-density lipoprotein cholesterol; SBP, systolic blood pressure, DBP, diastolic blood pressure, HOMA-IR, homeostatic model assessment of insulin resistance. Differences between means that share a letter are not statistically significant ($p < 0.05$).

Table 4. Characteristics of girls diagnosed of MetS according to the different diagnostic criteria.

Variables	IDF		Cook		de Ferranti		Weiss		Viner		Duncan		Rodríguez-Moran		Cruz & Goran	
	Mean	SD	Mean	SD	Mean	SD	Mean	SD	Mean	SD	Mean	SD	Mean	SD	Mean	SD
MetS (number)	32		58		97		18		21		134		86		171	
Age (years)	13.3 ^{a}	1.1	12.9 ^{a}	1.1	12.9 ^{a}	1.1	13.1 ^{a}	1.4	13.2 ^{a}	1.3	13.0 ^{a}	1.1	13.1 ^{a}	1.1	13.1 ^{a}	1.1
Weight (kg)	67.1 ^{a}	10.1	51.8 ^{b}	12.8	55.4 ^{bc}	11.9	57.0 ^{ab}	18.0	59.2 ^{ab}	16.6	54.1 ^{b}	10.4	60.3 ^{ac}	15.3	54.8 ^{b}	11.0
Fat (%)	38.1 ^{a}	6.6	30.0 ^{a}	8.4	32.6 ^{a}	8.0	31.9 ^{a}	11.3	33.0 ^{a}	9.9	31.9 ^{a}	7.5	31.3 ^{a}	7.8	32.0 ^{a}	7.6
BMI (kg/m^2)	25.8 ^{a}	3.5	21.1 ^{b}	4.3	22.5 ^{bc}	4.0	22.4 ^{ab}	5.9	23.1 ^{ab}	5.2	22.1 ^{bc}	3.6	23.4 ^{a}	4.5	22.1 ^{bc}	3.7
WC (cm)	83.2 ^{a}	7.5	70.5 ^{b}	10.4	75.2 ^{bc}	10.3	73.7 ^{bc}	14.8	75.5 ^{ab}	13.3	73.6 ^{b}	9.1	79.5 ^{ac}	12.4	73.7 ^{b}	9.5
Glucose (mg/dL)	132.0 ^{abc}	52.2	148.3 ^{b}	51.8	121.1 ^{a}	52.3	194.4 ^{d}	7.1	188.2 ^{d}	22.5	110.0 ^{c}	48.2	136.0 ^{ab}	56.2	104.5	43.9 ^{c}
TG (mg/dL)	196.2 ^{ab}	120.9	191.6 ^{ab}	114.9	164.5 ^{ab}	98.1	329.8 ^{c}	121.9	312.9 ^{c}	128.1	151.9 ^{a}	85.9	204.0 ^{b}	130.6	145.5 ^{a}	77.0
Chol (mg/dL)	132.3 ^{ab}	33.2	139.9 ^{a}	30.9	122.1 ^{b}	35.8	161.4 ^{a}	4.8	160.0 ^{a}	4.9	114.1 ^{c}	34.8	133.4 ^{a}	35.4	109.3 ^{c}	32.5
LDL-c (mg/dL)	106.3 ^{ab}	20.0	109.3 ^{a}	21.2	98.2 ^{b}	23.3	126.1 ^{a}	16.1	122.8 ^{a}	15.9	92.9 ^{c}	22.3	107.2 ^{a}	25.3	90.1 ^{c}	21.2
HDL-c (mg/dL)	35.3 ^{ab}	2.6	33.7 ^{a}	4.5	36.1 ^{b}	4.8	32.8 ^{a}	1.3	33.1 ^{a}	1.3	37.2 ^{c}	4.6	34.9	3.2 ^{a}	38.0	4.3 ^{c}
SBP (mmHg)	132.3 ^{a}	10.2	113.4 ^{b}	17.1	117.7 ^{bc}	17.0	116.4 ^{bc}	20.8	118.8 ^{ab}	19.5	117.2 ^{b}	15.5	124.0 ^{ac}	16.6	117.5 ^{b}	15.3
DBP mmHg)	70.7 ^{a}	8.8	62.1 ^{a}	8.8	62.6 ^{a}	9.5	64.4 ^{a}	10.2	64.4 ^{a}	10.1	63.0 ^{a}	9.0	66.3 ^{a}	8.7	63.7 ^{a}	8.9
Insulin (mU/mL)	11.0 ^{a}	8.0	8.4 ^{b}	6.6	7.1 ^{bc}	5.6	13.8 ^{a}	8.7	13.6 ^{a}	8.5	6.1 ^{b}	5.0	8.0 ^{ab}	5.0	5.8 ^{c}	4.6
HOMA-IR	32.5 ^{a}	15.8	22.0 ^{b}	12.2	23.6 ^{b}	12.3	28.8 ^{ab}	17.9	28.8 ^{ab}	17.1	21.7 ^{b}	10.4	24.9 ^{ab}	13.3	21.8 ^{b}	10.5

Notes: Fat (%), body fat percentage; BMI, body mass index; WC, waist circumference; TG, triglycerides; Chol, cholesterol; LDL-c, low-density lipoprotein cholesterol; HDL-c, high-density lipoprotein cholesterol; SBP, systolic blood pressure, DBP, diastolic blood pressure, HOMA-IR, homeostatic model assessment of insulin resistance. Differences between means that share a letter are not statistically significant ($p < 0.05$).

In girls, the variability in the number of diagnosed individuals was much higher. The criteria proposed by Weiss et al. [13] resulted in the diagnostic of only 18 individuals with MetS, while those proposed by Cruz and Goran [16] resulted in 171 individuals. The criteria proposed by the IDF consistently showed the highest mean values for weight, BMI, WC and SBP, while the lowest were found when the criteria by Cook et al. [12] were employed. Regarding mean biochemical parameters (glucose, triglycerides, cholesterol and LDL-cholesterol), the highest values were observed in individuals diagnosed using the criteria by Weiss et al. [13], while the lowest corresponded to individuals diagnosed using the criteria by Cruz and Goran [16]. Among the components of the MetS, the highest mean values for WC and SBP were 83.2 cm, and 132.3 mmHg, respectively (IDF), for HDL-cholesterol was 38.0 mg/dL (Cruz and Goran [16]) and for glucose and triglycerides, 194.4 mg/dL and 329.8 mg/dL, respectively (Weiss et al. [13]). The lowest mean values for WC and SBP were 70.5 cm and 113.4 mmHg, respectively (Cook et al. [12]), for HDL-cholesterol was 32.8 (Weiss et al. [13]) and for glucose and triglycerides, 104.5 mg/dL and 145.5 mg/dL, respectively (Cruz and Goran [16]). No significant differences were observed in age, fat content and DBP among girls with MetS regardless the criteria used.

3.2. Area under the Curve Values of the Anthropometric Indexes for the Diagnosis of Metabolic Syndrome

Tables 5 and 6 show the area under the curve (AUC) values obtained from ROC analyses of the different anthropometric indexes for predicting MetS in adolescent boys and girls, respectively, according to the different diagnostic criteria employed. In boys, only WC, AVI and BRI achieved AUC values above 0.8, thus showing a high predictive capacity. These values were obtained when the diagnosis of MetS was performed using the IDF criteria. When using any of the other criteria studied, AUC values were always below 0.8. The lowest AUC values observed, i.e., the lowest predictive capacity of all of the anthropometric indexes, were found when the criteria used for the diagnosis were those proposed by Weiss et al. [13] and Cook et al. [12].

In girls, fat content, BMI, WC, AVI, BRI and BAIp showed AUC values for MetS above 0.8 and in all cases when the diagnostic was carried out using the IDF criteria. WHR, ABSI and BAI were unable to predict the MetS in girls with a high level of certainty, as AUC values were below 0.8 for all diagnostic criteria employed. In particular, the highest AUC value for ABSI was obtained when the criteria proposed by de Ferranti et al. [15] were used, although it was only 0.590. The lowest AUC values observed corresponded to anthropometric indexes when using the criteria recommended by Weiss et al. [13].

The collinearity test for all anthropometric indexes that included WC for their calculation was found to be negative for WC and AVI (VIF < 3) and positive for, BRI and ABSI (VIF > 3).

Table 5. Area under the curve (AUC) in receiver-operator curve (ROC) analysis of different anthropometric indexes for predicting MetS components in boys according to diagnostic criteria.

Variables	IDF	Cook	De Ferranti	Weiss	Viner	Duncan	Rodríguez-Moran	Cruz & Goran	Maximum	Author	Minimum	Author
Fat (%)	0.757	0.582	0.696	0.576	0.612	0.666	0.666	0.666	0.757	IDF	0.576	Weiss
BMI	0.783	0.523	0.663	0.523	0.542	0.657	0.657	0.657	0.783	IDF	0.523	Weiss and Cook
WC	0.831	0.526	0.680	0.564	0.601	0.669	0.669	0.669	0.831	IDF	0.526	Cook
WHR	0.789	0.609	0.715	0.635	0.690	0.655	0.655	0.655	0.789	IDF	0.609	Cook
ABSI	0.663	0.559	0.652	0.564	0.617	0.615	0.615	0.615	0.663	IDF	0.559	Cook
BAI	0.686	0.559	0.689	0.496	0.512	0.664	0.664	0.664	0.689	de Ferranti	0.496	Weiss
AVI	0.831	0.524	0.678	0.562	0.599	0.668	0.668	0.668	0.831	IDF	0.524	Cook
BRI	0.800	0.590	0.728	0.572	0.615	0.700	0.700	0.700	0.800	IDF	0.572	Weiss
CI	0.767	0.577	0.706	0.593	0.644	0.675	0.675	0.675	0.767	IDF	0.577	Cook
BAIp	0.752	0.521	0.671	0.499	0.515	0.668	0.668	0.668	0.752	IDF	0.499	Weiss

Notes: ABSI, a body shape index; AVI, abdominal volume index; BAI, body adiposity index; BAIp, pediatric body adiposity index; BMI, body mass index; BRI, body roundness index; C-Index, conicity index; Fat (%), body fat percentage; WC, waist circumference; WHR, waist-to-hip ratio. Maximum and minimum indicate the highest and lowest AUC values observed, together with the corresponding author of the diagnostic criteria.

Table 6. Area under the curve (AUC) in receiver-operator curve (ROC) analysis of different anthropometric indexes for predicting MetS components in girls according to diagnostic criteria.

Variables	IDF	Cook	De Ferranti	Weiss	Viner	Duncan	Rodríguez-Moran	Cruz & Goran	Maximum	Author	Minimum	Author
Fat (%)	0.812	0.638	0.638	0.559	0.605	0.619	0.557	0.634	0.812	IDF	0.557	Rodriguez-Moran
BMI	0.855	0.635	0.635	0.517	0.607	0.627	0.557	0.636	0.855	IDF	0.517	Weiss
WC	0.866	0.645	0.645	0.535	0.614	0.616	0.554	0.626	0.866	IDF	0.535	Weiss
WHR	0.717	0.662	0.662	0.528	0.557	0.536	0.533	0.537	0.717	IDF	0.528	Weiss
ABSI	0.585	0.590	0.590	0.489	0.496	0.541	0.511	0.539	0.590	de Ferranti	0.489	Weiss
BAI	0.797	0.651	0.651	0.513	0.585	0.714	0.590	0.702	0.797	IDF	0.513	Weiss
AVI	0.867	0.643	0.643	0.535	0.616	0.619	0.554	0.629	0.867	IDF	0.535	Weiss
BRI	0.848	0.677	0.677	0.519	0.594	0.663	0.575	0.661	0.848	IDF	0.519	Weiss
CI	0.730	0.642	0.642	0.520	0.552	0.597	0.542	0.593	0.730	IDF	0.520	Weiss
BAIp	0.840	0.624	0.624	0.525	0.608	0.687	0.575	0.688	0.840	IDF	0.525	Weiss

Notes: ABSI, a body shape index; AVI, abdominal volume index; BAI, body adiposity index; BAIp, pediatric body adiposity index; BMI, body mass index; BRI, body roundness index; C-Index, conicity index; Fat (%), body fat percentage; WC, waist circumference; WHR, waist-to-hip ratio. Maximum and minimum indicate the highest and lowest AUC values observed, together with the corresponding author of the diagnostic criteria.

4. Discussion

In this study, eight different criteria for the diagnosis of MetS in adolescents were used, which resulted in a high variability in prevalence both in boys and girls, but no significant differences in age, fat content or in BMI, which is in agreement with Pergher et al. [8]. In boys, the number of diagnosed individuals ranged from 25 cases when the criteria of Viner et al. [18] were used, up to 68 cases when applying the criteria of Duncan et al. [14], Rodriguez-Moran et al. [17] and Cruz and Goran [16]. This variability could be explained by differences in the cut-off points of the components that make up each of the criteria to define MetS in the adolescent population [32]. There is also a high variability in terms of the components that are considered to be altered for each of the criteria used, which makes it difficult to establish comparisons [33]. Among the criteria used, those proposed by the IDF resulted in the highest average values for the variables weight, WC, HDL cholesterol, SBP, DBP and insulin and the lowest values for glucose, triglycerides, cholesterol and LDL cholesterol. These results differ partially from those obtained in other studies. Sarrafzadegan et al. [34], in their study of an Iranian adolescent population, used the criteria proposed by the IDF and found higher blood pressure levels but lower HDL-c levels compared with our study. On the other hand, Ramírez-Vélez et al. [35], in their study of adolescents from Colombia, also applying the criteria of the IDF, found that the most prevalent altered components were low levels of HDL-c and high levels of triglycerides, whereas the less prevalent components were elevated waist circumference and hyperglycemia. In our study, using the criteria proposed by Viner et al. [18], higher mean levels of glucose, triglycerides, cholesterol, LDL-c and HOMA-IR were obtained.

In girls, the variability of individuals diagnosed with MetS was even higher, ranging from 18 diagnosed subjects with the criteria of Weiss et al. [13] to 171 with the criteria of Cruz and Goran [16]. According to Nasreddine et al. [36], in their study of adolescents in Lebanon, the differences in the prevalence of MetS among boys and girls could be explained, in part, by the variations in the body composition of the human species, in particular due to a higher fat content in girls. This was also observed in our study, as girls presented a significantly higher fat content, expressed as percentage (Table 2). In addition, in line with Nasreddine et al. [36], the criteria proposed by the IDF showed higher mean values for the variables weight, BMI, WC and SBP in girls.

Regarding the discriminatory capacity for MetS of the anthropometric indexes studied and according to the different diagnostic criteria used, the ROC analysis showed that in boys, only WC, AVI and BRI reached AUC values higher than 0.8, indicating a high predictive capacity. Interestingly, this occurred only when the diagnosis of MetS was performed using the IDF criteria. Consequently, these results show the importance of these indices in the assessment of fat tissue distribution in the body and its relationship with the development of metabolic and cardiovascular disorders at an early age [37].

For the rest of the criteria studied, AUC values lower than 0.8 were obtained, indicating a lower predictive capacity of all anthropometric indexes. Values were particularly low when the criteria used for diagnosis were those proposed by Weiss et al. [13] and Cook et al. [12].

In girls, fat content, BMI, WC, AVI, BRI and BAIp showed values of AUC for the MetS above 0.8 and in all cases when the diagnosis was made using the criteria of the IDF, but not when other criteria were used. On the other hand, WHR, ABSI and BAI showed a lower predictive capacity against MetS in girls, with AUC values below 0.8 for all of the diagnostic criteria used. Based on these findings, it is worth noting the importance of using the IDF criteria for the diagnosis of MetS in adolescents compared to the other criteria in adolescents, in particular when trying to estimate the presence of MetS from anthropometric indexes. These results are in contrast with those obtained by Xu et al. [38], in Chinese male adolescents, who, using the criteria of Cook et al. [12], found AUC values of 0.79 for WHR, higher than those observed in our study. Similarly, Zaki et al. [39], in Egyptian adolescents and using the IDF criteria, found AUC values considerably higher than 0.80 for WHR, while in our study, values were slightly below 0.8 in both boys and girls. These results could suggest a possible influence of factors such as ethnicity and culture on the usefulness of the different criteria to define MetS in adolescents.

It is noteworthy that, for the ABSI index, the highest value of AUC was obtained only when the criteria proposed by de Ferranti et al. [15] were applied, and was lower than 0.6, indicating a very low predictive capacity. Consequently, and in line with previous studies in adults [40,41] and our previous report in adolescents [6], ABSI should not be used as a predictive index for MetS in adolescents of both genders. As with boys, the lowest values of AUC observed corresponded to the anthropometric indexes after using the criteria recommended by Weiss et al. [13]. At the same time, assuming that WC is used as a component of the MetS, the collinearity test for all the anthropometric indexes that included the WC for calculation showed negative results for WC and AVI (VIF <3) and positive for BRI and ABSI (VIF >3). These results show, once again, that WC and AVI are appropriate anthropometric indicators and of great clinical utility for the diagnosis of MetS in the adolescent population. Cutoff points obtained from ROC analysis for the diagnosis of MetS showed a high variability among the different criteria. Only the cutoff points for WHR and BRI showed a variation coefficient lower than 2% in boys (Supplementary Materials Table S1). In girls, variability was even higher, and Fat (%), BMI, BAI, BAIp and BRI showed variation coefficients above 10% (Supplementary Materials Table S2).

The present study has some strengths and limitations. To the best of our knowledge, this study is the first to use eight different criteria for the diagnosis of MetS in adolescents. In addition, we would like to emphasize the usefulness of the large sample size, which allowed us to obtain solid results that are comparable to those of other studies. Furthermore, the acquisition of a representative sample for the age groups contemplated in each region gave this study even greater epidemiological value. Moreover, the fact that all of the adolescents came from the same geographic area and shared the same culture, life style, and nutritional habits increased the homogeneity of sample. This study had various limitations, such as its transversal design, which does not permit causal inference. In addition, there is also a lack of information regarding the puberty status of the participants. For these reasons, the results should be interpreted with caution.

5. Conclusions

In conclusion, the results confirm that AVI and WC are the anthropometric indexes that best discriminate between MetS and non-MetS individuals when the criteria proposed by the IDF are used for diagnosis in adolescents. Importantly, the other seven diagnostic criteria were not helpful for this purpose, despite the fact that some of them (Duncan et al. [14] and Cruz and Goran [16], in particular) resulted in a large number of diagnosed individuals, especially in girls. These findings should be considered in future studies and in daily clinical practice, and health professionals should apply the criteria proposed by the IDF. The health authorities should promote the implementation of individual anthropometric indicators in the physical examination that takes place during periodic health checks in the adolescent population. At the same time, new studies with ethnically and culturally different populations are necessary in order to explore in greater depth the usefulness of the different criteria for the diagnosis of MetS and the predictive capacity of all the anthropometric indices studied.

Author Contributions: E.G.-J. and J.S.P. conceived and designed the study. M.C.-R. and A.F.-A. collected and analyzed the data. J.S.-R. and R.R.-V. interpreted the data. E.G.-J. and J.S.P. drafted the manuscript. All authors have revised and approved the submitted manuscript.

Acknowledgments: The authors are grateful to schools, parents, and guardians as well as to participant students for their collaboration in the development of this study. This work was supported by funds from Grant CEI2015-MP-BS23 from Campus of International Excellence CEIBioTic Granada and by funds from Ministry of Economy and Competitiveness (AGL2011-23810).

References

1. Eisenmann, J.C.; Laurson, K.R.; Dubose, K.D.; Smith, B.K.; Donnelly, J.E. Construct validity of a continuous metabolic syndrome score in children. *Diabetol. Metab. Syndr.* **2010**, *2*, 8. [CrossRef] [PubMed]
2. Costa, R.F.; Santos, N.S.; Goldraich, N.P.; Barski, T.F.; Andrade, K.S.; Kruel, L.F.M. Metabolic syndrome in obese adolescents: A comparison of three different diagnostic criteria. *J. Pediatr.* **2012**, *88*, 303–309. [CrossRef] [PubMed]
3. Kim, J.; Lee, I.; Lim, S. Overweight or obesity in children aged 0 to 6 and the risk of adultmetabolic-syndrome: A systematic review and meta-analysis. *J. Clin. Nurs.* **2017**, *26*, 3869–3880. [CrossRef] [PubMed]
4. Kaur, J. A comprehensive review on metabolic syndrome. *Cardiol. Res. Pract.* **2014**, *2014*, 1–21. [CrossRef] [PubMed]
5. Vanlancker, T.; Schaubroeck, E.; Vyncke, K.; Cadenas-Sanchez, C.; Breidenassel, C.; González-Gross, M.; Gottrand, F.; Moreno, L.A.; Beghin, L.; Molnár, D.; et al. Comparison of definitions for the metabolic syndrome in adolescents. The HELENA study. *Eur. J. Pediatr.* **2017**, *176*, 241–252. [CrossRef]
6. Perona, J.S.; Schmidt Rio-Valle, J.; Ramírez-Vélez, R.; Correa-Rodríguez, M.; Fernández-Aparicio, Á.; González-Jiménez, E. Waist circumference and abdominal volume index are the strongest anthropometric discriminators of metabolic syndrome in Spanish adolescents. *Eur. J. Clin. Investig.* **2019**, *49*, e13060. [CrossRef]
7. Zimmet, P.; Alberti, K.G.; Kaufman, F.; Tajima, N.; Silink, M.; Arslanian, S.; Wong, G.; Bennett, P.; Shaw, J.; Caprio, S. The metabolic syndrome in children and adolescents—An IDF consensus report. *Pediatr. Diabetes* **2007**, *8*, 299–306. [CrossRef]
8. Pergher, R.N.; Melo, M.E.; Halpern, A. Is a diagnosis of metabolic syndrome applicable to children? *J. Pediatr.* **2010**, *86*, 101–108. [CrossRef]
9. Weiss, R.; Bremer, A.; Lustig, R.H. What is metabolic syndrome, and why are children getting it? *Ann. N. Y. Acad. Sci.* **2013**, *1281*, 123–140. [CrossRef]
10. Goodman, E.; Daniels, S.R.; Meigs, J.B.; Dolan, L.M. Instability in the diagnosis of metabolic syndrome in adolescents. *Circulation* **2007**, *115*, 2316–2322. [CrossRef]
11. National Institutes of Health/National Heart, Lung, and Blood Institute. Third Report of the National Cholesterol Education Program (NCEP). In *Expert Panel on Detection, Evaluation, and Treatment of High Blood Cholesterol in Adults (Adult Treatment Panel III)*; Final Report; National Institutes of Health: Bethesda, MD, USA, 2002.
12. Cook, S.; Weitzman, M.; Auinger, P.; Nguyen, M.; Dietz, W.H. Prevalence of a metabolic syndrome phenotype in adolescents: Findings from the third National Health and Nutrition Examination Survey, 1988-1994. *Arch. Pediatr. Adolesc. Med.* **2003**, *157*, 821–827. [CrossRef] [PubMed]
13. Weiss, R.; Dziura, J.; Burgert, T.S.; Tamborlane, W.V.; Taksali, S.E.; Yeckel, C.W.; Allen, K.; Lopes, M.; Savoye, M.; Morrison, J.; et al. Obesity and the metabolic syndrome in children and adolescents. *N. Engl. J. Med.* **2004**, *350*, 2362–2374. [CrossRef] [PubMed]
14. Duncan, G.E.; Li, S.M.; Zhou, X.H. Prevalence and trends of a metabolic syndrome phenotype among U.S. adolescents, 1999–2000. *Diabetes Care* **2004**, *27*, 2438–2443. [CrossRef] [PubMed]
15. De Ferranti, S.D.; Gauvreau, K.; Ludwig, D.S.; Neufeld, E.J.; Newburger, J.W.; Rifai, N. Prevalence of the metabolic syndrome in American adolescents: Findings from the Third National Health and Nutrition Examination Survey. *Circulation* **2004**, *110*, 2494–2497. [CrossRef] [PubMed]
16. Cruz, M.L.; Goran, M.I. The metabolic syndrome in children and adolescents. *Curr. Diabetes Rep.* **2004**, *4*, 53–62. [CrossRef]
17. Rodríguez, M.; Salazar, B.; Violante, R.; Guerrero, F. Metabolic syndrome among children and adolescents aged 10–18 years. *Diabetes Care* **2004**, *27*, 2516–2517. [CrossRef] [PubMed]
18. Viner, R.M.; Segal, T.Y.; Lichtarowicz-Krynska, E.; Hindmarsh, P. Prevalence of the insulin resistance syndrome in obesity. *Arch. Dis. Child.* **2005**, *90*, 10–14. [CrossRef]
19. Alberti, K.G.; Zimmet, P.Z. Definition, diagnosis and classification of diabetes mellitus and its complications. Part 1: Diagnosis and classification of diabetes mellitus provisional report of a WHO consultation. *Diabetes Med.* **1998**, *15*, 539–553. [CrossRef]
20. Marfell-Jones, M.; Olds, T.; Stewart, A. *International Standards for Anthropometric Assessment*; ISAK: Potchefstroom, South Africa, 2006.

21. Brook, C.G.D. Determination of body composition of children from skinfold measurements. *Arch. Dis. Child.* **1971**, *46*, 182–184. [CrossRef]
22. Siri, W.E. Body composition from fluid spaces and density: Analysis of methods. In *Techniques for Measuring Body Composition*; Brozeck, J., Henschel, A., Eds.; National Academies Sciences National Research Council: Washington, DC, USA, 1961.
23. Guerrero-Romero, F.; Rodríguez-Morán, M. Abdominal volume index. An anthropometry-based index for estimation of obesity is strongly related to impaired glucose tolerance and type 2 diabetes mellitus. *Arch. Med. Res.* **2003**, *34*, 428–432. [CrossRef]
24. Thomas, D.M.; Bredlau, C.; Bosy-Westphal, A.; Mueller, M.; Shen, W.; Gallagher, D.; Maeda, Y.; McDougall, A.; Peterson, C.M.; Ravussin, E.; et al. Relationships between body roundness with body fat and visceral adipose tissue emerging from a new geometrical model. *Obesity* **2013**, *21*, 2264–2271. [CrossRef] [PubMed]
25. Bergman, R.N.; Stefanovski, D.; Buchanan, T.A.; Sumner, A.E.; Reynolds, J.C.; Sebring, N.G.; Xiang, A.H.; Watanabe, R.M. A better index of body adiposity. *Obesity* **2011**, *19*, 1083–1089. [CrossRef] [PubMed]
26. El Aarbaoui, T.; Samouda, H.; Zitouni, D.; di Pompeo, C.; de Beaufort, C.; Trincaretto, F.; Mormentyn, A.; Hubert, H.; Lemdani, M.; Guinhouya, B.C. Does the body adiposity index (BAI) apply to paediatric populations? *Ann. Hum. Biol.* **2013**, *40*, 451–458. [CrossRef] [PubMed]
27. Valdez, R. A simple model-based index of abdominal adiposity. *J. Clin. Epidemiol.* **1991**, *44*, 955–956. [CrossRef]
28. Krakauer, N.Y.; Krakauer, J.C. A new body shape index predicts mortality hazard independently of body mass index. *PLoS ONE* **2012**, *7*, e39504. [CrossRef] [PubMed]
29. Matthews, D.; Hosker, J.; Rudenski, A.; Naylor, B.; Treacher, D.; Turner, R. Homeostasis model assessment: Insulin resistance and B-cell function from fasting plasma glucose and insulin concentrations in man. *Diabetologia* **1985**, *28*, 412–419. [CrossRef] [PubMed]
30. Pickering, T.G.; Hall, J.E.; Appel, L.J.; Falkner, B.E.; Graves, J.; Hill, M.N.; Jones, D.W.; Kurtz, T.; Sheps, S.G.; Roccella, E.J. Subcommittee of Professional and Public Education of the American Heart Association Council on High Blood Pressure Research. Recommendations for blood pressure measurement in humans and experimental animals, part 1: Blood pressure measurement in humans: A statement for professionals from the Subcommittee of Professional and Public Education of the American Heart Association Council on High Blood Pressure Research. *Hypertension* **2005**, *45*, 142–161. [PubMed]
31. DeLong, E.R.; DeLong, D.M.; Clarke-Pearson, D.L. Comparing the areas under two or more correlated receiver operating characteristic curves: A nonparametric approach. *Biometrics* **1988**, *44*, 837–845. [CrossRef]
32. Braga-Tavares, H.; Fonseca, H. Prevalence of metabolic syndrome in a Portuguese obese adolescent population according to three different definitions. *Eur. J. Pediatr.* **2010**, *169*, 935–940. [CrossRef]
33. Saffari, F.; Jalilolghadr, S.; Esmailzadehha, N.; Azinfar, P. Metabolic syndrome in a sample of the 6- to 16-year-old overweight or obese pediatric population: A comparison of two definitions. *Ther. Clin. Risk Manag.* **2012**, *8*, 55–63. [CrossRef]
34. Sarrafzadegan, N.; Gharipour, M.; Sadeghi, M.; Nouri, F.; Asgary, S.; Zarfeshani, S. Differences in the prevalence of metabolic syndrome in boys and girls based on various definitions. *ARYA Atheroscler.* **2013**, *9*, 70–76. [PubMed]
35. Ramírez-Vélez, R.; Anzola, A.; Martinez-Torres, J.; Vivas, A.; Tordecilla-Sanders, A.; Prieto-Benavides, D.; Izquierdo, M.; Correa-Bautista, J.E.; Garcia-Hermoso, A. Metabolic Syndrome and Associated Factors in a Population-Based Sample of Schoolchildren in Colombia: The FUPRECOL Study. *Metab. Syndr. Relat. Disord.* **2016**, *14*, 455–462. [CrossRef] [PubMed]
36. Nasreddine, L.; Naja, F.; Tabet, M.; Habbal, M.; El-Aily, A.; Haikal, C.; Sidani, S.; Adra, N.; Hwalla, N. Obesity is associated with insulin resistance and components of the metabolic syndrome in Lebanese adolescents. *Ann. Hum. Biol.* **2012**, *39*, 122–128. [CrossRef] [PubMed]
37. Shashaj, B.; Bedogni, G.; Graziani, M.P.; Tozzi, A.E.; DiCorpo, M.L.; Morano, D.; Tacconi, L.; Veronelli, P.; Contoli, B.; Manco, M. Origin of cardiovascular risk in overweight preschool children: A cohort study of cardiometabolic risk factors at the onset of obesity. *JAMA Pediatr.* **2014**, *168*, 917–924. [CrossRef] [PubMed]
38. Xu, T.; Liu, J.; Liu, J.; Zhu, G.; Han, S. Relation between metabolic syndrome and body compositions among Chinese adolescents and adults from a large-scale population survey. *BMC Public Health* **2017**, *17*, 337. [CrossRef] [PubMed]

39. Zaki, M.E.; El-Bassyouni, H.T.; El-Gammal, M.; Kamal, S. Indicators of the metabolic syndrome in obese adolescents. *Arch. Med. Sci.* **2015**, *11*, 92–98. [CrossRef] [PubMed]
40. Haghighatdoost, F.; Sarrafzadegan, N.; Mohammadifard, N.; Asgary, S.; Boshtam, M.; Azadbakht, L. Assessing body shape index as a risk predictor for cardiovascular diseases and metabolic syndrome among Iranian adults. *Nutrition* **2014**, *30*, 636–644. [CrossRef]
41. Behboudi-Gandevani, S.; Ramezani Tehrani, F.; Cheraghi, L.; Azizi, F. Could, "a body shape index" and "waist to height ratio" predict insulin resistance and metabolic syndrome in polycystic ovary syndrome? *Eur. J. Obstet. Gynecol. Reprod. Biol.* **2016**, *205*, 110–114. [CrossRef]

7

Assessing and Managing the Metabolic Syndrome in Children and Adolescents

Mark D. DeBoer

Department of Pediatrics, University of Virginia, Charlottesville, VA 22908, USA; deboer@virginia.edu

Abstract: The metabolic syndrome (MetS) is a group of cardiovascular risk factors that are associated with insulin resistance and are driven by underlying factors, including visceral obesity, systemic inflammation, and cellular dysfunction. These risks increasingly begin in childhood and adolescence and are associated with a high likelihood of future chronic disease in adulthood. Efforts should be made at both recognition of this metabolic risk, screening for potential associated Type 2 diabetes, and targeting affected individuals for appropriate treatment with an emphasis on lifestyle modification. Effective interventions have been linked to reductions in MetS—and in adults, reductions in the severity of MetS have been linked to reduced diabetes and cardiovascular disease.

Keywords: metabolic syndrome; obesity; insulin resistance; risk; pediatric; adolescent

---

1. Introduction

The roots of cardiovascular disease—the most common cause of mortality among adults worldwide—begin in childhood [1], underscoring the need to identify and intervene in at-risk children [2]. These issues have become even more important in light of the global obesity epidemic, in which over 100 million children worldwide are obese [3], including in developing areas more commonly associated with food scarcity [4]. One predictor of future risk is the metabolic syndrome (MetS), a cluster of cardiovascular risk factors including central obesity (typically measured by high waist circumference or high BMI), hypertension, high fasting triglycerides, low high density lipoprotein (HDL) cholesterol and high fasting glucose [5]. These individual components of MetS occur together more often than would be expected by chance—as though they are driven by similar underlying processes that lead to insulin resistance, including cellular dysfunction in adipocytes, myocytes, and hepatocytes; oxidative stress; and cellular inflammation [6,7]. In addition to predicting cardiovascular disease (CVD), MetS is also a predictor of future Type 2 diabetes among children [8,9].

This review addresses means of assessing MetS in children and adolescents, the implications of altered metabolic status, and approaches toward intervening among affected children and adolescents.

2. What is MetS?

MetS, at its core, appears to be due to dysregulated cellular metabolism [7], leading to insulin resistance. A central driver appears to be an excess of central obesity, with visceral adipocytes releasing chemo-attractants, contributing to infiltration by macrophages and release of cytokines and an overall increase in systemic inflammation [6]. Further adipocyte dysfunction includes reduced production of the adipokine adiponectin (which appears to be in the causative pathway of insulin resistance) [10] and higher release of free fatty acids [11]. In peripheral tissues, these high levels of free fatty acids and triglycerides alter mitochondrial function and increase the degree of oxidative stress, with an overall effect of reductions in insulin's ability to stimulate glucose transporters to the cell surface [7]. The degree of insulin resistance results in heightened need for insulin production, and glucose levels rise as the resistance exceeds the ability of the pancreatic beta cells to release adequate amounts of insulin, ultimately contributing to risk for Type 2 diabetes [12]. Further downstream effects include hypertension and reduced levels of HDL cholesterol, both of which contribute additional risk to cardiovascular disease [2]. This multifaceted process has made it difficult to adequately target—though, as we will see, weight reduction to decrease the central adiposity and exercise to increase energy utilization have been effective in reducing the metabolic abnormalities.

3. Clinical Measures of MetS

3.1. Evaluation among Adults

The first observations regarding MetS were related to linking distinct abnormalities in the individual components [5], and this approach ultimately led to forming diagnostic criteria that identified individuals with several of these metabolic abnormalities. These criteria were first set for classifying MetS among adults, with the most commonly-used criteria being those of the National Cholesterol Education Program's Adult Treatment Panel III (ATP-III) [13]. Using ATP-III criteria, an individual is categorized as having MetS if they have measured values that are outside the adult normal range for at least three of the individual MetS components (WC, BP, triglycerides, HDL, glucose—with current diabetes qualifying as an abnormal glucose level even in the absence of an elevated value). Other organizations have proposed slightly different criteria; the World Health Organization criteria utilized results from oral glucose tolerance tests [14], while the International Diabetes Federation (IDF) initially required the presence of central obesity for MetS classification (regardless of how many other MetS abnormalities were present) [15]. The IDF criteria (later harmonized to be in line with ATP-III criteria [16]) also allow for use of separate cut-offs for elevated waist circumference by race/ethnicity, based on evidence demonstrating risk in a specific group [15].

Each of these sets of categories above diagnoses MetS on a dichotomous basis (i.e., you either have it or you do not). Among adults, there have been scoring systems that take into account that MetS abnormalities exist on a spectrum. Approaches to this have often consisted of a summation of standardized *z*-scores for each individual component among a defined population of interest. We formulated a score of MetS severity using confirmatory factor analysis that allowed for a weighted contribution of the individual criteria, with these weights varying by sex and racial/ethnicity based on how these components correlated together in each sex and racial/ethnic subgroup [17]. Because this was done using nationally-representative data, these MetS-*z* scores can be used to assess risk in other populations without reformulating the scores based on the distribution of abnormalities for the new population. As compared to dichotomous criteria, use of continuous scores such as this can provide improved power for statistical assessment of MetS-related risk [18]. In addition, whereas dichotomous criteria can only be used to follow for the presence or absence of MetS over time [19], continuous scores are also useful to follow for the risks associated with changes in MetS severity over time [20,21] and how an individual responds to intervention [22].

3.2. Evaluation among Children

Whereas assessment of MetS in adults relied on criteria established by national or international agencies, assessment among children and adolescents has not been as clear [23]. Most assessments have relied on adaptations that were based on adult criteria, with cut-off values for the individual components that were altered to reflect the more moderate values for these risk factors among adolescents (Table 1) [24–26]. The IDF proposed a set of criteria for children that was based on the adult IDF criteria, again requiring abnormal waist circumference for MetS classification [27]. Other criteria have acknowledged the gradual shift over the course of adolescence in normal ranges of the individual components, with cut-offs that change with time [28].

Table 1. Pediatric and adolescent metabolic syndrome (MetS) criteria adapted from the National Cholesterol Education Program Adult Treatment Panel III *.

Central Obesity (WC)	High BP (mmHg)	High Triglycerides (mg/dL)	Low HDL (mg/dL)	High Fasting Glucose
WC ≥ 90th percentile [25]	Systolic or diastolic DBP ≥ 90% for age, sex, height [26]	TG ≥ 110 mg/dL (≥1.24 mmol/L)	HDL ≤ 40 mg/dL (<1.03 mmol/L)	≥100 mg/dL (5.6 mmol/L) or known T2DM

* Individuals need to have at least three abnormalities in MetS components to be classified as having MetS.

As with the assessment of MetS-related risk in adults, continuous scores have frequently been used in pediatrics. There have been multiple approaches to this, again with most consisting of summation of *z*-scores for a particular underlying population [18]. We again used confirmatory factor analysis in a nationally-representative group of US adolescents age 12–19 to produce MetS severity scores that are weighted to how MetS was manifest by sex and racial/ethnic subgroup [29]. These scores appear to reflect the underlying metabolic disarray in correlating closely with markers of the processes underlying MetS, including C-reactive protein (CRP), uric acid, adiponectin, and insulin [29–32].

Continuous scores are also able to overcome a drawback to sets of criteria, namely, their apparent lack of durability, with a high occurrence of adolescents who toggle between having a diagnosis of MetS or not based on having individual components that are just above or below the cut-off [33,34]. The clinical use of these criteria would likely benefit from incorporation into the electronic medical record [35] but at this time remains less certain, and some researchers have lobbied for an approach that simply targets individual component risk factors [36].

4. Epidemiology

The underlying prevalence of MetS in adolescents depends on the set of MetS criteria used, with overall ranges in the US from 1.2%–9.8% using modified ATP-III [31,37] criteria to 4.5%–8.4% using the IDF adolescent criteria [38,39]. Assessments among school-aged children and early adolescents is lower (0.2%–1.2%) [37,40], which is likely because of the strong effects of puberty on insulin resistance. For example, insulin resistance as estimated by measures such as the homeostasis model of insulin resistance—which usually tracks closely with MetS [41]—at age 8 years is half that seen among those at 15 years, consistent with the concept that puberty itself may be involved with the progression of abnormal metabolic processes [42].

In addition to variation by age, the prevalence of MetS also varies significantly by sex, with male adolescents having a greater prevalence than females (Figure 1). Interestingly, there is also variation by race/ethnicity, being more common in whites and Hispanics compared to African Americans (Figure 1). This is surprising, given tight associations of MetS with insulin resistance, diabetes, and CVD mortality—all of which are more common in African Americans [38]. The reason for this appears to be more favorable lipid levels in African Americans, particularly lower triglyceride levels, which appear to have a lower baseline levels but do increase with worsening insulin resistance [43].

Not surprisingly, MetS varies by location, with one meta-analysis estimating a lower prevalence in Europe (2.1%) and the Far East (3.3%) compared to the Americas (4.5%) and the Middle East (6.5%) [44]. Even in the US, prevalence varies by geography, with higher prevalence in the Midwest and South of the US compared to the West and Northeast (Figure 2), with potential implications for allocation of resources by region toward improved lifestyle efforts [45]. While MetS has traditionally been thought of as a problem of developed countries, the increase in pediatric obesity across the globe has made MetS a concern in developing countries as well [46]. The prevalence of MetS in developing areas of the world is likely to worsen with changing diet patterns as calorie-dense foods become increasingly available [46]. Worldwide variation in MetS prevalence is compounded by an apparent increase in susceptibility for obesity and MetS by race/ethnicity [47].

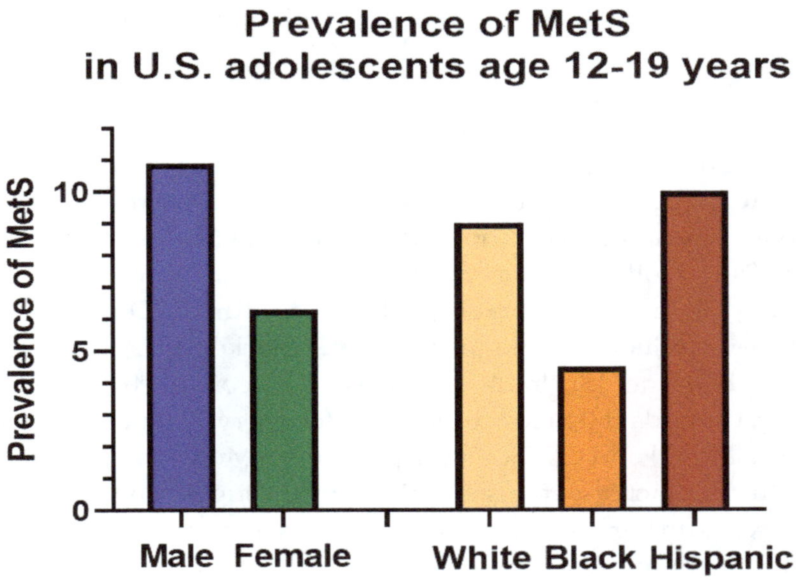

Figure 1. Prevalence of metabolic syndrome in adolescents by sex and race ethnicity. Data are for adolescent participants age 12–19 years from the National Health and Nutrition Examination Survey 1999–2012 as reported in Lee et al. [31].

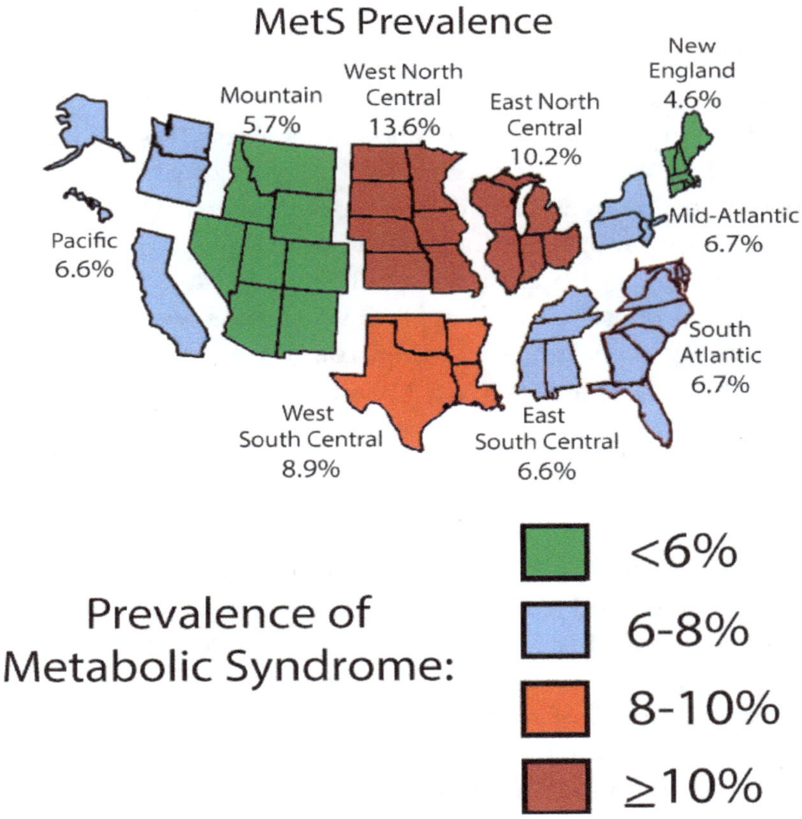

Figure 2. Geographic variation in MetS prevalence among US adolescents. Data are for adolescents age 12–19 years from National Health and Nutrition Examination Survey 1999–2014. (From, DeBoer et al. used with permission.) [45].

The high prevalence of MetS in adolescents coincides with the current obesity levels, and there has not been evidence of a decrease in the prevalence of MetS by classical criteria. However, there has been a recent decrease in the severity of MetS as assessed by a continuous score over time. This is surprising and appears to be due to decreases in triglycerides, potentially from lower consumption of saturated fat [31].

5. Long-Term Risks

The importance of considering MetS in ongoing patient care is driven home by the long-term associations between MetS and future disease. While the downstream sequelae of childhood MetS are usually greater than 10 years in development, studies that followed children for MetS-related characteristics in the 1970s and followed up in the 2000s have demonstrated strong links, with childhood MetS (vs. no MetS) carrying an odds ratio of 2.3–11.5 for future T2DM 14–31 years later [9,48], 2.0 for elevated carotid artery media thickness (a subclinical marker of CVD risk) 14–27 years later [48], and 14.6 for CVD 24–31 years later [8]. In utilizing a MetS Z-score in childhood to assess risk of adult disease 24–31 years later, the odds ratio of increased risk for every 1 standard deviation of the score was 2.7 and 9.8 for future T2DM [49] and CVD [50] (respectively). Moreover, the change in score over time was associated with a further increase in disease risk [49,50], suggesting potential utility in following an adolescent's MetS score during lifestyle modification treatment as a means of following ongoing risks and motivating further improvements.

It is notable that the prevalence of MetS in the 1970s was only 3.9% [9], compared to the prevalence of 9.8% today [31]. This underscores an enormous risk for future T2DM and CVD based on prevalence of risk factors in the current generation of US adolescents. In addition, MetS is also linked to other obesity-related disease processes, including non-alcoholic fatty liver disease (NAFLD) [51] and renal function [52], with implications for chronic kidney disease [53].

6. An Emphasis on Prevention

It should be noted that the best means of reducing the prevalence of MetS in the future is to prevent the occurrence of obesity among children and adolescents. This includes efforts at encouraging an active lifestyle from a young age and preserving of levels of physical activity among younger children (before the usual decline in activity during adolescence [54]). It also includes encouraging families to maintain consumption of fresh foods and avoid energy-dense foods, including as these are increasingly introduced to developed parts of the world [46]. As discussed below, after the development of overweight or obesity, it is difficult to lose excess weight, and stronger efforts should be made at preventing obesity and MetS, including from the standpoint of public policy, including availability of safe spaces for physical activity and healthy nutrition choices in schools [55].

7. Use of Criteria in Clinical Settings

Identify Individuals at Highest Need for Assessment

Given the potential long-term sequelae of MetS, the chief roles of MetS as a concept in pediatric clinical care is in-risk identification and patient motivation. However, while the sets of criteria described above provide a means of categorizing MetS and assessing related factors and long-term risk, there is a sense that these criteria are not commonly used in clinical settings [36]. This may be because of the potentially time-intensive nature of comparing measured values of each component with cut-off values. Clearly, the process would be improved by automatic assessments performed by electronic health record systems [35]—though such tools are not commonly available for assessment of pediatric and adolescent MetS. In all settings, including in developing areas in the world, attention should be given to obtaining accurate height and weight measures and assessing how a child's BMI compares to standardized percentiles for age, such as those of the World Health Organization [56].

Children and adolescents who present with obesity and/or findings associated with MetS should receive extra attention toward reducing long-term risks for future chronic disease. Many of the interventions against MetS (described below) are likely to also have benefits among all overweight children [57]; nevertheless, children classified as having MetS are likely to benefit from additional time and encouragement because of their additional CVD risk factors [36]. In the absence of formal screening for MetS itself (which requires a fasting blood draw and waist circumference measurement), other indicators of insulin resistance and long-term risk for chronic disease may offer alternative means of identifying patients at higher risk. This includes the presence of a strong family history of T2DM [58] or CVD [59] upon questioning or of acanthosis nigricans [60] or hypertension [36] upon physical exam. The presence of these factors in an overweight patient should prompt assessment for potential concurrent Type 2 diabetes, through assessment of symptoms such as polyuria, polydipsia, and unintended weight loss, and through testing HbA1c, with a HbA1c level of 5.7%–6.4% reflective of a pre-diabetes state and a level ≥6.5% consistent with Type 2 diabetes [61].

Discussion regarding how MetS influences a child's or adolescent's risk and how reductions in MetS severity may improve their chances of disease development [22] may assist in motivation toward change [2]. Use of such risk identification as a motivator is a key consideration, as the difficulty in care for adolescents with MetS-related risk for future T2D and CVD is not usually in the identification of at-risk adolescents—using either accepted algorithms or looking at higher-risk groups based on epidemiology—or even in advising interventions but in achieving adherence to these interventions, discussed in the following section.

8. Intervention

Because of the strong connection between MetS and obesity, most interventions for MetS have paralleled those for pediatric obesity in general, namely interventions aimed at altering unhealthy lifestyle factors that likely contributed to the metabolic problems in the first place. This includes diets that are high in saturated fat and carbohydrates (and ultimately an excess of overall calories) [31] and physical activity levels that fall far short of recommendations [54]. In addition, further abnormalities in the components of MetS should be addressed if present. In some cases, this could include, for example, treating hypertension with medication. However, because the predominant "lesion" in MetS is the central obesity, the majority of approaches have focused on lifestyle approaches, as addressed in the following section.

Interventions that have been assessed for efficacy in reducing the proportion of children with MetS have thus focused on altering dietary choices, increasing physical activity, and a combination of both. The goal of these is to thus decrease the ratio of energy ingested vs. energy expended, primarily to reduce the degree of central obesity that drives the metabolic abnormalities. Unfortunately, the unfavorable balance of energy ingested vs. expended has occurred because many children and adolescents have developed suboptimal lifestyle practices due to ease, availability or palatability, and it can be difficult to motivate pediatric patients (and adults as well) to overcome the draw toward these unhealthy lifestyle choices. Effective approaches have included efforts at exploring the motivation of adolescents using techniques such as motivational interviewing, which involves assessments of an individual patient's readiness to change [62]. These approaches are thus tailored to the individual patient and require the time to probe the patient's current food choices and level of physical activity—and a degree of flexibility in working out a treatment plan to which the child/adolescent is willing to commit. This kind of approach is able to increase the adherence rate of adolescents to a treatment plan [62].

8.1. Dietary Changes

The main approach for dietary changes for children and adolescents as recommended by the American Academy of Pediatrics, the American Heart Association, and the World Health Organization has been an increase in vegetable and fruit consumption and a reduced intake of saturated fat in lieu of unsaturated fat (e.g., olive oil and other vegetable oils), as well as a reduction in sugar intake [56]. A meta-analysis of studies that recommended these changes (though usually as part of an approach combined with changes in physical activity, as compared to no change) demonstrated decreases in BMI. One helpful way of achieving these changes has been through implementation of the Mediterranean diet, which incorporates vegetables and olive oil. With respect to MetS itself, a 16-week trial of the

Mediterranean diet among children and adolescents revealed a decrease in MetS prevalence (16% to 5%) among those on the Mediterranean diet compared to no change or worsening in the control group (Velazquez-Lopez). Other studies have supported additional concepts such as that intake of highly-processed food was associated with a 2.5-fold increased risk of MetS [63], and intake of sugar-sweetened beverages (vs. not) is associated with >5-fold risk of MetS [64].While intervention studies assessing effects of eliminating sugar-sweetened beverages on MetS have not been performed, randomized trials have shown some efficacy of sugar-sweetened beverage elimination on improved weight status [55,65], which clearly contributes to risk of MetS. Overall, among patients with MetS, efforts should be made toward reducing consumption of sugar-sweetened beverages, saturated fat, and calorie-dense food (e.g., fast food) and toward increasing consumption of oils and vegetables—likely through negotiating individual changes with adolescents and their families.

8.2. Physical Activity Changes

Increases in physical activity serve to maintain or increase total energy expenditure in the face of reduced caloric intake. The US Center for Disease Control and Prevention and the World Health Organization recommend at least 60 minutes of moderate to vigorous physical activity among school-age children and adolescents [66]—though adolescents do particularly poorly in meeting these goals, with <30% engaging in this much activity [54]. As expected, lower levels of physical activity are associated with a greater risk for MetS, including higher levels of a MetS *z*-score [67,68]. Physical activity is particularly good at increasing insulin sensitivity [69].

A goal of increasing physical activity in clinical practice has been through incorporating these activities into a child's or adolescent's usual routine. One research group assessed the likelihood of MetS among children and adolescents who rode their bicycle to school (vs. not), finding lower odds of MetS associated with bicycle use [70]. Other approaches have involved providing pedometers to patients and negotiating a daily goal for total steps taken—which the child can document and take personal pride in achieving. Increased walks with family, friends or pets can be a way to ensure continued activity. Finally, participation in sports, either through schools, clubs or regular meetings with friends, can further sustain physical activity and maintain higher energy expenditure. There is a tendency toward declining physical activity with age [54], so encouragement at continuing activity starting at younger ages may be more successful.

8.3. Combined Intervention Approaches

The most effective interventions are likely to include a combined approach incorporating reducing calorie intake while increasing energy expenditure. This is because isolated increased physical activity may lead to a compensatory increase in food intake [71], while isolated caloric restriction results in a lowering of basal metabolic rate [72]—while a combination of these approaches aims to prevent these counterproductive reactions. Combined interventions to reduce MetS have focused on nutritional counselling with specific goals for physical activity—usually consisting of at least three weekly exercise sessions [73,74]. This kind of approach can produce dramatic reductions in MetS over time, with one group reporting a decrease from 27% at baseline to 8.3% after one year of combined nutrition and activity interventions [73].

While it is more difficult among children and adolescents to demonstrate the long-term benefits of approaches like this, we evaluated adults in the Diabetes Prevention Program, revealing that the degree of decrease in MetS severity among adults randomized to intensive lifestyle change (compared to those randomized to usual care) was associated with reductions in further odds of developing diabetes or CVD [22]. This underscores the potential utility in following for MetS changes over time during intervention—potentially as a motivator for patients [2] to track changes in future risk.

Thus, in most clinical intervention care, the medical team makes recommendations for improvements in dietary choices and physical activity concurrently [75] with follow-up to encourage ongoing adherence [76]. Success rates in clinical settings have not always been stellar [77], but children and adolescents who make these changes are likely to improve their metabolic status, with likely long-term health benefits.

9. Conclusions

Overall, the high prevalence that we see of MetS currently and the strong associations of MetS with future diabetes and CVD is a great cause of concern that should alarm practitioners who care for children and adolescents. This is particularly true with worsening obesity prevalence worldwide, including in developing areas. Prevention of childhood obesity is critical to reducing future MetS. Screening for obesity and MetS should be incorporated in multiple aspects of pediatric clinical care. Finally, recognizing the presence of MetS and intervening with targeted lifestyle recommendations—with repeated follow-up to encourage adherence—is likely to improve the future health of these children.

Author Contributions: M.D.D. researched and wrote the paper.

References

1. Berenson, G.S.; Srinivasan, S.R.; Bao, W.; Newman, W.P.; Wattigney, W.A. Association between multiple cardiovascular risk factors and atherosclerosis in children and young adults. The Bogalusa Heart Study. *N. Engl. J. Med.* **1998**, *338*, 1650–1656. [CrossRef] [PubMed]
2. DeBoer, M.D. Obesity, systemic inflammation, and increased risk for cardiovascular disease and diabetes among adolescents: A need for screening tools to target interventions. *Nutrition* **2013**, *29*, 379–386. [CrossRef] [PubMed]
3. Afshin, A.; Forouzanfar, M.H.; Reitsma, M.B.; Sur, P.; Estep, K.; Lee, A.; Marczak, L.; Mokdad, A.H.; Moradi-Lakeh, M.; Naghavi, M.; et al. Health Effects of Overweight and Obesity in 195 Countries over 25 Years. *N. Engl. J. Med.* **2017**, *377*, 13–27.
4. Kelishadi, R. Childhood overweight, obesity, and the metabolic syndrome in developing countries. *Epidemiol. Rev.* **2007**, *29*, 62–76. [CrossRef] [PubMed]
5. Reaven, G.M. Banting lecture 1988. Role of insulin resistance in human disease. *Diabetes* **1988**, *37*, 1595–1607. [CrossRef]
6. Tilg, H.; Moschen, A.R. Inflammatory mechanisms in the regulation of insulin resistance. *Mol. Med.* **2008**, *14*, 222–231. [CrossRef] [PubMed]
7. Shulman, G.I. Ectopic fat in insulin resistance, dyslipidemia, and cardiometabolic disease. *N. Engl. J. Med.* **2014**, *371*, 2237–2238. [CrossRef]
8. Morrison, J.A.; Friedman, L.A.; Gray-McGuire, C. Metabolic syndrome in childhood predicts adult cardiovascular disease 25 years later: The Princeton Lipid Research Clinics follow-up study. *Pediatrics* **2007**, *120*, 340–345. [CrossRef]
9. Morrison, J.A.; Friedman, L.A.; Wang, P.; Glueck, C.J. Metabolic syndrome in childhood predicts adult metabolic syndrome and type 2 diabetes mellitus 25 to 30 years later. *J. Pediatr.* **2008**, *152*, 201–206. [CrossRef]
10. Kadowaki, T.; Yamauchi, T.; Kubota, N.; Hara, K.; Ueki, K.; Tobe, K. Adiponectin and adiponectin receptors in insulin resistance, diabetes, and the metabolic syndrome. *J. Clin. Investig.* **2006**, *116*, 1784–1792. [CrossRef]
11. de Ferranti, S.; Mozaffarian, D. The perfect storm: Obesity, adipocyte dysfunction, and metabolic consequences. *Clin. Chem.* **2008**, *54*, 945–955. [CrossRef] [PubMed]
12. Defronzo, R.A. Banting Lecture. From the triumvirate to the ominous octet: A new paradigm for the treatment of type 2 diabetes mellitus. *Diabetes* **2009**, *58*, 773–795. [CrossRef] [PubMed]
13. Grundy, S.M.; Cleeman, J.I.; Daniels, S.R.; Donato, K.A.; Eckel, R.H.; Franklin, B.A.; Gordon, D.J.; Krauss, R.M.; Savage, P.J.; Smith, S.C.J.; et al. Diagnosis and management of the metabolic syndrome—An American Heart Association/National Heart, Lung, and Blood Institute Scientific Statement. *Circulation* **2005**, *112*, 2735–2752. [CrossRef] [PubMed]

14. Alberti, K.G.; Zimmet, P.Z. Definition, diagnosis and classification of diabetes mellitus and its complications. Part 1: Diagnosis and classification of diabetes mellitus provisional report of a WHO consultation. *Diabet. Med.* **1998**, *15*, 539–553. [CrossRef]
15. Alberti, K.G.; Zimmet, P.; Shaw, J. Metabolic syndrome-a new world-wide definition. A Consensus Statement from the International Diabetes Federation. *Diabet. Med.* **2006**, *23*, 469–480. [CrossRef] [PubMed]
16. Alberti, K.G.; Eckel, R.H.; Grundy, S.M.; Zimmet, P.Z.; Cleeman, J.I.; Donato, K.A.; Fruchart, J.C.; James, W.P.T.; Loria, C.M.; Smith, S.C.J. Harmonizing the metabolic syndrome: A joint interim statement of the International Diabetes Federation Task Force on Epidemiology and Prevention; National Heart, Lung, and Blood Institute; American Heart Association; World Heart Federation; International Atherosclerosis Society; and International Association for the Study of Obesity. *Circulation* **2009**, *120*, 1640–1645. [PubMed]
17. Gurka, M.J.; Lilly, C.L.; Norman, O.M.; DeBoer, M.D. An Examination of Sex and Racial/Ethnic Differences in the Metabolic Syndrome among Adults: A Confirmatory Factor Analysis and a Resulting Continuous Severity Score. *Metabolism* **2014**, *63*, 218–225. [CrossRef]
18. Eisenmann, J.C. On the use of a continuous metabolic syndrome score in pediatric research. *Cardiovasc. Diabetol.* **2008**, *7*, 17. [CrossRef]
19. Vishnu, A.; Gurka, M.J.; DeBoer, M.D. The severity of the metabolic syndrome increases over time within individuals, independent of baseline metabolic syndrome status and medication use: The Atherosclerosis Risk in Communities Study. *Atherosclerosis* **2015**, *243*, 278–285. [CrossRef]
20. DeBoer, M.D.; Gurka, M.J.; Golden, S.H.; Musani, S.K.; Sims, M.; Vishnu, A.; Guo, Y.; Cardel, M.; Pearson, T.A. Independent Associations between Metabolic Syndrome Severity & Future Coronary Heart Disease by Sex and Race. *J. Am. Coll. Card.* **2017**, *69*, 1204–1205.
21. Gurka, M.J.; Golden, S.H.; Musani, S.K.; Sims, M.; Vishnu, A.; Guo, Y.; Cardel, M.; Pearson, T.A.; DeBoer, M.D. Independent associations between a metabolic syndrome severity score and future diabetes by sex and race: The Atherosclerosis Risk in Communities Study and Jackson Heart Study. *Diabetologia* **2017**, *60*, 1261–1270. [CrossRef] [PubMed]
22. DeBoer, M.D.; Filipp, S.L.; Gurka, M.J. Use of a Metabolic Syndrome Severity Z Score to Track Risk During Treatment of Prediabetes: An Analysis of the Diabetes Prevention Program. *Diabetes Care* **2018**, *41*, 2421–2430. [CrossRef] [PubMed]
23. Reinehr, T.; de Sousa, G.; Toschke, A.M.; Andler, W. Comparison of metabolic syndrome prevalence using eight different definitions: A critical approach. *Arch. Dis. Child.* **2007**, *92*, 1067–1072. [CrossRef] [PubMed]
24. Ford, E.S.; Li, C.; Cook, S.; Choi, H.K. Serum concentrations of uric acid and the metabolic syndrome among US children and adolescents. *Circulation* **2007**, *115*, 2526–2532. [CrossRef] [PubMed]
25. Fernandez, J.R.; Redden, D.T.; Pietrobelli, A.; Allison, D.B. Waist circumference percentiles in nationally representative samples of African-American, European-American, and Mexican-American children and adolescents. *J. Pediatr.* **2004**, *145*, 439–444. [CrossRef] [PubMed]
26. National High Blood Pressure Education Program Working Group. The fourth report on the diagnosis, evaluation, and treatment of high blood pressure in children and adolescents. *Pediatrics* **2004**, *114*, 555–576. [CrossRef]
27. Zimmet, P.; Alberti, K.G.M.; Kaufman, F.; Tajima, N.; Silink, M.; Arslanian, S.; Wong, G.; Bennett, P.; Shaw, J.; Caprio, S.; et al. The metabolic syndrome in children and adolescents—An IDF consensus report. *Pediatr. Diabetes* **2007**, *8*, 299–306. [CrossRef]
28. Jolliffe, C.J.; Janssen, I. Development of age-specific adolescent metabolic syndrome criteria that are linked to the Adult Treatment Panel III and International Diabetes Federation criteria. *J. Am. Coll. Cardiol.* **2007**, *49*, 891–898. [CrossRef]
29. Gurka, M.J.; Ice, C.L.; Sun, S.S.; DeBoer, M.D. A confirmatory factor analysis of the metabolic syndrome in adolescents: An examination of sex and racial/ethnic differences. *Cardiovasc. Diabetol.* **2012**, *11*, 128. [CrossRef]
30. DeBoer, M.D.; Gurka, M.J.; Morrison, J.A.; Woo, J.G. Inter-relationships between the severity of metabolic syndrome, insulin and adiponectin and their relationship to future type 2 diabetes and cardiovascular disease. *Int. J. Obes.* **2016**, *40*, 1353–1359. [CrossRef]
31. Lee, A.M.; Gurka, M.J.; DeBoer, M.D. Trends in Metabolic Syndrome Severity and Lifestyle Factors Among Adolescents. *Pediatrics* **2016**, *137*, 1–9. [CrossRef] [PubMed]

32. Lee, A.M.; Fermin, C.R.; Filipp, S.L.; Gurka, M.J.; DeBoer, M.D. Examining trends in prediabetes and its relationship with the metabolic syndrome in US adolescents, 1999–2014. *Acta Diabetol.* **2017**, *54*, 373–381. [CrossRef] [PubMed]
33. Gustafson, J.K.; Yanoff, L.B.; Easter, B.D.; Brady, S.M.; Keil, M.F.; Roberts, M.D.; Sebring, N.G.; Han, J.C.; Yanovski, S.Z.; Hubbard, V.S.; et al. The Stability of Metabolic Syndrome in Children and Adolescents. *J. Clin. Endocrinol. Metab.* **2009**, *94*, 4828–4834. [CrossRef] [PubMed]
34. Li, C.; Ford, E.S.; Huang, T.T.-K.; Sun, S.S.; Goodman, E. Patterns of change in cardiometabolic risk factors associated with the metabolic syndrome among children and adolescents: The Fels Longitudinal Study. *J. Pediatr.* **2009**, *155*, S5.e9–S5.e16. [CrossRef] [PubMed]
35. Scheitel, M.R.; Kessler, M.E.; Shellum, J.L.; Peters, S.G.; Milliner, D.S.; Liu, H.; Elayavilli, R.K.; Poterack, K.A.; Miksch, T.A.; Boysen, J.J.; et al. Effect of a Novel Clinical Decision Support Tool on the Efficiency and Accuracy of Treatment Recommendations for Cholesterol Management. *Appl. Clin. Inform.* **2017**, *8*, 124–136. [CrossRef] [PubMed]
36. Magge, S.N.; Goodman, E.; Armstrong, S.C. The Metabolic Syndrome in Children and Adolescents: Shifting the Focus to Cardiometabolic Risk Factor Clustering. *Pediatrics* **2017**, *140*, e20171603. [CrossRef] [PubMed]
37. Messiah, S.E.; Arheart, K.L.; Luke, B.; Lipshultz, S.E.; Miller, T.L. Relationship between body mass index and metabolic syndrome risk factors among US 8-to 14-year-olds, 1999 to 2002. *J. Pediatr.* **2008**, *153*, 215–221. [CrossRef] [PubMed]
38. Walker, S.E.; Gurka, M.J.; Oliver, M.N.; Johns, D.W.; DeBoer, M.D. Racial/ethnic discrepancies in the metabolic syndrome begin in childhood and persist after adjustment for environmental factors. *Nutr. Metab. Cardiovasc. Dis.* **2012**, *22*, 141–148. [CrossRef] [PubMed]
39. Ford, E.S.; Li, C.; Zhao, G.; Pearson, W.S.; Mokdad, A.H. Prevalence of the metabolic syndrome among U.S. adolescents using the definition from the International Diabetes Federation. *Diabetes Care* **2008**, *31*, 587–589. [CrossRef] [PubMed]
40. Morrison, J.A.; Friedman, L.A.; Harlan, W.R.; Harlan, L.C.; Barton, B.A.; Schreiber, G.B.; Klein, D.J. Development of the metabolic syndrome in black and white adolescent girls: A longitudinal assessment. *Pediatrics* **2005**, *116*, 1178–1182. [CrossRef] [PubMed]
41. DeBoer, M.D.; Gurka, M.J. Ability among adolescents for the metabolic syndrome to predict elevations in factors associated with type 2 diabetes and cardiovascular disease: Data from the national health and nutrition examination survey 1999-2006. *Metab. Syndr. Relat. Disord.* **2010**, *8*, 343–353. [CrossRef] [PubMed]
42. Aradillas-García, C.; Rodríguez-Morán, M.; Garay-Sevilla, M.E.; Malacara, J.M.; Rascon-Pacheco, R.A.; Guerrero-Romero, F. Distribution of the homeostasis model assessment of insulin resistance in Mexican children and adolescents. *Eur. J. Endocrinol.* **2012**, *166*, 301–306. [CrossRef] [PubMed]
43. DeBoer, M.D. Underdiagnosis of Metabolic Syndrome in Non-Hispanic Black Adolescents: A Call for Ethnic-Specific Criteria. *Curr. Cardiovasc. Risk Rep.* **2010**, *4*, 302–310. [CrossRef] [PubMed]
44. Friend, A.; Craig, L.; Turner, S. The prevalence of metabolic syndrome in children: A systematic review of the literature. *Metab. Syndr. Relat. Disord.* **2013**, *11*, 71–80. [CrossRef] [PubMed]
45. DeBoer, M.D.; Filipp, S.L.; Gurka, M.J. Geographical variation in the prevalence of obesity and metabolic syndrome among US adolescents. *Pediatr. Obes.* **2019**, *14*, e12483. [CrossRef] [PubMed]
46. Gupta, N.; Goel, K.; Shah, P.; Misra, A. Childhood obesity in developing countries: Epidemiology, determinants, and prevention. *Endocr. Rev.* **2012**, *33*, 48–70. [CrossRef] [PubMed]
47. Cossrow, N.; Falkner, B. Race/ethnic issues in obesity and obesity-related comorbidities. *J. Clin. Endocrinol. Metab.* **2004**, *89*, 2590–2594. [CrossRef]
48. Magnussen, C.G.; Koskinen, J.; Chen, W.; Thomson, R.; Schmidt, M.D.; Srinivasan, S.R.; Kivimaki, M.; Mattsson, N.; Kähönen, M.; Laitinen, T.; et al. Pediatric metabolic syndrome predicts adulthood metabolic syndrome, subclinical atherosclerosis, and type 2 diabetes mellitus but is no better than body mass index alone: The Bogalusa Heart Study and the Cardiovascular Risk in Young Finns Study. *Circulation* **2010**, *122*, 1604–1611. [CrossRef]
49. DeBoer, M.D.; Gurka, M.J.; Woo, J.G.; Morrison, J.A. Severity of the metabolic syndrome as a predictor of type 2 diabetes between childhood and adulthood: The Princeton Lipid Research Cohort Study. *Diabetologia* **2015**, *58*, 2745–2752. [CrossRef]

50. DeBoer, M.D.; Gurka, M.J.; Woo, J.G.; Morrison, J.A. Severity of Metabolic Syndrome as a Predictor of Cardiovascular Disease Between Childhood and Adulthood: The Princeton Lipid Research Cohort Study. *J. Amer. Coll. Card.* **2015**, *66*, 755–757. [CrossRef]
51. Deboer, M.D.; Wiener, R.C.; Barnes, B.H.; Gurka, M.J. Ethnic differences in the link between insulin resistance and elevated ALT. *Pediatrics* **2013**, *132*, e718–e726. [CrossRef] [PubMed]
52. Lee, A.M.; Charlton, J.R.; Carmody, J.B.; Gurka, M.J.; DeBoer, M.D. Metabolic risk factors in nondiabetic adolescents with glomerular hyperfiltration. *Nephrol. Dial. Transpl.* **2016**, *32*, 1517–1524. [CrossRef] [PubMed]
53. DeBoer, M.D.; Filipp, S.L.; Musani, S.K.; Sims, M.; Okusa, M.D.; Gurka, M.J. Metabolic Syndrome Severity and Risk of CKD and Worsened GFR: The Jackson Heart Study. *Kidney Blood Press. Res.* **2018**, *43*, 555–567. [CrossRef] [PubMed]
54. Nader, P.R.; Bradley, R.H.; Houts, R.M.; McRitchie, S.L.; O'Brien, M. Moderate-to-vigorous physical activity from ages 9 to 15 years. *JAMA* **2008**, *300*, 295–305. [CrossRef] [PubMed]
55. Scharf, R.J.; DeBoer, M.D. Sugar-Sweetened Beverages and Children's Health. *Annu. Rev. Public Health* **2016**, *37*, 273–293. [CrossRef] [PubMed]
56. World Health Organization. *Interim Report of the Commission on Ending Childhood Obesity*; World Health Organization: Geneva, Switzerland, 2015.
57. O'Connor, E.A.; Evans, C.V.; Burda, B.U.; Walsh, E.S.; Eder, M.; Lozano, P. Screening for Obesity and Intervention for Weight Management in Children and Adolescents: Evidence Report and Systematic Review for the US Preventive Services Task Force. *JAMA* **2017**, *317*, 2427–2444. [CrossRef] [PubMed]
58. Morrison, J.A.; Glueck, C.J.; Horn, P.S.; Wang, P. Childhood predictors of adult type 2 diabetes at 9 and 26-year follow-ups. *Arch. Pediatr. Adolesc. Med.* **2010**, *164*, 53–60. [CrossRef] [PubMed]
59. Daniels, S.R.; Greer, F.R. Lipid screening and cardiovascular health in childhood. *Pediatrics* **2008**, *122*, 198–208. [CrossRef] [PubMed]
60. Brickman, W.J.; Huang, J.; Silverman, B.L.; Metzger, B.E. Acanthosis nigricans identifies youth at high risk for metabolic abnormalities. *J. Pediatr.* **2010**, *156*, 87–92. [CrossRef]
61. American Diabetes Association. 2. Classification and Diagnosis of Diabetes. *Diabetes Care* **2018**, *41*, S13–S27. [CrossRef]
62. Bean, M.K.; Powell, P.; Quinoy, A.; Ingersoll, K.; Wickham, E.P., III; Mazzeo, S.E. Motivational interviewing targeting diet and physical activity improves adherence to paediatric obesity treatment: Results from the MI Values randomized controlled trial. *Pediatr. Obes.* **2015**, *10*, 118–125. [CrossRef] [PubMed]
63. Tavares, L.F.; Fonseca, S.C.; Garcia Rosa, M.L.; Yokoo, E.M. Relationship between ultra-processed foods and metabolic syndrome in adolescents from a Brazilian Family Doctor Program. *Public Health Nutr.* **2012**, *15*, 82–87. [CrossRef] [PubMed]
64. Chan, T.-F.; Lin, W.-T.; Huang, H.-L.; Lee, C.-Y.; Wu, P.-W.; Chiu, Y.-W.; Huang, C.-C.; Tsai, S.; Lin, C.-L.; Lee, C.-H. Consumption of sugar-sweetened beverages is associated with components of the metabolic syndrome in adolescents. *Nutrients* **2014**, *6*, 2088–2103. [CrossRef] [PubMed]
65. Ebbeling, C.B.; Ludwig, D.S. Sugar-sweetened beverages, genetic risk, and obesity. *N. Engl. J. Med.* **2013**, *368*, 287. [PubMed]
66. CDC. 2008 Physical Activity Guidelines Americans. Available online: https://health.gov/paguidelines/pdf/paguide.pdf (accessed on 1 August 2019).
67. Ekelund, U.; Anderssen, S.A.; Froberg, K.; Sardinha, L.B.; Andersen, L.B.; Brage, S. Independent associations of physical activity and cardiorespiratory fitness with metabolic risk factors in children: The European youth heart study. *Diabetologia* **2007**, *50*, 1832–1840. [CrossRef] [PubMed]
68. Stabelini Neto, A.; de Campos, W.; Dos Santos, G.C.; Junior, O.M. Metabolic syndrome risk score and time expended in moderate to vigorous physical activity in adolescents. *BMC Pediatr.* **2014**, *14*, 42. [CrossRef] [PubMed]
69. Guinhouya, B.C.; Samouda, H.; Zitouni, D.; Vilhelm, C.; Hubert, H. Evidence of the influence of physical activity on the metabolic syndrome and/or on insulin resistance in pediatric populations: A systematic review. *Int. J. Pediatr. Obes.* **2011**, *6*, 361–388. [CrossRef] [PubMed]
70. Ramírez-Vélez, R.; García-Hermoso, A.; Agostinis-Sobrinho, C.A.; Mota, J.; Santos, R.; Correa-Bautista, J.E.; Amaya-Tambo, D.C.; Villa-González, E. Cycling to School and Body Composition, Physical Fitness, and Metabolic Syndrome in Children and Adolescents. *J. Pediatr.* **2017**, *188*, 57–63. [CrossRef] [PubMed]

71. Blundell, J.E.; Stubbs, R.J.; Hughes, D.A.; Whybrow, S.; King, N.A. Cross talk between physical activity and appetite control: Does physical activity stimulate appetite? *Proc. Nutr. Soc.* **2003**, *62*, 651–661. [CrossRef]
72. Martin, C.K.; Heilbronn, L.K.; De Jonge, L.; Delany, J.P.; Volaufova, J.; Anton, S.D.; Redman, L.M.; Smith, S.R.; Ravussin, E.; Jonge, L. Effect of calorie restriction on resting metabolic rate and spontaneous physical activity. *Obesity* **2007**, *15*, 2964–2973. [CrossRef]
73. Caranti, D.A.; De Mello, M.T.; Prado, W.L.; Tock, L.; Siqueira, K.O.; De Piano, A.; Lofrano, M.C.; Cristofalo, D.M.; Lederman, H.; Tufik, S.; et al. Short and long-term beneficial effects of a multidisciplinary therapy for the control of metabolic syndrome in obese adolescents. *Metabolism* **2007**, *56*, 1293–1300. [CrossRef]
74. Leite, N.; Milano, G.; Cieslak, F.; Lopes, W.; Rodacki, A.; Radominski, R. Effects of physical exercise and nutritional guidance on metabolic syndrome in obese adolescents. *Braz. J. Phys. Ther.* **2009**, *12*, 73–81. [CrossRef]
75. WHO. Global Strategy on Diet, Physical Activity and Health. Available online: http://www.who.int/dietphysicalactivity/factsheet_young_people/en/ (accessed on 1 August 2019).
76. Walker, S.E.; Smolkin, M.E.; O'Leary, M.L.; Cluett, S.B.; Norwood, V.F.; DeBoer, M.D.; Gurka, M.J. Predictors of Retention and BMI Loss or Stabilization in Obese Youth Enrolled in a Weight Loss Intervention. *Obes. Res. Clin. Pract.* **2012**, *6*, e330–e339. [CrossRef]
77. Wu, T.; Gao, X.; Chen, M.; Van Dam, R.M. Long-term effectiveness of diet-plus-exercise interventions vs. diet-only interventions for weight loss: A meta-analysis. *Obes. Rev.* **2009**, *10*, 313–323. [CrossRef]

8

The Effects of a Mediterranean Diet Intervention on Targeted Plasma Metabolic Biomarkers among US Firefighters

Mercedes Sotos-Prieto [1,2,3,*], Miguel Ruiz-Canela [4,5], Yiqing Song [6], Costas Christophi [3,7], Steven Mofatt [8], Fernando Rodriguez-Artalejo [1,2,9] and Stefanos N. Kales [3,10]

1. Department of Preventive Medicine and Public Health, School of Medicine, Universidad Autónoma de Madrid, IdiPaz (Instituto de Investigación Sanitaria Hospital Universitario La Paz), Calle del Arzobispo Morcillo 4, 28029 Madrid, Spain; fernando.artalejo@uam.es
2. Biomedical Research Network Centre of Epidemiology and Public Health (CIBERESP), Carlos III Health Institute, 28029 Madrid, Spain
3. Department of Environmental Health, Harvard T.H. Chan School of Public Health, Boston, MA 02115, USA; costas.christophi@cut.ac.cy (C.C.); stefokali@aol.com (S.N.K.)
4. Department of Preventive Medicine and Public Health, IdiSNA, University of Navarra, 31009 Pamplona, Spain; mcanela@unav.es
5. Biomedical Research Network Centre for Pathophysiology of Obesity and Nutrition (CIBEROBN), Carlos III Health Institute, 28029 Madrid, Spain
6. Department of Epidemiology, Richard M. Fairbanks School of Public Health, Indiana University, Indianapolis, IN 46202, USA; yiqsong@iu.edu
7. Cyprus International Institute for Environmental and Public Health, Cyprus University of Technology, 30 Archbishop Kyprianou Str., 3036 Lemesos, Cyprus
8. National Institute for Public Safety Health, Indianapolis, IN 46204, USA; steven.mofatt@ascension.org
9. IMDEA-Food Institute, CEI UAM+CSIC, 28049 Madrid, Spain
10. Department of Occupational Medicine, Cambridge Health Alliance, Harvard Medical School, Cambridge, MA 02145, USA

* Correspondence: mercedes.sotos@uam.es

Abstract: Metabolomics is improving the understanding of the mechanisms of the health effects of diet. Previous research has identified several metabolites associated with the Mediterranean Diet (MedDiet), but knowledge about longitudinal changes in metabolic biomarkers after a MedDiet intervention is scarce. A subsample of 48 firefighters from a cluster-randomized trial at Indianapolis fire stations was randomly selected for the metabolomics study at 12 months of follow up (time point 1), where Group 1 (n = 24) continued for another 6 months in a self-sustained MedDiet intervention, and Group 2 (n = 24), the control group at that time, started with an active MedDiet intervention for 6 months (time point 2). A total of 225 metabolites were assessed at the two time points by using a targeted NMR platform. The MedDiet score improved slightly but changes were non-significant (intervention: 24.2 vs. 26.0 points and control group: 26.1 vs. 26.5 points). The MedDiet intervention led to favorable changes in biomarkers related to lipid metabolism, including lower LDL-C, ApoB/ApoA1 ratio, remnant cholesterol, M-VLDL-CE; and higher HDL-C, and better lipoprotein composition. This MedDiet intervention induces only modest changes in adherence to the MedDiet and consequently in metabolic biomarkers. Further research should confirm these results based on larger study samples in workplace interventions with powerful study designs.

Keywords: Mediterranean Diet; metabolites; clinical trial; lipoprotein composition; biomarkers

1. Introduction

Currently, the understanding of diet-health relationships has gradually shifted from individual dietary components to overall dietary patterns that beneficially modulate metabolic physiology [1]. In this regard, several epidemiological and clinical studies have shown that the traditional Mediterranean-style eating pattern (characterized by high intake of fruits and vegetables, olive oil, legumes, whole grains, and fish and moderate consumption of white meat, dairy and wine during meals) has many health benefits [2,3], including beneficial changes in biomarkers of CVD risk [4,5] and lower risk of cardiovascular disease (CVD) [6–8].

However, the exact mechanisms of the benefits of the Mediterranean-style dietary pattern have yet to be understood. The application of metabolomics to measure changes in biological variables in response to dietary interventions has been proposed as a potential tool to discover biomarkers associated with healthier eating [9–13]. There is observational epidemiological evidence that acylcarnitines, Trimethylamine N-oxide (TMAO), some amino acids such as phenylalanine, glutamate as well as several lipid classes are associated with CVD risk [14]. While the effects of individual dietary ingredients on metabolome have been reported [15–20], only a few studies have focused on overall dietary patterns [21–26]. Some cross-sectional studies such as the Whitehall II study showed that a healthy diet was associated with specific fatty acids that reduced the risk of CVD [27]. In a British population, the association between the adherence to the MedDiet and cardiometabolic outcomes was mediated by baseline levels of acylcarnitines, sphingolipids, and phospholipids [24]. In the Supplementation en Vitamines et Mineraux Antioxydants (SU.VI.MAX) study, some metabolites were also cross-sectionally associated with dietary recommendations [28]. More recently, a metabolic signature of the Mediterranean Diet has been consistently identified in two large cohorts [26].

Importantly, studies analyzing changes in metabolites levels in response to MedDiet interventions are still scarce and inconclusive. In the Metabolic Syndrome Reduction in Navarra (RESMENA)study, after 2 months of an energy restricted MedDiet intervention, some significant changes in metabolites were shown but they were no longer observed after 6 months [22]. Additional evidence comes from the Prevention with Mediterranean Diet (PREDIMED) study, where several a priori-designed analyses found that the MedDiet may reduce the deleterious effect on cardiovascular or type-2 diabetes risk associated with 1 year changes in branched-chain amino acids [29,30], carnitines [31] and other metabolites. However, in most of these analyses, the 1 year metabolite changes were similar between the intervention and the control group, suggesting that the observed protective effect of the MedDiet could be due to other mechanisms.

Therefore, the objective of this study is to identify changes in plasma metabolic biomarkers associated with a MedDiet intervention within a subsample of a cluster-randomized controlled trial (Feeding America's Bravest) among firefighters. We hypothesize that the MedDiet intervention induces changes in metabolites within clinically relevant pathways.

2. Materials and Methods

2.1. Study Design and Participants

The overall study design, intervention strategies and primary outcomes of the Feeding America's Bravest trial have been previously reported [32]. Briefly, Feeding America's Bravest is a step-wedge cluster-randomized controlled trial within the 44 stations of Indianapolis Fire Department, which aims to compare a MedDiet Nutritional Intervention vs. an ad libitum Midwestern-style diet (control or no intervention) during 12 months. Group 1 (or the intervention group for 12 months) continued under a self-sustained continuation phase for another 12 months. Group 2 (initially controls) crossed over (at 12 months) to receive the active Mediterranean Diet Nutritional Intervention for 6 months followed by another 6 months of a self-sustained intervention phase. For this nested study, we randomly selected a sub-group of participants ($n = 48$) whose fire stations had been assigned to the MedDiet intervention ($n = 24$) or the control group ($n = 24$) for the previous 12 months. At that time (time point 1 for our study and 12 months follow up of the parent study), the intervention group (Group 1) continued under a self-sustained phase for another 6 months (time point 2 for our study or 18 months of the parent study) and the control group underwent the active MedDiet intervention for 6 months. Plasma metabolic biomarkers were analyzed at the two time points (Figure 1). The overarching Feeding America's Bravest protocol was approved by the Harvard Institutional Review Board (IRB16-0170) and is registered at Clinical Trials (NCT02941757). All participants provided informed consent for participation.

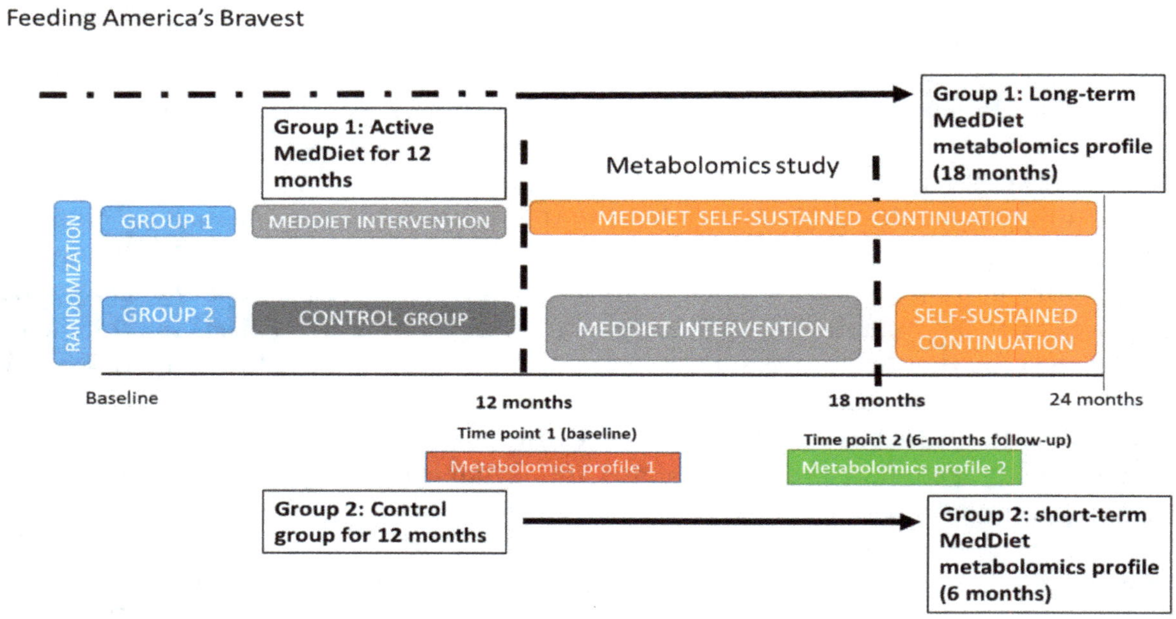

Figure 1. Study design and timeline of the metabolomics study within Feeding America´s Bravest parent study (step-wedge cluster-randomized control trial).

2.2. Mediterranean Diet Intervention

At the two time points of this study, data on sociodemographic characteristics, physical activity, sleep behaviors (a modified Pittsburgh Sleep Quality Index, where on a scale from 0 to 7 participants were asked to identify the statement which option best described their habitual level of physical activity over the past month [33]), food consumption based on a self- reported validated food frequency questionnaire [34] and a modified Mediterranean Diet scale [35], and anthropometric and clinical variables were assessed.

The MedDiet intervention has been described in detail elsewhere [32]. Briefly, it consisted of educational sessions and videos created by a certified nutritionist, leaflet and recommendations about the Mediterranean Dietand lifestyle, firefighter-tailored Mediterranean recipes (by modifying Firefighters´ favorite recipes according to the MedDiet principles by a chef and a nutritionist), in-site chef cooking demonstration, a firefighters' food pyramid, Mediterranean food samples and discount coupons to a large supermarket chain for specific Mediterranean Diet-compatible foods [32].

Adherence to the MedDiet was assessed by the validated modified Mediterranean Diet Score (mMDS) [35,36] and the PREDIMED score. (36) The mMDS range from 0 (lowest) to 51 (highest conformity to the MedDiet) [36] and consists of 13 domains including consumption of fast food, fruits, vegetables, legumes, nuts, sweet desserts, fried foods, ocean fish, breads and starches (consumed at home and the fire station), the type and frequency of alcoholic beverages, non-alcoholic beverages (consumed at home and the fire station) and the type of cooking oil or fat (consumed at home and the fire station). Each component ranged from 0 (less adherence) to 4 points (better adherence) except the type of alcohol (wine; 0–2 points) and the type of cooking oil or fat (0–5 points). Weighted scores was considered for domains evaluated at both the homes and fire stations based on the percentage of meals consumed at each location [36].

The PREDIMED score [37] consists of 14 questions; 12 of them are about food consumption frequency (olive oil consumption, vegetables, fruits, red/processed meats, butter/margarine, soda drinks, wine, legumes, fish/seafood, nuts, commercial sweets, sofrito consumption), and another two about food intake habits considered characteristic of the Spanish Mediterranean Diet (preference of poultry consumption instead of red meats, use of olive oil as main culinary fat). Each question was scored 0 or 1, with a total possible range of 0 to 14; higher scores indicate greater adherence to the MedDiet.

2.3. Collection of Plasma Samples

In this nested study, 12 h fasting blood samples were collected at time point 1 (baseline for this metabolomics study and 12 months for the trial) and time point 2 (6 months follow up for this metabolomics study and 18 months for the trial) of follow up; samples were kept cold and immediately processed to separate the plasma with a refrigerated centrifuge. Next, the 200 μL cryovials were placed at −80 °C.

2.4. Plasma Biomarkers Measurements

Metabolites were quantified in plasma samples from 83 individuals that had optimal values using high-throughput proton Nuclear Magnetic Resonance (NMR) metabolomics (Nightingale Health Ltd., Helsinki, Finland). This method provides simultaneous quantification of routine lipids, lipoprotein subclass profiling with lipid concentrations within 14 subclasses, fatty acid composition, and various low-molecular metabolites including amino acids, ketone bodies and glycolysis-related metabolites. Details of the experimentation and applications of the NMR metabolomics platform have been described previously [38]. All measured metabolites fall in the range of detection; representative coefficients of variations (CVs) for the metabolic biomarkers were published previously [39,40].

2.5. Statistical Analysis

Differences in baseline characteristics between the two groups were examined by *t*-test ANOVA for continuous variables (means ± standard deviation [SD]) or Chi-square for categorical data (percentages). Statistical analyses of the metabolites were performed on log-transformed data that were scaled to SD units to facilitate comparisons across metabolites. The effect of the MedDiet intervention between point 1 and point 2 in this analysis (6 months) was assessed using a linear mixed-effects model adjusted for age and sex. As many of the metabolites are biologically correlated, applying a multiple testing correction using all the 225 biomarkers would be too strict. Thus, account for multiple testing, Bonferroni correction was applied with significance level defined as $0.05/21 = 0.002$, with 21 being the number of principal components that explained 99% of the variation in the NMR data.

Cross-sectional linear associations between the adherence to the mMDS score and metabolite concentrations at both time points for both the MedDiet intervention and control groups were obtained using a linear regression model adjusted for age and sex. The analyses were performed using ggforestplot R package (version 0.0.2) and the linear mixed-effects model was fitted with the nlme R package (version 3.1.-144).

3. Results

3.1. Participant Characteristics

Characteristics of the 48 participants at time point 1, and changes after 6 months follow up (time point 2), are summarized in Table 1. Of the 48 participants at time point 1, 44 (92%) were followed up and provided dietary information and anthropometric measures at time point 2. Information for the plasma metabolites were available for $n = 47$ at baseline and $n = 36$ at the end of follow up (Supplementary Materials Figure S1). There were no statistically significant differences in the adherence to the mMDS or PREDIMED score at time 1 and after the 6 months follow up within and between groups. Similarly, no differences were seen for age or sex (Table 1).

Table 1. Characteristics of the firefighters participating in the Feeding America's Bravest intervention study.

	Time Point 1 (n = 48)			Time Point 2 (n = 44 *)				
	12 Months MedDiet Intervention (n = 24)	**Control Group (n = 24)**	***p*-Value**	**18 Months MedDiet Intervention (n = 22)**	**Control Group After a 6 Months of Active MedDiet Intervention (n = 22)**	***p*-Value**	***p*-Value (Follow Up-Baseline) Intervention Group**	***p*-Value (Follow Up-Baseline) Control Group**
Sex, male (%)	91.7	95.8	0.55	84.6	94.1	0.39	N/A	N/A
Age (years)	47.5 (6.7)	47.6 (8.6)	0.95	45.9 (6.7)	49.9 (8.4)	0.17	N/A	N/A
PREDIMED score (0–14 points)	6.1 (2.1)	6.6 (2.1)	0.31	6.4 (1.9)	6.7 (1.9)	0.64	0.48	0.64
mMDs score (0–51 points)	24.2 (6.5)	26.1 (4.9)	0.27	26.0 (6.5)	26.5 (5.6)	0.81	0.23	0.52
Fast food consumption (0–4 points)	2.8 (0.94)	3 (0.61)	0.47	2.76 (0.83)	2.69 (0.63)	0.79	0.06	0.13
Fruit (0–4 points)	1.56 (0.61)	1.65 (0.79)	0.70	1.62 (0.56)	1.71 (0.69)	0.693	0.62	0.71
Vegetable (0–4 points)	1.8 (0.93)	2.11 (0.69)	0.314	1.70 (0.85)	2.06 (0.56)	0.16	0.07	0.11
Sweet desserts (0–4 points)	1 (0.69)	1.24 (0.75)	0.340	0.85 (0.69)	1.35 (0.61)	0.04	0.05	0.84
Cooking oil or fat use at home (0–5 points)	3.0 (2.20)	2.88 (1.99)	0.57	3.85 (1.77)	3.59 (1.87)	0.70	0.07	0.56
Fried food consumption (0–4 points)	0.12 (0.47)	0.35 (0.78)	0.27	0.46 (0.88)	0.71 (0.98)	0.49	0.33	0.33
Breads and starches at home (0–4 points)	2.70 (1.82)	2.39 (1.97)	0.63	1.15 (1.80)	1.41 (1.62)	0.92	0.07	0.21
Ocean fish (0–4 points)	0.78 (0.88)	0.53 (0.72)	0.37	0.39 (0.87)	0.65 (0.86)	0.42	0.09	0.33
Non-alcoholic beverage at home	2.61 (1.72)	3.06 (1.39)	0.41	2.85 (1.41)	3.11 (1.45)	0.61	0.12	0.38
Alcoholic beverages (0–4 points)	1.06 (1.26)	0.94 (1.14)	0.78	1.31 (1.43)	1.12 (1.22)	0.61	1.0	0.58
Wine (0–2 points)	1.58 (0.51)	1.89 (0.31)	0.03	1.61 (0.51)	1.82 (0.39)	0.22	0.35	0.33
Legumes (0–4 points)	3.05 (0.87)	3.06 (0.87)	0.99	3.15 (1.28)	2.53 (1.12)	0.17	0.04	0.04
Nuts (0–4 points)	2.40 (1.09)	2.6 (0.9)	0.57	2.69 (1.11)	2.47 (0.71)	0.61	0.09	0.29

Pairwise comparisons over time include only those participants with complete information at baseline and at the end of follow up (n = 23). * At the end of follow up, 44 participants provided information about diet, n = 36 plasma serum and diet information, and 30 participants were assessed for anthropometric and other cardiovascular risk factors (Figure S1). Thus, mMDS and PREDIMED included n = 44 for the analysis at the end of follow up and for the comparisons.

3.2. The 6 Month Effect of the MedDiet Intervention

Figure 2 shows the 6 months effects of the intervention in the most relevant metabolites pathways. Data on the effect of the intervention in all the metabolites studied by group are presented in Table S1. The main subgroups affected by the intervention were the lipids and lipoproteins. Specifically, we observed a reduction in LDL-C, ApoB/ApoA1 ratio, remnant cholesterol, and higher HDL-C, and other subfractions such as lower cholesterol in L-VLDL-C, S-VLDL-C, L-LDL-C, M-LDL-C, S-LDL-C lipoproteins, and the composition of the lipoproteins after 6 months of intervention. Of note, these associations did not reach statistical significance after correcting the *p*-values for multiple testing (except for a decrease in M-VLDL-CE and an increase in lactate).

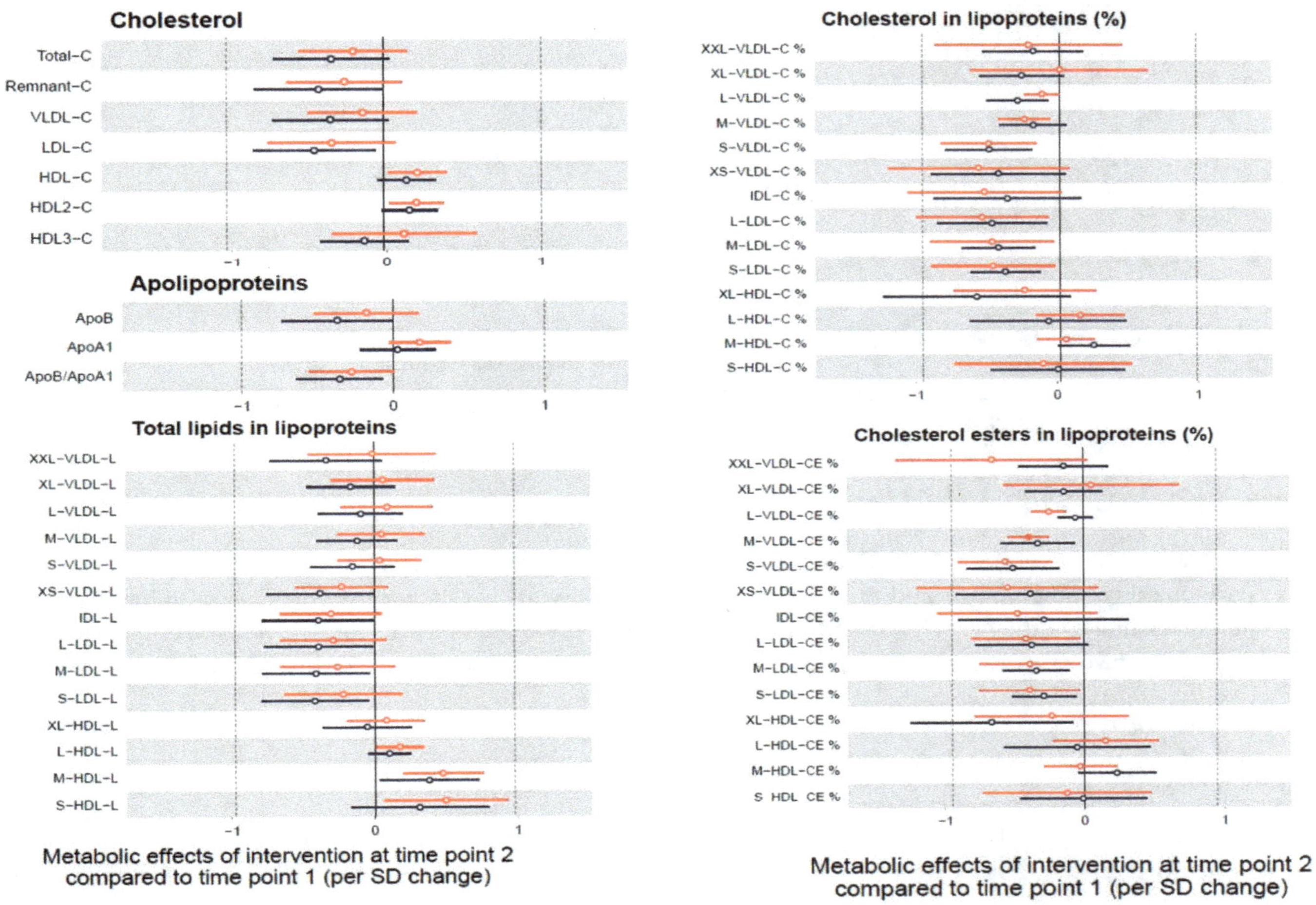

Figure 2. Metabolic effects of the intervention after 6 months follow up (time point 2) compared to baseline (time point 1) (linear mixed models adjusted by age and sex). Results show changes by SD in each metabolite per unit change in mMDS score and are displayed by hollow points. Only those significant results (after correction of multiple testing) are indicated by filled points along with their 95% confidence intervals. In black is shown Group 1 (the intervention group for 12 months) that continued under a self-sustained continuation phase for another 6 months. In red is shown Group 2 (control) that received the active Mediterranean Diet Nutritional Intervention for 6 months.

3.3. Cross-Sectional Association between Mediterranean Diet Adherence and Biomarkers

We also examined the cross-sectional linear association between biomarkers and adherence to the MedDiet at point 1 and 2 of this study, regardless of the participant's group at baseline and follow up. Results were similar at both time points, although somewhat higher effect sizes where observed at time 2 where all participants had received at least 6 months of the MedDiet intervention (Figure 3). A 1 unit difference in mMDS score was associated with lower total lipids in lipoproteins of different sizes (VLDL, LDL) and ApoB/ApoA1 ratio, lower concentrations of a marker of inflammation (Glyc A), lower concentrations of branched chain amino acids and higher polyunsaturated fatty acids (PUFAs) and Docosahexaenoic acid (DHA) (Figure 3). We further included all the participants grouped together and analyzed the association between unit changes in the MedDiet score and SD changes in metabolic markers. We found a similar pattern in the results, but not significant, with a tendency to higher lipoprotein particle size with higher MedDiet scores (Figure S2).

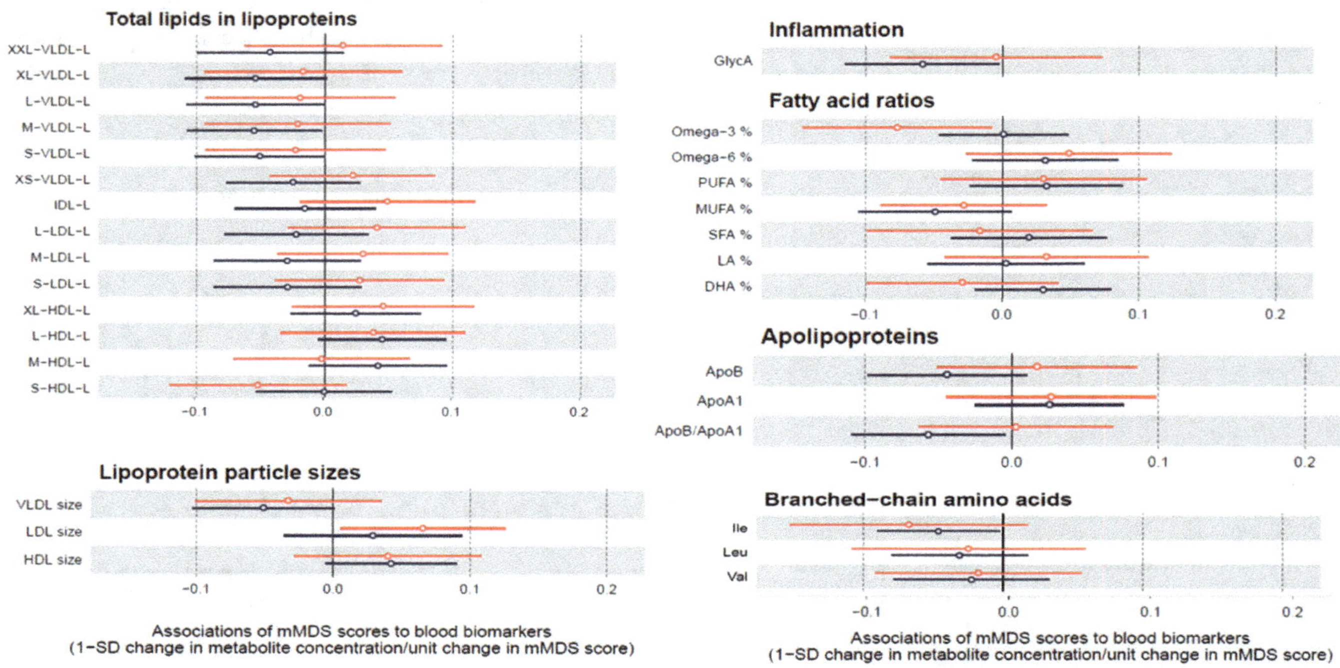

Figure 3. Cross-sectional association between biomarkers and adherence to the MedDiet for all participants at time point 1 and time point 2. Red lines show the results for the participants at baseline and black lines for the participants at follow up. Results show changes by SD in each biomarker per unit change in mMDS score and are displayed by hollow points along with their 95% confidence intervals.

Similar results were found when we used the PREDIMED score instead of the mMDS (Figure S3).

4. Discussion

In this sub-study of firefighters in Indianapolis participating in a cluster-randomized MedDiet intervention trial, we found that the MedDiet intervention was associated with favorable changes in markers of cardiovascular risk, specifically those related to the lipid metabolism (cholesterol, lipid composition, or cholesterol esters in the VLDL, IDL, and LDL lipoprotein subclasses, and ApoB/ApoA ratio) that were non-significant after correcting for multiple testing (except for a decrease in M-VLDL-CE). When the adherence to the MedDiet was measured with a self-reported scale (mMDS), the direction of the association with metabolites was similar at both time points (baseline and 6 months after the follow up).

Our results highlighting the changes in plasma metabolites related to lipid metabolism are in line with other studies [20,26]. A recent investigation that identified a metabolic signature of adherence to the MedDiet showed that out of 67 metabolites, 45 were lipids followed by 19 amino acids, 2 vitamins and 1 xenobiotic [26]. Although we used a different methodology and a different set of biomarkers, and thus we could not replicate this metabolic signature, our results support that the MedDiet may induce changes in relevant lipid species and subclasses related to atherogenic risk. In fact, the MedDiet is high in healthy fats (>35–40% of the total energy) mostly from monounsaturated fatty acids (MUFAs) (olive oil mostly) and PUFAs (from nuts and fish), and therefore the results are not surprising. In the firefighter population, we previously reported good correlation between nutrient intake from the food frequency questionnaire and the corresponding plasma biomarkers (omega-3, Eicosapentaenoic acid (EPA), and DHA) [36]. In line with these results, we found that changes in the MedDiet scores showed some tendency to be associated with fatty acids (an increase in PUFA% specifically DHA% in the expense of MUFA%). Although olive oil is a main component of the MedDiet, previous research found that higher consumption of this oil was linked to changes in omega 3, but not MUFA concentrations [36,41,42]. In addition, the average olive oil consumption in the firefighters is only approximately 0.5 tbsp/day, which is similar to other US cohorts [43] but much lower than in a Spanish cohort (4 tbsp/day) [44]. Nonetheless, it looks like changes in omega 3 to fatty acid ratio, PUFA to FA ratio and DHA to FA ratio increase with changes in the adherence to the MedDiet. This is in line with other studies [20,36], and suggests that those biomarkers could serve as indicators of adherence to the MedDiet.

We found that the MedDiet intervention induced a decrease in total cholesterol, remnant-C, VLDL-C and LDL-C and an increase in HDL-C and HDL2-C. Many studies have already demonstrated the effect of the MedDiet on total lipid metabolism, especially reducing total cholesterol and increasing HDL-C [45]. For example, the PREDIMED study, a randomized control trial, found that those in the MedDiet intervention (with olive oil or nuts) over 6 months had an increase in HDL-C but not a reduction in LDL-C [45]. Other studies support that replacing dietary saturated fatty acids (SFAs) with PUFA reduces the plasma LDL-C and subsequently the risk of cardiovascular disease [46–48].

In our study, we also observed a decrease in large, medium and small LDL fractions such as total lipids, cholesterol, particle concentration or cholesterol esters. Similarly, the MedDiet intervention decreased total cholesterol and cholesterol esters in the large, medium and small VLDL. Literature shows that VLDL concentrations are related directly or indirectly in the development of atherosclerosis [49]; for example the fatty acid composition of VLDL is critical for the activity of lipoprotein lipase and the formation of proatherogenic LDL and VLDL remnants [50]. In the FINRISK cohort, increased risk of cardiovascular disease was associated with all VLDL, IDL, and LDL subclasses, while the L- and M-HDL subclasses were associated with lower risk [51]. Despite the evidence of the role of these metabolites in CVD development, few studies have studied the effect of a MedDiet intervention in different lipids composition of lipoproteins or its subfractions. Interestingly, our results on lipid subfractions agree with a recent publication using the same metabolomic approach, where 47 participants were randomized to a SFA-rich diet, a MUFA-rich diet or a MED diet for 8 weeks. Additionally, in another study, compared to the control group, those participants that replaced SFAs with PUFAs reduced the lipoprotein particle concentration [52]. Finally, olive oil consumption modifies the lipid composition of VLDL [53] as well as the lipoprotein subfractions [54].

In our study, the effect was consistently shown in both groups, usually being stronger in the group undergoing a longer MedDiet intervention/exposure (MedDiet intervention + a self-sustained continuation phase), suggesting that the MedDiet induces favorable changes in metabolites related to CVD disease while the adherence to the MedDiet is sustained. For example, in our study, the ApoB/ApoA1 ratio was decreased in both groups after the intervention and also by adherence to the mMDS, which agrees with other short-term randomized trial with the MedDiet supplemented with olive oil, suggesting that these ratios may predict CVD beyond conventional lipid measures [55]. Finally, we found a significant association with lactate, a metabolite that was previously shown to increase the diabetes risk in the PREDIMED study [56]. However, we found that it occurs in the opposite direction.

Study Limitations

This was a pilot study with a small sample size. Possibly because of this, most associations lost statistical significance after correcting for multiple testing. However, results were in line with previous research, suggesting that a larger sample size would have retrieved significant results. In addition, the fact that we did not find differences in the mMDS adherence between groups may reflect selection bias since this is a sub-study within 400 firefighters participating in the Feeding America's Bravest trial, and participants willing to participate could potentially be healthier and more health conscious. Moreover, the control group had higher scores of mMDS at baseline and their scores were slightly improved during the intervention; however, the results were consistent in the cross-sectional analysis. We only adjusted for age and sex, since it was a randomized study with no significant differences between this sub-study and the parent study for the rest of the variables which suggests the need to perform a study that includes larger metabolites. In addition, we did not analyze other metabolites included in other studies nor at baseline for the parent study. In this pilot trial, Group 2 could be considered as the intervention group but Group 1 was not a pure control group because they already finished an active MedDiet intervention and began their self-sustained MedDiet phase. The changes in biomarkers in Group 1 (between time point 1 and 2) are more likely to reflect both residual effects of the MedDiet and continued effects from self-sustained diet intervention. Additionally, most of our participants were male and thus generalizability should be explored. In any case, the results in this study should be corroborated in larger clinical studies with longer follow up due to the pilot study nature and with a powerful study design.

5. Conclusions

This MedDiet intervention induces only modest changes in adherence to the MedDiet and consequently in metabolic biomarkers related to lipid metabolism. Further research should confirm these results based on larger study samples in workplace interventions with powerful study designs.

Supplementary Materials:
Figure S1: Flowchart of participants at time point 1 and 2 of the Feeding America's Bravest trial, Figure S2: Associations of unit changes in mMDS score by SD changes in plasma biomarkers between month 6 (time point 2) and baseline (time point 1) in all participants grouped together, Figure S3: Association between biomarkers and the PREDIMED score adherence (cross-sectional analysis), Table S1: The 6 months effect of the Mediterranean Diet intervention on metabolic biomarkers (linear mixed model analysis with p-values corrected for multiple testing).

Author Contributions: All authors have participated sufficiently and meaningfully to the research study and the preparation of this manuscript. M.S.-P. formulated the study question and design, interpreted the results, and drafted the manuscript. M.S.-P. and M.R.-C. were involved in statistical modeling. M.S.-P., S.N.K., Y.S. and S.M. contributed to the conception and design of the study and acquisition of the data. All authors contributed to the interpretation of data and critical revision of the manuscript and approved the final version. M.S.P., M.R.-C. and S.N.K. share primary responsibility for the final content. All authors have read and agreed to the published version of the manuscript.

Acknowledgments: We appreciate the participation of the Indianapolis Fire Departments as well as the firefighters and their spouses. We also thank Noora Kanerva and Heli Julkunen for their help with data analysis, as well as the Indiana Clinical and Translational Science Institute for helping with sample processing, the Kroger Company (coupons and customer loyalty discounts), Barilla America (Barilla Plus Products), Arianna Trading Company, Innoliva and Molino de Zafra, Spain (extra virgin olive oil samples and discounts) and the Almond Board of California (free samples of roasted unsalted almonds) for study support. The sponsors had no involvement in the overall study design; collection, analysis and interpretation of data; writing of the report; or the decision to submit the report for publication.

References

1. Cespedes, E.M.; Hu, F.B. Dietary patterns: From nutritional epidemiologic analysis to national guidelines. *Am. J. Clin. Nutr.* **2015**, *101*, 899–900. [CrossRef] [PubMed]
2. Martínez-González, M.A.; Gea, A.; Ruiz-Canela, M. The Mediterranean Diet and Cardiovascular Health. *Circ. Res.* **2019**, *124*, 779–798. [CrossRef]

3. Dinu, M.; Pagliai, G.; Casini, A.; Sofi, F. Mediterranean diet and multiple health outcomes: An umbrella review of meta-analyses of observational studies and randomised trials. *Eur. J. Clin. Nutr.* **2017**. [CrossRef]
4. Godos, J.; Zappala, G.; Bernardini, S.; Giambini, I.; Bes-Rastrollo, M.; Martinez-Gonzalez, M. Adherence to the Mediterranean diet is inversely associated with metabolic syndrome occurrence: A meta-analysis of observational studies. *Int. J. Food Sci. Nutr.* **2017**, *68*, 138–148. [CrossRef] [PubMed]
5. Mattei, J.; Sotos-Prieto, M.; Bigornia, S.J.; Noel, S.E.; Tucker, K.L. The Mediterranean Diet Score Is More Strongly Associated with Favorable Cardiometabolic Risk Factors over 2 Years Than Other Diet Quality Indexes in Puerto Rican Adults. *J. Nutr.* **2017**, *147*, 661–669. [CrossRef]
6. Rosato, V.; Temple, N.J.; La Vecchia, C.; Castellan, G.; Tavani, A.; Guercio, V. Mediterranean diet and cardiovascular disease: A systematic review and meta-analysis of observational studies. *Eur. J. Nutr.* **2017**. [CrossRef]
7. Sotos-Prieto, M.; Bhupathiraju, S.N.; Mattei, J.; Fung, T.T.; Li, Y.; Pan, A.; Willett, W.C.; Rimm, E.B.; Hu, F.B. Changes in Diet Quality Scores and Risk of Cardiovascular Disease Among US Men and Women. *Circulation* **2015**, *132*, 2212–2219. [CrossRef]
8. Sotos-Prieto, M.; Bhupathiraju, S.N.; Mattei, J.; Fung, T.T.; Li, Y.; Pan, A.; Willett, W.C.; Rimm, E.B.; Hu, F.B. Association of Changes in Diet Quality with Total and Cause-Specific Mortality. *N. Engl. J. Med.* **2017**, *377*, 143–153. [CrossRef]
9. Guasch-Ferré, M.; Bhupathiraju, S.N.; Hu, F.B. Use of Metabolomics in Improving Assessment of Dietary Intake. *Clin. Chem.* **2018**, *64*, 82–98. [CrossRef]
10. Brennan, L.; Hu, F.B. Metabolomics Based Dietary Biomarkers in Nutritional Epidemiology-Current Status and Future Opportunities. *Mol. Nutr. Food Res.* **2018**, 1701064. [CrossRef]
11. Hardin, D.S. Validating dietary intake with biochemical markers. *J. Am. Diet. Assoc.* **2009**, *109*, 1698–1699. [CrossRef] [PubMed]
12. Garcia-Perez, I.; Posma, J.M.; Gibson, R.; Chambers, E.S.; Hansen, T.H.; Vestergaard, H.; Hansen, T.; Beckmann, M.; Pedersen, O.; Elliott, P.; et al. Objective assessment of dietary patterns by use of metabolic phenotyping: A randomised, controlled, crossover trial. *Lancet Diabetes Endocrinol.* **2017**, *5*, 184–195. [CrossRef]
13. Scalbert, A.; Brennan, L.; Manach, C.; Andres-Lacueva, C.; Dragsted, L.O.; Draper, J.; Rappaport, S.M.; van der Hooft, J.J.; Wishart, D.S. The food metabolome: A window over dietary exposure. *Am. J. Clin. Nutr.* **2014**, *99*, 1286–1308. [CrossRef] [PubMed]
14. Ruiz-Canela, M.; Hruby, A.; Clish, C.B.; Liang, L.; Martinez-Gonzalez, M.A.; Hu, F.B. Comprehensive Metabolomic Profiling and Incident Cardiovascular Disease: A Systematic Review. *J. Am. Heart Assoc.* **2017**, *6*. [CrossRef] [PubMed]
15. Cheung, W.; Keski-Rahkonen, P.; Assi, N.; Ferrari, P.; Freisling, H.; Rinaldi, S.; Slimani, N.; Zamora-Ros, R.; Rundle, M.; Frost, G.; et al. A metabolomic study of biomarkers of meat and fish intake. *Am. J. Clin. Nutr.* **2017**, *105*, 600–608. [CrossRef]
16. Papandreou, C.; Hernández-Alonso, P.; Bulló, M.; Ruiz-Canela, M.; Yu, E.; Guasch-Ferré, M.; Toledo, E.; Dennis, C.; Deik, A.; Clish, C.; et al. Plasma Metabolites Associated with Coffee Consumption: A Metabolomic Approach within the PREDIMED Study. *Nutrients* **2019**, *11*, 32. [CrossRef] [PubMed]
17. Hernández-Alonso, P.; Papandreou, C.; Bulló, M.; Ruiz-Canela, M.; Dennis, C.; Deik, A.; Wang, D.D.; Guasch-Ferré, M.; Yu, E.; Toledo, E.; et al. Plasma Metabolites Associated with Frequent Red Wine Consumption: A Metabolomics Approach within the PREDIMED Study. *Mol. Nutr. Food Res.* **2019**, *63*, e1900140. [CrossRef] [PubMed]
18. Schmidt, J.A.; Rinaldi, S.; Ferrari, P.; Carayol, M.; Achaintre, D.; Scalbert, A.; Cross, A.J.; Gunter, M.J.; Fensom, G.K.; Appleby, P.N.; et al. Metabolic profiles of male meat eaters, fish eaters, vegetarians, and vegans from the EPIC-Oxford cohort. *Am. J. Clin. Nutr.* **2015**, *102*, 1518–1526. [CrossRef]
19. Edmands, W.M.B.; Beckonert, O.P.; Stella, C.; Campbell, A.; Lake, B.G.; Lindon, J.C.; Holmes, E.; Gooderham, N.J. Identification of human urinary biomarkers of cruciferous vegetable consumption by metabonomic profiling. *J. Proteome Res.* **2011**, *10*, 4513–4521. [CrossRef]
20. Michielsen, C.C.J.R.; Hangelbroek, R.W.J.; Feskens, E.J.M.; Afman, L.A. Disentangling the Effects of Monounsaturated Fatty Acids from Other Components of a Mediterranean Diet on Serum Metabolite Profiles: A Randomized Fully Controlled Dietary Intervention in Healthy Subjects at Risk of the Metabolic Syndrome. *Mol. Nutr. Food Res.* **2019**, *63*, e1801095. [CrossRef]

21. Jin, Q.; Black, A.; Kales, S.N.; Vattem, D.; Ruiz-Canela, M.; Sotos-Prieto, M. Metabolomics and Microbiomes as Potential Tools to Evaluate the Effects of the Mediterranean Diet. *Nutrients* **2019**, *11*, 207. [CrossRef] [PubMed]
22. Bondia-Pons, I.; Martinez, J.A.; de la Iglesia, R.; Lopez-Legarrea, P.; Poutanen, K.; Hanhineva, K.; Zulet, M.d.l.Á. Effects of short- and long-term Mediterranean-based dietary treatment on plasma LC-QTOF/MS metabolic profiling of subjects with metabolic syndrome features: The Metabolic Syndrome Reduction in Navarra (RESMENA) randomized controlled trial. *Mol. Nutr. Food Res.* **2015**, *59*, 711–728. [CrossRef]
23. Playdon, M.C.; Moore, S.C.; Derkach, A.; Reedy, J.; Subar, A.F.; Sampson, J.N.; Albanes, D.; Gu, F.; Kontto, J.; Lassale, C.; et al. Identifying biomarkers of dietary patterns by using metabolomics. *Am. J. Clin. Nutr.* **2017**, *105*, 450–465. [CrossRef] [PubMed]
24. Tong, T.Y.N.; Koulman, A.; Griffin, J.L.; Wareham, N.J.; Forouhi, N.G.; Imamura, F. A Combination of Metabolites Predicts Adherence to the Mediterranean Diet Pattern and Its Associations with Insulin Sensitivity and Lipid Homeostasis in the General Population: The Fenland Study, United Kingdom. *J. Nutr.* **2020**, *150*, 568–578. [CrossRef] [PubMed]
25. Rebholz, C.M.; Lichtenstein, A.H.; Zheng, Z.; Appel, L.J.; Coresh, J. Serum untargeted metabolomic profile of the Dietary Approaches to Stop Hypertension (DASH) dietary pattern. *Am. J. Clin. Nutr.* **2018**, *108*, 243–255. [CrossRef] [PubMed]
26. Li, J.; Guasch-Ferré, M.; Chung, W.; Ruiz-Canela, M.; Toledo, E.; Corella, D.; Bhupathiraju, S.N.; Tobias, D.K.; Tabung, F.K.; Hu, J.; et al. The Mediterranean diet, plasma metabolome, and cardiovascular disease risk. *Eur. Heart J.* **2020**. [CrossRef] [PubMed]
27. Akbaraly, T.; Würtz, P.; Singh-Manoux, A.; Shipley, M.J.; Haapakoski, R.; Lehto, M.; Desrumaux, C.; Kähönen, M.; Lehtimäki, T.; Mikkilä, V.; et al. Association of circulating metabolites with healthy diet and risk of cardiovascular disease: Analysis of two cohort studies. *Sci. Rep.* **2018**, *8*, 8620. [CrossRef]
28. Lécuyer, L.; Dalle, C.; Micheau, P.; Pétéra, M.; Centeno, D.; Lyan, B.; Lagree, M.; Galan, P.; Hercberg, S.; Rossary, A.; et al. Untargeted plasma metabolomic profiles associated with overall diet in women from the SU.VI.MAX cohort. *Eur. J. Nutr.* **2020**. [CrossRef]
29. Ruiz-Canela, M.; Guasch-Ferré, M.; Toledo, E.; Clish, C.B.; Razquin, C.; Liang, L.; Wang, D.D.; Corella, D.; Estruch, R.; Hernáez, Á.; et al. Plasma branched chain/aromatic amino acids, enriched Mediterranean diet and risk of type 2 diabetes: Case-cohort study within the PREDIMED Trial. *Diabetologia* **2018**, *61*, 1560–1571. [CrossRef]
30. Ruiz-Canela, M.; Toledo, E.; Clish, C.B.; Hruby, A.; Liang, L.; Salas-Salvadó, J.; Razquin, C.; Corella, D.; Estruch, R.; Ros, E.; et al. Plasma Branched-Chain Amino Acids and Incident Cardiovascular Disease in the PREDIMED Trial. *Clin. Chem.* **2016**, *62*, 582–592. [CrossRef]
31. Guasch-Ferré, M.; Ruiz-Canela, M.; Li, J.; Zheng, Y.; Bulló, M.; Wang, D.D.; Toledo, E.; Clish, C.; Corella, D.; Estruch, R.; et al. Plasma Acylcarnitines and Risk of Type 2 Diabetes in a Mediterranean Population at High Cardiovascular Risk. *J. Clin. Endocrinol. Metab.* **2019**, *104*, 1508–1519. [CrossRef] [PubMed]
32. Sotos-Prieto, M.; Cash, S.B.; Christophi, C.A.; Folta, S.; Moffatt, S.; Muegge, C.; Korre, M.; Mozaffarian, D.; Kales, S.N. Rationale and design of feeding America's bravest: Mediterranean diet-based intervention to change firefighters' eating habits and improve cardiovascular risk profiles. *Contemp. Clin. Trials* **2017**, *61*, 101–107. [CrossRef] [PubMed]
33. Jackson, A.S.; Blair, S.N.; Mahar, M.T.; Wier, L.T.; Ross, R.M.; Stuteville, J.E. Prediction of functional aerobic capacity without exercise testing. *Med. Sci. Sport. Exerc.* **1990**, *22*, 863–870. [CrossRef] [PubMed]
34. Salvini, S.; Hunter, D.J.; Sampson, L.; Stampfer, M.J.; Colditz, G.A.; Rosner, B.; Willett, W.C. Food-based validation of a dietary questionnaire: The effects of week-to-week variation in food consumption. *Int. J. Epidemiol.* **1989**, *18*, 858–867. [CrossRef] [PubMed]
35. Gong, Y.; Yang, J.; Farioli, A.; Korre, M.; Kales, S.N. Modified Mediterranean Diet Score and Cardiovascular Risk in a North American Working Population. *PLoS ONE* **2014**, *9*, e87539. [CrossRef]
36. Sotos-Prieto, M.; Christophi, C.; Black, A.; Furtado, J.D.; Song, Y.; Magiatis, P.; Papakonstantinou, A.; Melliou, E.; Moffatt, S.; Kales, S.N. Assessing Validity of Self-Reported Dietary Intake within a Mediterranean Diet Cluster Randomized Controlled Trial among US Firefighters. *Nutrients* **2019**, *11*, 2250. [CrossRef]
37. Schroder, H.; Fito, M.; Estruch, R.; Martinez-Gonzalez, M.A.; Corella, D.; Salas-Salvado, J.; Lamuela-Raventos, R.; Ros, E.; Salaverria, I.; Fiol, M.; et al. A short screener is valid for assessing Mediterranean diet adherence among older Spanish men and women. *J. Nutr.* **2011**, *141*, 1140–1145. [CrossRef]

38. Soininen, P.; Kangas, A.J.; Würtz, P.; Suna, T.; Ala-Korpela, M. Quantitative serum nuclear magnetic resonance metabolomics in cardiovascular epidemiology and genetics. *Circ. Cardiovasc. Genet.* **2015**, *8*, 192–206. [CrossRef]
39. Kettunen, J.; Demirkan, A.; Würtz, P.; Draisma, H.H.M.; Haller, T.; Rawal, R.; Vaarhorst, A.; Kangas, A.J.; Lyytikäinen, L.-P.; Pirinen, M.; et al. Genome-wide study for circulating metabolites identifies 62 loci and reveals novel systemic effects of LPA. *Nat. Commun.* **2016**, *7*, 11122. [CrossRef]
40. Würtz, P.; Kangas, A.J.; Soininen, P.; Lawlor, D.A.; Davey Smith, G.; Ala-Korpela, M. Quantitative Serum Nuclear Magnetic Resonance Metabolomics in Large-Scale Epidemiology: A Primer on -Omic Technologies. *Am. J. Epidemiol.* **2017**, *186*, 1084–1096. [CrossRef]
41. Hebestreit, K.; Yahiaoui-Doktor, M.; Engel, C.; Vetter, W.; Siniatchkin, M.; Erickson, N.; Halle, M.; Kiechle, M.; Bischoff, S.C. Validation of the German version of the Mediterranean Diet Adherence Screener (MEDAS) questionnaire. *BMC Cancer* **2017**, *17*, 341. [CrossRef] [PubMed]
42. Barceló, F.; Perona, J.S.; Prades, J.; Funari, S.S.; Gomez-Gracia, E.; Conde, M.; Estruch, R.; Ruiz-Gutiérrez, V. Mediterranean-style diet effect on the structural properties of the erythrocyte cell membrane of hypertensive patients: The Prevencion con Dieta Mediterranea Study. *Hypertension* **2009**, *54*, 1143–1150. [CrossRef] [PubMed]
43. Guasch-Ferré, M.; Hu, F.B.; Martínez-González, M.A.; Fitó, M.; Bulló, M.; Estruch, R.; Ros, E.; Corella, D.; Recondo, J.; Gómez-Gracia, E.; et al. Olive oil intake and risk of cardiovascular disease and mortality in the PREDIMED Study. *BMC Med.* **2014**, *12*, 78. [CrossRef] [PubMed]
44. Guasch-Ferré, M.; Liu, G.; Li, Y.; Sampson, L.; Manson, J.E.; Salas-Salvadó, J.; Martínez-González, M.A.; Stampfer, M.J.; Willett, W.C.; Sun, Q.; et al. Olive Oil Consumption and Cardiovascular Risk in U.S. Adults. *J. Am. Coll. Cardiol.* **2020**, *75*, 1729–1739. [CrossRef]
45. Estruch, R.; Martínez-González, M.A.; Corella, D.; Salas-Salvadó, J.; Ruiz-Gutiérrez, V.; Covas, M.I.; Fiol, M.; Gómez-Gracia, E.; López-Sabater, M.C.; Vinyoles, E.; et al. Effects of a Mediterranean-style diet on cardiovascular risk factors: A randomized trial. *Ann. Intern. Med.* **2006**, *145*, 1–11. [CrossRef]
46. Mensink, R.P.; Zock, P.L.; Kester, A.D.M.; Katan, M.B. Effects of dietary fatty acids and carbohydrates on the ratio of serum total to HDL cholesterol and on serum lipids and apolipoproteins: A meta-analysis of 60 controlled trials. *Am. J. Clin. Nutr.* **2003**, *77*, 1146–1155. [CrossRef]
47. Sacks, F.M.; Lichtenstein, A.H.; Wu, J.H.Y.; Appel, L.J.; Creager, M.A.; Kris-Etherton, P.M.; Miller, M.; Rimm, E.B.; Rudel, L.L.; Robinson, J.G.; et al. Dietary Fats and Cardiovascular Disease: A Presidential Advisory From the American Heart Association. *Circulation* **2017**, *136*, e1–e23. [CrossRef]
48. Stone, N.J.; Robinson, J.G.; Lichtenstein, A.H.; Bairey Merz, C.N.; Blum, C.B.; Eckel, R.H.; Goldberg, A.C.; Gordon, D.; Levy, D.; Lloyd-Jones, D.M.; et al. 2013 ACC/AHA guideline on the treatment of blood cholesterol to reduce atherosclerotic cardiovascular risk in adults: A report of the American College of Cardiology/American Heart Association Task Force on Practice Guidelines. *J. Am. Coll. Cardiol.* **2014**, *63*, 2889–2934. [CrossRef]
49. Wilhelm, M.G.; Cooper, A.D. Induction of atherosclerosis by human chylomicron remnants: A hypothesis. *J. Atheroscler. Thromb.* **2003**, *10*, 132–139. [CrossRef]
50. Liu, J.; Sempos, C.T.; Donahue, R.P.; Dorn, J.; Trevisan, M.; Grundy, S.M. Non-high-density lipoprotein and very-low-density lipoprotein cholesterol and their risk predictive values in coronary heart disease. *Am. J. Cardiol.* **2006**, *98*, 1363–1368. [CrossRef]
51. Metabolite Profiling and Cardiovascular Event Risk: A Prospective Study of 3 Population-Based Cohorts—PubMed. Available online: https://pubmed.ncbi.nlm.nih.gov/25573147/?from_single_result=Metabolite+profiling+and+cardiovascular+event+risk%3A+a+prospective+study+of+3+population-based+cohorts (accessed on 3 June 2020).
52. Ulven, S.M.; Christensen, J.J.; Nygård, O.; Svardal, A.; Leder, L.; Ottestad, I.; Lysne, V.; Laupsa-Borge, J.; Ueland, P.M.; Midttun, Ø.; et al. Using metabolic profiling and gene expression analyses to explore molecular effects of replacing saturated fat with polyunsaturated fat-a randomized controlled dietary intervention study. *Am. J. Clin. Nutr.* **2019**, *109*, 1239–1250. [CrossRef] [PubMed]
53. Perona, J.S.; Cañizares, J.; Montero, E.; Sánchez-Domínguez, J.M.; Pacheco, Y.M.; Ruiz-Gutierrez, V. Dietary virgin olive oil triacylglycerols as an independent determinant of very low-density lipoprotein composition. *Nutrition* **2004**, *20*, 509–514. [CrossRef]

54. Damasceno, N.R.T.; Sala-Vila, A.; Cofán, M.; Pérez-Heras, A.M.; Fitó, M.; Ruiz-Gutiérrez, V.; Martínez-González, M.-Á.; Corella, D.; Arós, F.; Estruch, R.; et al. Mediterranean diet supplemented with nuts reduces waist circumference and shifts lipoprotein subfractions to a less atherogenic pattern in subjects at high cardiovascular risk. *Atherosclerosis* **2013**, *230*, 347–353. [CrossRef] [PubMed]
55. Solá, R.; Fitó, M.; Estruch, R.; Salas-Salvadó, J.; Corella, D.; de La Torre, R.; Muñoz, M.A.; López-Sabater, M.d.C.; Martínez-González, M.-A.; Arós, F.; et al. Effect of a traditional Mediterranean diet on apolipoproteins B, A-I, and their ratio: A randomized, controlled trial. *Atherosclerosis* **2011**, *218*, 174–180. [CrossRef] [PubMed]
56. Guasch-Ferré, M.; Santos, J.L.; Martínez-González, M.A.; Clish, C.B.; Razquin, C.; Wang, D.; Liang, L.; Li, J.; Dennis, C.; Corella, D.; et al. Glycolysis/gluconeogenesis- and tricarboxylic acid cycle-related metabolites, Mediterranean diet, and type 2 diabetes. *Am. J. Clin. Nutr.* **2020**, *111*, 835–844. [CrossRef] [PubMed]

9

Metabolic Syndrome—Role of Dietary Fat Type and Quantity

Peter Clifton

School of Pharmacy and Medical Sciences, University of South Australia, Adelaide SA 5000, Australia; peter.clifton@unisa.edu.au

Abstract: Background: Metabolic syndrome increases the risk of cardiovascular disease (CVD) over and above that related to type 2 diabetes. The optimal diet for the treatment of metabolic syndrome is not clear. Materials and Methods: A review of dietary interventions in volunteers with metabolic syndrome as well as studies examining the impact of dietary fat on the separate components of metabolic syndrome was undertaken using only recent meta-analyses, if available. Results: Most of the data suggest that replacing carbohydrates with any fat, but particularly polyunsaturated fat, will lower triglyceride(TG), increase high density lipoprotein (HDL) cholesterol, and lower blood pressure, but have no effects on fasting glucose in normal volunteers or insulin sensitivity, as assessed by euglycemic hyperinsulinemic clamps. Fasting insulin may be lowered by fat. Monounsaturated fat (MUFA) is preferable to polyunsaturated fat (PUFA) for fasting insulin and glucose lowering. The addition of 3–4 g of N3 fats will lower TG and blood pressure (BP) and reduce the proportion of subjects with metabolic syndrome. Dairy fat (50% saturated fat) is also related to a lower incidence of metabolic syndrome in cohort studies.

Keywords: carbohydrate; polyunsaturated fat; monounsaturated fat; saturated fat; fish oil; meta-analyses; lipids; glucose; blood pressure; insulin resistance

---

1. Introduction

The metabolic syndrome is associated with an increased risk of cardiovascular disease and type 2 diabetes and enhances the risk of CVD in people with diabetes [1]. There are currently four definitions of metabolic syndrome, three of which require insulin resistance, as evidenced by central obesity, or fasting hyperinsulinemia or a disturbance in glucose homeostasis, plus two other abnormalities [2]. The National Cholesterol Education Program Adult Treatment Panel (NCEP ATP-III (revision 2005) guidelines does not require this, but demands 3 of 5 possible abnormalities—central obesity, impaired fasting glucose, hypertriglyceridemia, low HDL cholesterol, and blood pressure (>130 systolic or >85 diastolic). The other criteria vary with different levels of blood pressure (140/90), with a combination of high TG and low HDL as one criterion, and varying levels of fasting TG—either 1.7 or 2 mmol/L—and varying levels of HDL cholesterol. This review will focus on the components of the metabolic syndrome and where there are data on the presence or absence of metabolic syndrome, the criterion used will be mentioned. The aim of this review is to systematically examine meta-analyses that summarise the evidence from interventions on fat amount and type in metabolic syndrome or its separate components. Some evidence from individual trials that are illustrative will be included.

2. Aim

To systematically review meta-analyses of interventions that replace carbohydrates with fat in people with metabolic syndrome and interventions that examine these effects on the individual components of the syndrome.

3. Methods

Pubmed was searched (all years available) with the terms "meta-analysis AND dietary fat AND carbohydrate AND intervention AND (TG, OR, HDL, OR blood pressure, OR glucose, OR weight)". We reviewed 102 titles.

4. Results

4.1. Lipids

A large amount of evidence has accumulated that replacing carbohydrates (usually quality unspecified) with fat of any sort will lower fasting triglyceride and increase HDL cholesterol. A meta-analysis by Mensink and Katan [3] found that a 1% increase in fat calories in place of carbohydrates led to a fall in TG of 0.026 mmol/L (95% confidence intervals: 0.020–0.031) with polyunsaturated fat, 0.021 (0.015–0.027) with saturated fat, and 0.019 (0.014–0.024) with monounsaturated fat from 100 studies with 45 diets. For HDL cholesterol the same diets led to an increase in HDL cholesterol of 0.006 (0.003–0.009) mmol/L, 0.010 (0.007–0.013), and 0.008 (0.005–0.011), respectively. Overall saturated fat is about 30% more effective than the other two fats in the combined lowering of TG and HDL cholesterol. However, differences in HDL cholesterol from genetic variance have not been associated with differences in coronary heart disease (CHD) risk [4], whereas TG lowering genetically has been associated with CVD reduction, with the same degree of benefit per mg/dL apoB lowering as a reduction in LDL cholesterol [5]. Thus, PUFA is preferred to other fat types for carbohydrate replacement. In a small study of 39 men with metabolic syndrome, PUFA produced greater TG lowering than MUFA (both 5–30% of energy). Overall, 25% (4 of 16) assigned to PUFA and 13% (3 of 23) to MUFA did not have metabolic syndrome after the intervention [6]. Metabolic syndrome in this study was based on NCEP-III (2001). A high total dairy intake (and, presumably, a lower carbohydrate diet) is associated with a 6% reduced risk of metabolic syndrome per additional serving of dairy [7]. Most studies in this meta-analysis of 16 case-control/cross-sectional studies used the NCEP-III criteria.

The relationship between carbohydrate intake and TG has been controversial for many years with arguments about the persistence of the TG elevation effect [8,9], with the moderating or even nullifying effect of fibre on TG elevation [10], the contrasting effects of higher versus lower sugar with sugars replacing starch [11,12], and the absence of TG elevation in Pima Indians with type 2 diabetes mellitus (DM) with increased carbohydrates [13]. Just when the landscape was reasonably predictable from interventions, the TOSCA.IT showed in 18,785 people with type 2 DM that increasing fat intake from <25% to >35% increased TG, while increasing carbohydrate intake from <45% to >65% decreased TG [14]. TG was lower in the highest tertile of the relative Mediterranean diet score, which had lower added sugars, more fibre, but less fat and more carbohydrates. [15]. However, the TOSCA-IT is a large cohort study and its results may well be confounded as they do not match the results from dietary intervention studies in people with type 2 DM. The Qian meta-analysis [16] of 24 studies with 1460 participants showed that fasting TG was reduced by 0.31 mmol/L (95% confidence interval −0.44, −0.18) with replacement of carbohydrates with MUFA. A high fibre intake is associated with a 30% lowering in the risk of metabolic syndrome [17].

In a meta-analysis of high-fat versus low-fat diets in people with obesity, but no overt metabolic disturbance, Lu et al. (2018) [18] found a significantly higher level of TG (WMD: 11.68 mg/dL (0.13 mmol/l), 95 % CI 5.90, 17.45; $p < 0.001$) and a lower level of HDL-cholesterol (WMD: −2.57 mg/dL (−0.07 mmol/l); 95 % CI −3.85, −1.28; $p < 0.001$) after the low-fat diets, compared with high-fat diets in 20 studies with 2016 participants.

4.2. Fish Oil Fatty Acids

Guo et al. [19] performed a meta-analysis of seven case-control and 20 cross-sectional studies and found that a higher level of plasma/serum n-3 PUFAs was associated with a lower metabolic syndrome risk (pooled OR = 0.63, 95% CI: 0.49, 0.81). The plasma/serum n-3 PUFAs in controls were significantly higher than in metabolic syndrome cases (WMD: 0.24; 95% CI: 0.04, 0.43), especially docosapentaenoic acid and docosahexaenoic acid.

The addition of fish oil fatty acids of at least 1 g/day lowers fasting TG and a metanalysis performed by Eslick et al. [20] of 47 studies showed that taking fish oils (weighted average daily intake of 3.25 g of EPA and/or DHA) produced a clinically significant reduction of TG (−0.34 mmol/L, 95% CI: −0.41 to −0.27), with a very slight increase in HDL (0.01 mmol/L, 95% CI: 0.00 to 0.02) and LDL cholesterol (0.06 mmol/L, 95% CI: 0.03 to 0.09). The reduction of TG correlated with EPA plus DHA intake and initial TG level.

4.3. Glucose

Fasting glucose lowering by reducing carbohydrate and replacing it with fat is far more controversial. A recent meta-analysis by Wanders et al. [21] showed no effect in normal subjects of replacing carbohydrate with polyunsaturated fat, even though fasting insulin was reduced. A 5% increase in energy from PUFA significantly reduced insulin by 5.8 pmol/L (95% CI −10.2 to −1.3 pmol/L), but not glucose (change −0.07, 95% CI −0.17 to 0.04 mmol/L) and even in the group with the highest intake of PUFA, glucose was still not significant (−0.09, 95% CI −0.18 to 0.01 mmol/L). Imamura et al. [22] found that replacing 5% energy from carbohydrates with SFA had no significant effect on fasting glucose (+0.02 mmol/L, 95% CI = −0.01, +0.04; n trials = 99), but lowered fasting insulin (−1.1 pmol/L; −1.7, −0.5; n = 90). Replacing saturated fat with PUFA lowered fasting glucose (0.04mmol/L; 0.01, 0.07). Thus, PUFA is clearly the better fat for replacing carbohydrates in normal people. In people with type 2 diabetes [16], high MUFA diets compared with high carbohydrate diets lowered fasting plasma glucose (WMD −0.57 mmol/L [95% CI −0.76, −0.39]) in 24 studies containing 1460 participants. HDL cholesterol was increased by 0.06 mmol/L (0.02, 0.10) [16]. Surprisingly, in this study, replacing PUFA with MUFA lowered fasting glucose by a large amount (−0.87 mmol/L (−1.67, −0.07)) but the data are much less reliable, taken from only four studies and 44 participants.

4.4. Blood Pressure

There are much less data on blood pressure and carbohydrate replacement with fat in non-diabetics and the effects are relatively small. A meta-analysis performed by Shah et al. [23] found that diets rich in carbohydrates resulted in significantly higher systolic blood pressure (difference: 2.6 (95% CI: 0.4, 4.7) mm Hg; $p = 0.02$) and diastolic blood pressure (1.8 (0.01, 3.6) mm Hg; $p = 0.05$) than did diets rich in cis-monounsaturated fat. Huntress et al. [24] examined low carbohydrate diets in people with type 2 diabetes from data at one year. Eighteen trials were included in the meta-analysis, which found that the low carbohydrate diet lowered systolic blood pressure (estimated effect = −2.74 mmHg, 95% CI −5.27 to −0.20), but diastolic BP was not significant. In the meta-analysis from Qian et al. [16], MUFA lowered systolic blood pressure (−2.31 mmHg (−4.13, −0.49)) when it replaced carbohydrates.

4.5. Diet Composition During Weight Loss and Lipid Changes

Mansoor et al. [25] performed a meta-analysis of 11 weight loss trials with 1369 participants with a low carbohydrate level being defined as <20% carbohydrates. Compared with participants on low fat diets, participants on low carbohydrate diets experienced a greater reduction in body weight (weighted mean difference [WMD] −2.17 kg; 95% CI −3.36, −0.99) and TG (WMD −0.26 mmol/L; 95% CI −0.37, −0.15), but a greater increase in HDL-cholesterol (WMD 0·14 mmol/l; 95% CI 0.09, 0.19) and LDL-cholesterol (WMD 0·16 mmol/L; 95% CI 0.003, 0.33). Most of the low carbohydrate diets followed an Atkins style diet with an increase in saturated fat, which accounted for the rise in LDL cholesterol. If carbohydrates are replaced by unsaturated fat and not saturated fat, no rise in LDL cholesterol is seen in either six months [26], or one- [27] or two-year follow ups [28].

4.6. Insulin Resistance

Insulin resistance is a key and essential element of the metabolic syndrome (except the NCEP111 criteria), usually assumed on the basis of central adiposity. As noted by Wanders et al. [21], replacing carbohydrates with PUFA led to a lowering of fasting insulin, as did saturated fat, suggesting reduced insulin resistance, at least in the liver. There have been a small number of formal hyperinsulemic euglycemic clamp studies, but no meta-analysis. Tardy et al. [29] compared high dairy and industrial trans fatty acids with low trans fat diets in 63 healthy women with abdominal obesity. After four weeks of 60 g low-TFA lipids/day (0.54 g/day; $n = 21$), ruminant TFA-rich lipids (4.86 g/day; $n = 21$), or industrial TFA-rich lipids (5.58 g/day; $n = 21$), no changes in peripheral insulin sensitivity were seen. Bendtsen et al. [30] found no effect either of 15 g/day of trans fat in partially hydrogenated soybean oil for 16 weeks in 52 overweight postmenopausal women. Fasching et al. [31] found no effect of exchanging 200 g of carbohydrates with 90 g of PUFA, MUFA, or saturated fat for one week in a randomised crossover study in eight men with insulin sensitivity, assessed with a euglycemic hyperinsulinemic clamp. Borkmann et al. [32] found no effect of substituting saturated fat for carbohydrates on insulin sensitivity in eight non-diabetic subjects, despite large changes in LDL and TG (the latter down 33%.) The KANWU study [33] showed that a high MUFA diet for three months reduced insulin resistance, compared with a high saturated fat diet in 162 healthy subjects, but carbohydrate levels were not examined. Fish oil had no effect and the effect of MUFA was lost when fat intake was >37% of energy. In a very small study in patients with fatty liver disease, a high MUFA Mediterranean diet improved insulin sensitivity, compared with a high carbohydrate diet ($p = 0.03$) accompanied by a reduction in liver fat [34]

A contrary result was found in the Lipgene study [35] where 472 volunteers with metabolic syndrome were randomised to one diet for 12 weeks: High MUFA or high saturated fat diets or high carbohydrate diets with and without fish oil (1.2 g/day). In the highest HOMA-IR tertile, MUFA and n3 fats lowered insulin significantly, compared with saturated fat. In the lowest HOMA-IR tertile, insulin and glucose rose with all diets, but it rose less with MUFA and N3 fats compared with saturated fat. There is regression to the mean in both these tertiles and there is no statistical contrast between the effect of diets in the different tertiles, so we don't actually know if there is a tertile/diet interaction. Triglycerides fell with N3 fats in tertiles 1 and 2, but surprisingly, not in the highest tertile with the highest TG level. Replacing carbohydrates with MUFA or saturated fat had no effect on TG in any tertile, which is contrary to the much bigger meta-analysis of Mensink et al. (3) and there is no good explanation other than strong time-related changes.

In another report from the same study, in 337 volunteers [36], the prevalence of metabolic syndrome (NECP-III) fell by 20.5% after the n-3 diet (blood pressure and TG fell), compared with the high saturated fat diet (10.6%), high MUFA diet (12%) diet, and high carbohydrate diet (10.4%) ($p < 0.028$).

5. Conclusions

Most meta-analyses show that replacement of carbohydrates with fat lowers fasting TG and glucose and blood pressure, and increases HDL cholesterol with some differences, depending on whether the population has type 2 diabetes or not. There are some large intervention and cohort studies that show the opposite results, but these are in the minority. PUFA is probably superior to MUFA, while fish oil is superior to both.

References

1. Reaven, G.M. Banting lecture 1988. Role of insulin resistance in human disease. *Diabetes* **1988**, *37*, 1595–1607. [CrossRef] [PubMed]

2. Kassi, E.; Pervanidou, P.; Kaltsas, G.; Chrousos, G. Metabolic syndrome: Definitions and controversies. *BMC Med.* **2011**, *9*, 48. [CrossRef] [PubMed]
3. Mensink, R.P.; Zock, P.L.; Kester, A.D.; Katan, M.B. Effects of dietary fatty acids and carbohydrates on the ratio of serum total to HDL cholesterol and on serum lipids and apolipoproteins: A meta-analysis of 60 controlled trials. *Am. J. Clin. Nutr.* **2003**, *77*, 1146–1155. [CrossRef] [PubMed]
4. Vitali, C.; Khetarpal, S.A.; Rader, D.J. Cholesterol Metabolism and the Risk of CHD: New Insights from Human Genetics. *Curr. Cardiol. Rep.* **2017**, *19*, 132. [CrossRef] [PubMed]
5. Ference, B.A.; Kastelein, J.J.P.; Ray, K.K.; Ginsberg, H.N.; Chapman, M.J.; Packard, C.J.; Laufs, U.; Oliver-Williams, C.; Wood, A.M.; Butterworth, A.S.; et al. Association of Triglyceride-Lowering LPL Variants and LDL-C-Lowering LDLR Variants with Risk of Coronary Heart Disease. *JAMA* **2019**, *321*, 364–373. [CrossRef] [PubMed]
6. Miller, M.; Sorkin, J.D.; Mastella, L.; Sutherland, A.; Rhyne, J.; Donnelly, P.; Simpson, K.; Goldberg, A.P. Poly is more effective than monounsaturated fat for dietary management in the metabolic syndrome: The muffin study. *J. Clin. Lipidol.* **2016**, *10*, 996–1003. [CrossRef] [PubMed]
7. Chen, G.C.; Szeto, I.M.; Chen, L.H.; Han, S.F.; Li, Y.J.; van Hekezen, R.; Qin, L.Q. Dairy products consumption and metabolic syndrome in adults: Systematic review and meta-analysis of observational studies. *Sci. Rep.* **2015**, *5*, 14606. [CrossRef]
8. Coulston, A.M.; Hollenbeck, C.B.; Reaven, G.M.; Swislocki, A.L.M. Persistence of Hypertriglyceridemic Effect of Low-Fat High-Carbohydrate Diets in NIDDM Patients. *Diabetes Care* **1989**, *12*, 94–101. [CrossRef]
9. Hollenbeck, C.B.; Coulston, A.M. Effects of dietary carbohydrate and fat intake on glucose and lipoprotein metabolism in individuals with diabetes mellitus. *Diabetes Care* **1991**, *14*, 774–785. [CrossRef]
10. Riccardi, G.; Rivellese, A.A.; Mokdad, A.H.; Ford, E.S.; Bowman, B.A.; Nelson, D.E.; Engelgau, M.M.; Vinicor, F.; Marks, J.S. Effects of Dietary Fiber and Carbohydrate on Glucose and Lipoprotein Metabolism in Diabetic Patients. *Diabetes Care* **1991**, *14*, 1115–1125. [CrossRef]
11. Te Morenga, L.A.; Howatson, A.J.; Jones, R.M.; Mann, J. Dietary sugars and cardiometabolic risk: Systematic review and meta-analyses of randomized controlled trials of the effects on blood pressure and lipids. *Am. J. Clin. Nutr.* **2014**, *100*, 65–79. [CrossRef] [PubMed]
12. Gibson, S.; Gunn, P.; Wittekind, A.; Cottrell, R. The Effects of Sucrose on Metabolic Health: A Systematic Review of Human Intervention Studies in Healthy Adults. *Crit. Rev. Food Sci. Nutr.* **2013**, *53*, 591–614. [CrossRef] [PubMed]
13. Howard, B.V.; Abbott, W.G.; A Swinburn, B. Evaluation of Metabolic Effects of Substitution of Complex Carbohydrates for Saturated Fat in Individuals with Obesity and NIDDM. *Diabetes Care* **1991**, *14*, 786–795. [CrossRef] [PubMed]
14. Vitale, M.; Masulli, M.; Rivellese, A.A.; Babini, A.C.; Boemi, M.; Bonora, E.; Buzzetti, R.; Ciano, O.; Cignarelli, M.; Cigolini, M.; et al. Influence of dietary fat and carbohydrates proportions on plasma lipids, glucose control and low-grade inflammation in patients with type 2 diabetes-The TOSCA.IT Study. *Eur. J. Nutr.* **2016**, *55*, 1645–1651. [CrossRef] [PubMed]
15. Vitale, M.; Masulli, M.; Calabrese, I.; Rivellese, A.A.; Bonora, E.; Signorini, S.; Perriello, G.; Squatrito, S.; Buzzetti, R.; Sartore, G.; et al. Impact of a Mediterranean Dietary Pattern and Its Components on Cardiovascular Risk Factors, Glucose Control, and Body Weight in People with Type 2 Diabetes: A Real-Life Study. *Nutrients* **2018**, *10*, 1067. [CrossRef]
16. Qian, F.; Korat, A.A.; Malik, V.; Hu, F.B. Metabolic Effects of Monounsaturated Fatty Acid–Enriched Diets Compared with Carbohydrate or Polyunsaturated Fatty Acid–Enriched Diets in Patients with Type 2 Diabetes: A Systematic Review and Meta-analysis of Randomized Controlled Trials. *Diabetes Care* **2016**, *39*, 1448–1457. [CrossRef]
17. Chen, J.P.; Chen, G.C.; Wang, X.P.; Qin, L.; Bai, Y. Dietary Fiber and Metabolic Syndrome: A Meta-Analysis and Review of Related Mechanisms. *Nutrients* **2017**, *10*, 24. [CrossRef]
18. Lu, M.; Wan, Y.; Yang, B.; Huggins, C.E.; Li, D. Effects of low-fat compared with high-fat diet on cardiometabolic indicators in people with overweight and obesity without overt metabolic disturbance: A systematic review and meta-analysis of randomised controlled trials. *Br. J. Nutr.* **2018**, *119*, 96–108. [CrossRef]

19. Guo, X.F.; Li, X.; Shi, M.; Li, D. n-3 Polyunsaturated Fatty Acids and Metabolic Syndrome Risk: A Meta-Analysis. *Nutrients* **2017**, *9*, 703. [CrossRef]
20. Eslick, G.D.; Howe, P.R.; Smith, C.; Priest, R.; Bensoussan, A. Benefits of fish oil supplementation in hyperlipidemia: A systematic review and meta-analysis. *Int. J. Cardiol.* **2009**, *136*, 4–16. [CrossRef]
21. Wanders, A.J.; Blom, W.A.M.; Zock, P.L.; Geleijnse, J.M.; A Brouwer, I.; Alssema, M. Plant-derived polyunsaturated fatty acids and markers of glucose metabolism and insulin resistance: A meta-analysis of randomized controlled feeding trials. *BMJ Open Diabetes Res. Care* **2019**, *7*, e000585. [CrossRef] [PubMed]
22. Imamura, F.; Micha, R.; Wu, J.H.; de Oliveira Otto, M.C.; Otite, F.O.; Abioye, A.I.; Mozaffarian, D. Effects of Saturated Fat, Polyunsaturated Fat, Monounsaturated Fat, and Carbohydrate on Glucose-Insulin Homeostasis: A Systematic Review and Meta-analysis of Randomised Controlled Feeding Trials. *PLoS Med.* **2016**, *13*, e1002087. [CrossRef] [PubMed]
23. Shah, M.; Adams-Huet, B.; Garg, A. Effect of high-carbohydrate or high-cis-monounsaturated fat diets on blood pressure: A meta-analysis of intervention trials. *Am. J. Clin. Nutr.* **2007**, *85*, 1251–1256. [CrossRef] [PubMed]
24. Huntriss, R.; Campbell, M.; Bedwell, C. The interpretation and effect of a low-carbohydrate diet in the management of type 2 diabetes: A systematic review and meta-analysis of randomised controlled trials. *Eur. J. Clin. Nutr.* **2018**, *72*, 311–325. [CrossRef] [PubMed]
25. Mansoor, N.; Vinknes, K.J.; Veierød, M.B.; Retterstøl, K. Effects of low-carbohydrate diets v. low-fat diets on body weight and cardiovascular risk factors: A meta-analysis of randomised controlled trials. *Br. J. Nutr.* **2016**, *115*, 466–479. [CrossRef]
26. Luscombe-Marsh, N.D.; Noakes, M.; Buckley, J.; Wittert, G.A.; Yancy, W.S.; Brinkworth, G.D.; Tay, J.; Thompson, C.H. A Very Low-Carbohydrate, Low–Saturated Fat Diet for Type 2 Diabetes Management: A Randomized Trial. *Diabetes Care* **2014**, *37*, 2909–2918. [CrossRef]
27. Tay, J.; Luscombe-Marsh, N.D.; Thompson, C.H.; Noakes, M.; Buckley, J.; Wittert, G.A.; Yancy, W.S., Jr.; Brinkworth, G.D. Comparison of low- and high-carbohydrate diets for type 2 diabetes management: A randomized trial. *Am. J. Clin. Nutr.* **2015**, *102*, 780–790. [CrossRef]
28. Tay, J.; Thompson, C.H.; Luscombe-Marsh, N.D.; Wycherley, T.P.; Noakes, M.; Buckley, J.D.; Wittert, G.A.; Yancy, W.S., Jr.; Brinkworth, G.D. Effects of an energy-restricted low-carbohydrate, high unsaturated fat/low saturated fat diet versus a high-carbohydrate, low-fat diet in type 2 diabetes: A 2-year randomized clinical trial. *Diabetes Obes. Metab.* **2018**, *20*, 858–871. [CrossRef]
29. Tardy, A.L.; Lambert-Porcheron, S.; Malpuech-Brugère, C.; Giraudet, C.; Rigaudière, J.P.; Laillet, B.; Leruyet, P.; Peyraud, J.L.; Boirie, Y.; Laville, M.; et al. Dairy and industrial sources of trans fat do not impair peripheral insulin sensitivity in overweight women. *Am. J. Clin. Nutr.* **2009**, *90*, 88–94. [CrossRef]
30. Bendsen, N.T.; Haugaard, S.B.; Larsen, T.M.; Chabanova, E.; Stender, S.; Astrup, A. Effect of trans-fatty acid intake on insulin sensitivity and intramuscular lipids–a randomized trial in overweight postmenopausal women. *Metabolism* **2011**, *60*, 906–913. [CrossRef]
31. Fasching, P.; Ratheiser, K.; Schneeweiss, B.; Rohac, M.; Nowotny, P.; Waldhäusl, W. No effect of short-term dietary supplementation of saturated and poly-and monounsaturated fatty acids on insulin secretion and sensitivity in healthy men. *Ann. Nutr. Metab.* **1996**, *40*, 116–122. [CrossRef] [PubMed]
32. Borkman, M.; Campbell, L.V.; Chisholm, D.J.; Storlien, L.H. Comparison of the effects on insulin sensitivity of high carbohydrate and high fat diets in normal subjects. *J. Clin. Endocrinol. Metab.* **1991**, *72*, 432–437. [CrossRef] [PubMed]
33. Vessby, B.; Uusitupa, M.; Hermansen, K.; Riccardi, G.; Rivellese, A.A.; Tapsell, L.C.; Nälsén, C.; Berglund, L.; Louheranta, A.; Rasmussen, B.M.; et al. Substituting dietary saturated for monounsaturated fat impairs insulin sensitivity in healthy men and women: The KANWU Study. *Diabetologia* **2001**, *44*, 312–319. [CrossRef] [PubMed]
34. Ryan, M.C.; Itsiopoulos, C.; Thodis, T.; Ward, G.; Trost, N.; Hofferberth, S.; O'Dea, K.; Desmond, P.V.; Johnson, N.A.; Wilson, A.M. The Mediterranean diet improves hepatic steatosis and insulin sensitivity in individuals with non-alcoholic fatty liver disease. *J. Hepatol.* **2013**, *59*, 138–143. [CrossRef] [PubMed]

35. Yubero-Serrano, E.M.; Delgado-Lista, J.; Tierney, A.C.; Perez-Martinez, P.; Garcia-Rios, A.; Alcala-Diaz, J.F.; Castaño, J.P.; Tinahones, F.J.; A Drevon, C.; Defoort, C.; et al. Insulin resistance determines a differential response to changes in dietary fat modification on metabolic syndrome risk factors: The LIPGENE study. *Am. J. Clin. Nutr.* **2015**, *102*, 1509–1517. [CrossRef] [PubMed]
36. Paniagua, J.A.; Pérez-Martinez, P.; Gjelstad, I.M.; Tierney, A.C.; Delgado-Lista, J.; Defoort, C.; Blaak, E.E.; Risérus, U.; Drevon, C.A.; Kiec-Wilk, B.; et al. A low-fat high-carbohydrate diet supplemented with long-chain n-3 PUFA reduces the risk of the metabolic syndrome. *Atherosclerosis* **2011**, *218*, 443–450. [CrossRef] [PubMed]

10

Metabolic Syndrome and its Associated Early-Life Factors among Chinese and Spanish Adolescents

Jiao Wang [1], Javier S. Perona [2], Jacqueline Schmidt-RioValle [3,*], Yajun Chen [1,*], Jin Jing [1] and Emilio González-Jiménez [3]

1 Department of Maternal and Child Health Care, School of Public Health, Sun Yat-Sen University, Guangzhou 510080, China

2 Instituto de la Grasa (CSIC), Campus Universidad Pablo de Olavide, Edificio 46, 41013 Seville, Spain

3 Departamento de Enfermería, CTS-436 Adscrito al Centro de Investigación Mente, Cerebro y Comportamiento (CIMCYC), University of Granada, Av/Ilustración 60, 18016 Granada, Spain

* Correspondence: jschmidt@ugr.es (J.S.-R.V.); chenyj68@mail.sysu.edu.cn (Y.C.)

Abstract: Metabolic syndrome (MetS) is a growing problem worldwide in adolescents. This study compared two sample populations of young people in Spain and China, and analyzed the association of birth weight and breastfeeding duration with MetS. A cross-sectional study was conducted in adolescents (10–15 years old); 1150 Chinese and 976 Spanish adolescents. The variables analyzed were anthropometric characteristics, biochemical markers, and demographic characteristics using the same methodology and data collection protocol. Also, birth weight and breastfeeding were retrospectively analyzed during the first year of life. The results showed statistically significant differences between the two groups in reference to body mass index (BMI), blood pressure, triglyceride, glucose, and high-density lipoprotein cholesterol (HDL-C) levels. The MetS prevalence was higher in Spanish adolescents (2.5%) than in the Chinese group (0.5%). Breastfeeding duration was inversely associated with hypertriglyceridemia, low HDL-C, and MetS, whereas higher birth weight was associated with hyperglycemia, low HDL-C, hypertriglyceridemia, and abdominal obesity. Spanish adolescents showed more altered MetS components, and consequently, a higher MetS prevalence than the Chinese adolescents. This made them more vulnerable to cardiometabolic risk. Our results highlight the need for interventions designed by health professionals, which would encourage pregnant women to breastfeed their children.

Keywords: metabolic syndrome; adolescents; breastfeeding duration; birth weight

---

1. Introduction

Metabolic syndrome (MetS) involves a cluster of risk factors. Subjects with MetS typically have at least three of the following conditions; abdominal obesity, hyperglycemia, hypertension, hypertriglyceridemia, and low HDL-cholesterol (HDL-C) levels [1]. MetS has been found to be strongly associated with a higher risk of cardiovascular disease in adults [2,3]. Unfortunately, there is a lack of data regarding MetS and its associated factors in childhood and adolescence. This is particularly the case in emerging countries such as China [4].

The prevalence of MetS in adolescents is currently increasing throughout the world [5]. In a Spanish population of 976 adolescents, 10–15 years of age, González-Jiménez et al. [6] observed a MetS prevalence of 3.9% in girls and 5.4% in boys. In contrast, Xu et al. [7] obtained a prevalence of 0.8% in Chinese adolescents over 10 years old. Similarly, in a study of 1770 Chinese adolescents by Wang et al. [8], the overall prevalence was 1.1%, though boys were more affected by MetS than girls. In these three studies, MetS was defined following to the criteria proposed by the International Diabetes Federation (IDF) for children and adolescents. According to these studies carried out in China and Spain it might be expected that MetS would be less frequent in Chinese adolescents. However, to date there has been no comparative study of MetS in sample populations in Spain and China.

It is crucial to identify the risk factors leading to the development of MetS in young people so that this disorder can be rapidly detected and prevented [9]. Accordingly, it has been suggested that a higher birth weight may be associated with an early development of insulin resistance and MetS [10]. An excessively short period (or absence) of breastfeeding during the first year of childhood seems to be another risk factor for MetS [11]. In González-Jiménez et al. [6] and Wang et al. [8], a high birth weight was significantly associated with MetS, whereas breastfeeding for longer than six months was inversely associated with the syndrome. Nevertheless, there is no consensus of opinion on this issue since the absence of conclusive results in Western and Chinese populations [12] has generated a certain controversy regarding the influence of these variables [13].

The initial hypothesis of this research was that the difference in MetS prevalence in China and Spain was probably related to differences in birth weight and breastfeeding duration. To confirm this hypothesis, our objectives were to compare the prevalence of MetS in Chinese and Spanish adolescents, and then analyze the associations of MetS with birth weight and breastfeeding duration (first year of life).

2. Materials and Methods

2.1. Study Design and Participants

Accordingly, we decided to conduct a comparative analysis of two cross-sectional studies. The first study was of a sample of Chinese adolescents, and the second study was of a sample of Spanish adolescents. In China, the research was carried out in the city of Guangzhou (southern China). Four districts were randomly selected, which comprised a total of ten schools. A letter of invitation was sent to the school principals along with an information sheet and an explanation of the research methodology and objectives. All parents, tutors, and legal guardians of the minors gave their written informed consent. The study had been previously approved by the Ethics Committee of the School of Public Health in Sun Yat-sen University.

In each of the ten schools, two classes per course were randomly selected and invited to participate in the study. A total of 1150 adolescents (554 boys and 596 girls), 10–15 years of age, were finally recruited for the study. All participants had a medium socioeconomic status and the response rate was 87%.

In Spain, the study was conducted in the province of Granada (southeastern Spain), a total of eighteen schools throughout the province were randomly selected. The study had been previously approved by the Board of Education of the Andalusian Regional Government (Granada Delegation), and authorized by the school directors. It had also been approved by the Ethics Committee of the University of Granada. All parents, tutors, and guardians had explicitly authorized the participation of their children.

In each of the schools, two classes per course were randomly selected and invited to participate in the study. Finally, a total of 976 adolescents, (457 boys and 519 girls), 10–15 years of age, were recruited. All of the subjects were Spanish and had a medium socioeconomic status.

Both in the Chinese and Spanish groups, adolescents with serious physical handicaps or psychological conditions (e.g., congenital disorder and cognitive dysfunction) were excluded from the study. The flow diagram (Figure 1) describes the selection process followed in both countries.

All procedures used in this study were in accordance with the ethical standards of the institutional and/or national research committee and with the 1964 Helsinki declaration and its later amendments or comparable ethical standards.

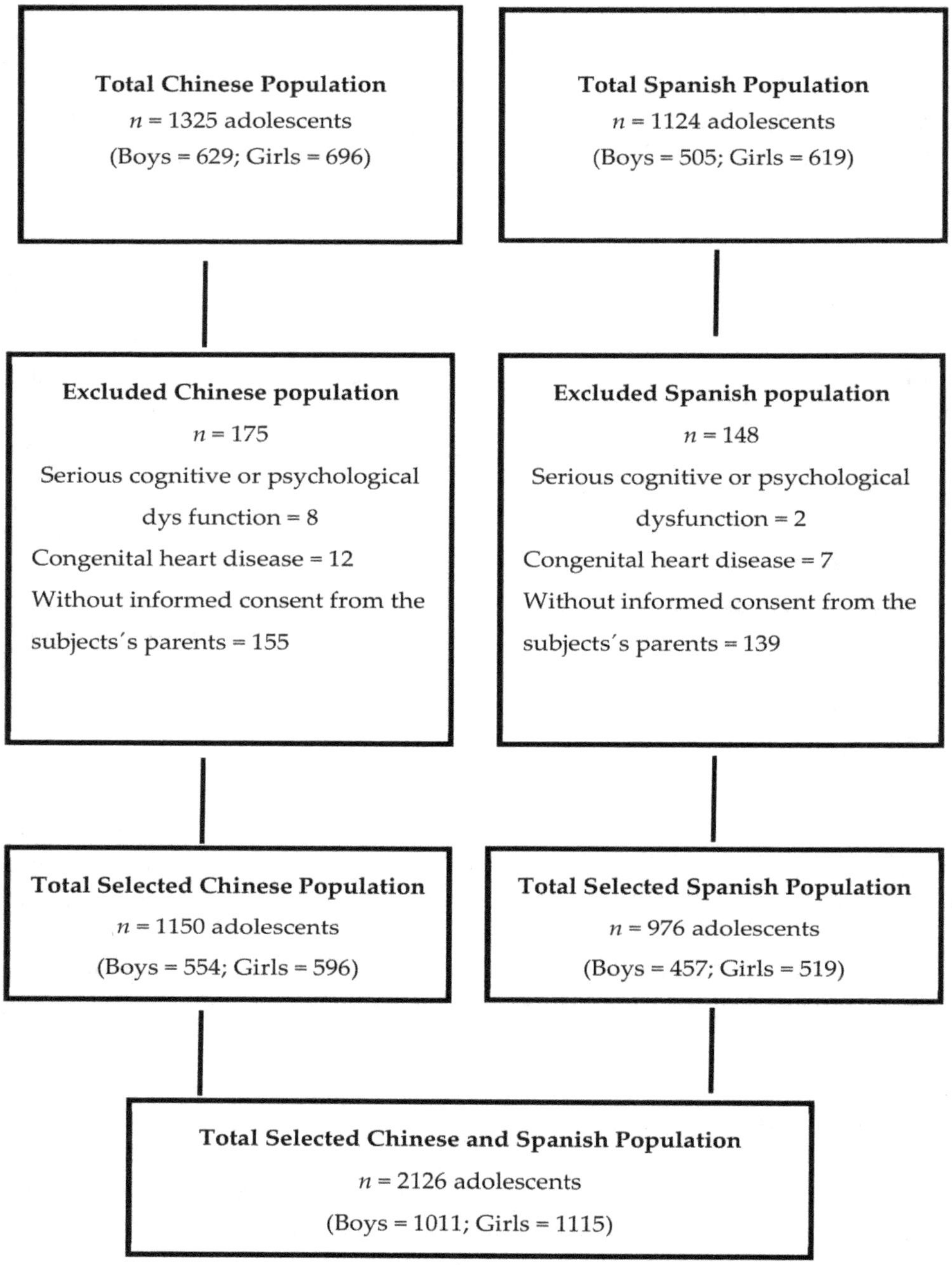

Figure 1. Flow diagram of the recruitment progress.

2.2. Data Collection and Measurements

The instrument used for data collection was a standard questionnaire elaborated ad hoc. The questionnaire was filled out during a face-to-face interview with one of the parents or guardians. The average questionnaire completion time was 20–25 min.

Questionnaire items focused on the collection of demographic data and information regarding birth weight and breastfeeding during the subjects' first year of life. All of this information was collected retrospectively. Furthermore, in order to guarantee the accuracy of the answers, parents were asked to bring the Child Health Record of their son/daughter. This document had been previously filled out by health professionals and contained accurate birth-weight and breastfeeding information. The completed questionnaires were reviewed by trained staff and uploaded into the database.

All participants underwent a complete anthropometric evaluation in accordance with the guidelines of the International Society for the Advancement of Kinanthropometry [14]. The variables assessed were weight, height, waist circumference (WC), hip circumference (HC), and BMI (weight (kg)/height (m)^2). In the Chinese sample, fasting body weight was measured to the nearest 0.1 kg on a double ruler scale (RGT-140, Wujin Hengqi Co. Ltd, Changzhou, China). During this assessment, participants were wearing light clothing and no shoes. In the Spanish sample, the subjects (also in light clothing and no shoes) were weighed on a self-calibrating Seca 861 Class (III) Digital Floor Scale (Hamburg, Germany) with a precision of up to 0.1 kg.

In the Chinese sample, height was measured to an accuracy of 1mm with a freestanding stadiometer mounted on a rigid tripod (GMCS-I; Xindong Huateng Sports Equipment Co. Ltd, Beijing, China) by trained interviewers following a standardized protocol. Participants were asked to stand erect with their back, buttocks, and heels in continuous contact with the vertical height rod of the stadiometer and their head orientated in the Frankfurt plane. The horizontal headpiece was then placed on top of their head to measure their height. The height of the Spanish children was measured with a Seca 214* portable stadiometer (seca gmbh & co., Hamburg, Germany), following the same procedure as in the Chinese study.

WC was measured with a Seca automatic roll-up measuring tape (precision of 1 mm) using the horizontal plane midway between the lowest rib and the upper border of the iliac crest at the end of a normal inspiration/expiration. HC was measured at the maximum extension of the buttocks as viewed from the right side. The average of two consecutive measurements was the value used in the analyses. In both samples, waist-to-height ratio was calculated as WC (cm) divided by height (cm), whereas waist-to-hip ratio was calculated by dividing WC by HC. The corresponding intraobserver technical error (reliability) of the measurements was 0.95%.

In the Chinese sample, blood pressure levels were calculated with a previously calibrated aneroid sphygmomanometer and a Littmann® stethoscope (3M Health Care, Saint Paul, MI, USA) after each participant had rested for at least 15 min in a sitting position, according to the BP measurement guidelines of the Subcommittee of Professional and Public Education of the American Heart Association Council on High Blood Pressure Research [15]. Diastolic pressure was defined as the point of disappearance of the Korotkoff sounds (fifth phase). Blood pressure was taken twice on the right arm with an appropriately sized cuff. The average of two readings obtained at a minimum interval of 5 min was recorded. In the Spanish sample, blood pressure levels were calculated with the same equipment and following the same procedure as the research team in China.

2.3. Serum Biochemical Examination

The biochemical variables analyzed were fasting glucose (FG), HDL-C, and triglycerides (TG). At 8 a.m., after a 12 h overnight fast, 10 mL of blood was extracted by venipuncture from the antecubital fossa of the right arm with a disposable vacuum blood collection tube. In the 4 hours after extraction, all samples were centrifuged at 3500 rpm for 15 min (Z400 K, Hermle, Wehingen, Germany). Red blood cells were separated and serum was finally frozen at −80 °C for its subsequent analysis. FG was measured with a colorimetric enzymatic method (GOD-PAP Method, Human Diagnostics, Germany). HDL-C and TG were also calculated by means of a colorimetric enzymatic method with an Olympus analyzer (GmbH company, Hamburg, Germany). The techniques and equipment employed in the biochemical analysis were the same in both samples. The precision performance of these assays was within the manufacturer's specifications. In both populations, blood samples were taken at the educational center in a classroom especially designated for this purpose and on different days in order to guarantee the fasting of the participants.

2.4. Diagnostic Criteria of Metabolic Syndrome according to the International Diabetes Federation, IDF

The definition of MetS was based on the criteria of the IDF, adapted for children and adolescents. These criteria were abdominal obesity (defined by WC adult ethnicity-specific cutoffs: ≥94 cm in men and ≥80 cm in women for the Spanish and ≥90 cm in men and ≥80 cm in women for the Chinese) and the presence of two or more clinical features, including TG ≥1.7 mmol/L, HDL-C <1.03 mmol/L, systolic blood pressure (SBP) ≥130 mmHg and/or diastolic blood pressure (DBP) ≥85 mmHg, and serum FG ≥5.6 mmol/L [16].

2.5. Statistical Analysis

Descriptive statistics were calculated for all of the variables, including continuous variables (reported as mean and standard deviation) and categorical variables (reported as number and percentage). A *p*-value of 0.05 and a power of 80% were used to determine sample sizes. The differences between sexes, ages, and countries for the variables studied were evaluated using Student's *t*-test, ANOVA, nonparametric test, or the χ^2 test, as appropriate. Pearson/Spearman's correlation coefficients between MetS components and their associated factors were also calculated. In the total sample and separated sample, multivariable logistic regression analyses (Enter method) were employed to identify the relationship between MetS and its features in the form of outcomes (abdominal obesity, low HDL-C, hyperglycemia, hypertriglyceridemia, hypertension), and associated factors. The multivariable logistic analysis in the country of origin (China), breastfeeding duration (months), and birth weight (100 g) was sex-adjusted and age-adjusted to control the influence of puberty. The prevalence odds ratios and the corresponding 95% confidence intervals were calculated as well. All statistical analyses were performed with the statistical software package SPSS version 21.0 (IBM, Armonk, NY, USA). In this study, *p*-values of less than 0.05 were regarded as statistically significant.

3. Results

Table 1. shows the data collected from the participants, including demographic information, anthropometry, MetS features, and early-life factors. It was observed that Spanish children had higher mean values for height, weight, BMI, WC, TG, and SBP than Chinese children. Generally speaking, the Spanish sample had also been breastfed for a longer period of time in their first year of life (9 months on average).

Table 1. Demographic and clinical characteristics of Chinese and Spanish adolescents.

Variable	Chinese Adolescents	Spanish Adolescents	*p*-Value
Demographic information			
n	1150	976	
Boys (%)	554 (48.2)	457 (45.7)	0.28
Age (years)	12.9 ± 1.8	13.1 ± 1.2	0.09
Anthropometry			
Height (m)	1.55 ± 0.14	1.59 ± 0.10	<0.01 **
Weight (kg)	46.28 ± 14.01	54.77 ± 12.71	<0.01 **
BMI (kg/m^2)	19.24 ± 7.25	21.22 ± 3.79	<0.01 **
HC (cm)	81.06 ± 16.91	83.82 ± 9.35	0.21
WHR	0.84 ± 0.09	0.87 ± 0.16	<0.01 **
WHtR	0.44 ± 0.07	0.45 ± 0.07	0.01 *
Metabolic syndrome features			
WC (cm)	66.7 ± 10.6	72.3 ± 10.8	<0.01 **
FG (mmol/L)	4.62 ± 0.49	4.77 ± 1.68	0.01 *
HDL-C (mmol/L)	1.4 ± 0.3	1.0 ± 0.1	<0.01 **
TG (mmol/L)	0.97 ± 0.51	1.43 ± 0.60	<0.01 **
SBP (mmHg)	99.9 ± 23.2	118.0 ± 15.5	<0.01 **
DBP (mmHg)	63.6 ± 15.7	64.1 ± 9.0	0.35
Information of early-life factors			
Breastfeeding duration (month)	4.2 ± 3.7	9.2 ± 2.7	<0.01 **
Breastfeeding duration range (month)	0~13	0~13	
Birth weight (kg)	3.23 ± 0.47	3.20 ± 0.50	0.09
Birth weight range (kg)	1.4~4.9	2.0~5.7	

Notes: BMI, body mass index; HC, hip circumference; WHR, waist-to-hip ratio; WHtR, waist-to-height ratio; WC, waist circumference; FG, fasting glucose; HDL-C, high-density lipoprotein cholesterol; TG, triglyceride; SBP, systolic blood pressure; DBP, diastolic blood pressure. Values are expressed as mean ± SD. The *p*-value was calculated by chi-square test for category variables and two-sample *t*-test for continuous variables. * $p < 0.05$, ** $p < 0.01$.

Regarding the prevalence of MetS and its components, Table 2 shows statistically significant differences between the two cohorts. As can be observed, the Spanish adolescents had a higher prevalence of abdominal obesity, hyperglycemia, and hypertension. In contrast, Chinese adolescents were more prone to hypertriglyceridemia though TG mean values were higher in the Spanish cohort. Consequently, the prevalence of MetS was 2.5% in the Spanish adolescents in comparison to 0.5% in the Chinese group.

Table 2. Prevalence of metabolic syndrome and its components in Chinese and Spanish adolescents.

Characteristics	Chinese Adolescents (n = 1150)	Spanish Adolescents (n = 976)
Abdominal obesity	65 (5.5)	128 (13.1) **
Hypertension	11 (1.0)	256 (26.2) **
Hyperglycemia	23 (2.0)	65 (6.7) **
Low HDL-C	160 (13.9)	176 (18.0) *
Hypertriglyceridemia	84 (7.3)	32 (3.3) **
Pattern of risk factors clustering		
0 Component	886 (77.0)	568 (58.2) **
1 Component	193 (16.8)	234 (24.0) **
2 Components	61 (5.6)	120 (12.3) **
≥3 Components	7 (0.6)	54 (5.5) **
MetS	6 (0.5)	24 (2.5) **

Notes: HDL-C, high-density lipoprotein cholesterol; MetS, metabolic syndrome. Values are expressed as numbers of individuals (%). p-value was calculated by chi-square; * $p < 0.05$, ** $p < 0.01$.

Generally, the correlations of breastfeeding duration or birth weight with MetS and its components (Table 3) differed in Chinese and Spanish individuals. In Chinese adolescents correlations were weak. In the case of the Spaniards, the duration of breastfeeding correlated positively with HDL-C (0.81) and negatively with FG (−0.89) and TG (−0.64). In contrast, birth weight correlated negatively with HDL-C (−0.58) and positively with FG (0.65) and TG (0.48). In the Chinese cohort, birth weight was found to be positively associated with WC (0.15), SBP (0.08), and DBP (0.07).

Table 3. The association of metabolic syndrome features and early-life factors in Chinese and Spanish adolescents.

	Chinese Adolescents (n = 1150)		Spanish Adolescents (n = 976)	
	Breastfeeding Duration	Birth Weight	Breastfeeding Duration	Birth Weight
WC	−0.04	0.15 **	0.05	0.10 **
FG	0.03	0.01	−0.89 **	0.65 **
HDL-C	−0.04	−0.01	0.81 **	−0.58 **
TG	0.09 **	−0.04	−0.64 **	0.48 **
SBP	0.03	0.08 *	−0.03	0.06
DBP	−0.02	0.07 *	−0.02	0.07 *

Notes: WC, waist circumference; FG, fasting glucose; HDL-C, high-density lipoprotein cholesterol; TG, triglyceride; SBP, systolic blood pressure; DBP, diastolic blood pressure; MetS, metabolic syndrome. Data are presented as Pearson/Spearman's correlation coefficients. * $p < 0.05$ ** $p < 0.01$.

Table 4 shows the adjusted associations of Mets features with early life factors including breastfeeding duration and birth weight in Chinese and Spanish adolescents. In the Spanish adolescents, breastfeeding duration had stronger associations with low HDL-C (OR 0.18), hyperglycemia (OR 0.17), hypertriglyceridemia (OR 0.52), and MetS (0.62) than in the Chinese adolescents. However, birth weight had closer associations with abdominal obesity (OR 1.09) in Chinese subjects and closer associations with hyperglycemia (OR 6.65) in Spanish subjects.

Table 4. Risk of MetS features based on associated factors from multivariable logistic regression in two sample.

	Chinese Adolescents (n = 1150)		Spanish Adolescents (n = 976)	
	Breastfeeding Duration (month)	**Birth Weight (100 g)**	**Breastfeeding Duration (month)**	**Birth Weight (100 g)**
	OR (95% CI)	OR (95% CI)	OR (95% CI)	OR (95% CI)
Abdominal obesity	0.95 (0.88, 1.02)	1.09 (1.03, 1.16)	0.98 (0.90, 1.07)	1.04 (0.99, 1.10)
Low HDL-C	1.03 (0.98, 1.08)	1.17 (0.98, 1.06)	0.18 (0.13, 0.26)	1.06 (0.93, 1.21)
Hyperglycemia	0.96 (0.86, 1.08)	0.96 (0.88, 1.05)	0.17 (0.04, 0.72)	6.65 (1.83, 24.19)
Hypertriglyceridemia	1.03 (0.97, 1.10)	0.99 (0.94, 1.04)	0.52 (0.40, 0.70)	1.09 (0.93, 1.27)
Hypertension	1.10 (0.91, 1.32)	1.07 (0.92, 1.23)	0.96 (0.90, 1.03)	1.02 (0.99, 1.07)
MetS	1.07 (0.87, 1.32)	0.93 (0.80, 1.08)	0.62 (0.51, 0.76)	0.98 (0.86, 1.12)

Note: Age and gender were adjusted in all above models.

Furthermore, the combined multivariable analysis of MetS and its components showed that girls were more likely to develop abdominal obesity than boys (Table 5). In addition, there was a strong association of MetS and its components with the participants' country of origin. In general, Spanish participants were at greater risk of MetS or of the alteration of certain MetS components. In this regard, the Spaniards had a higher risk of hypertension (OR 45.05), hyperglycemia (OR 26.85), and MetS (OR 13.6) than the Chinese adolescents. For the early-life factors, breastfeeding duration was negatively associated with hypertriglyceridemia (OR 0.87), low HDL-C (OR 0.81), hyperglycemia (OR 0.60), and MetS (OR 0.74), whereas higher birth weight was positively associated with MetS components such as hyperglycemia (OR 1.96) and abdominal obesity (OR 1.15) in the total sample. We also performed analyses to assess the interaction of breastfeeding duration and the country of origin and birth weight with the country of origin, using China as reference. When the interaction of breastfeeding duration and the country of origin was assessed, we observed that the effect was significant for low HDL-C, hyperglycemia and hypertriglyceridemia. In contrast, the interaction of birth weight with the country of origin was significant only for hyperglycemia. The results of the sensitivity analysis showed that breastfeeding duration (longer than 6 months) was a protective factor for MetS (Supplementary Table S1).

Table 5. Risk of MetS features based on associated factors from multivariable logistic regression.

Variables (Reference)	Abdominal Obesity	Low HDL-C	Hyperglycemia	Hypertriglyceridemia	Hypertension	MetS
	OR (95% CI)	OR (95% CI)	OR (95% CI)	OR (95% CI)	OR (95% CI)	OR (95% CI)
Age	1.20 (1.09, 1.32)	1.07 (0.99, 1.15)	0.96 (0.80, 1.16)	0.92 (0.83, 1.02)	1.04 (0.93, 1.17)	1.01 (0.80, 1.28)
Gender (Boy)	2.40 (1.72, 3.35)	0.78 (0.58,1.07)	0.30 (0.12, 0.73)	0.79 (0.53, 1.20)	0.77 (0.58, 1.02)	1.76 (0.79, 3.89)
Country (China)	12.04 (0.58, 24.23)	3.84 (2.68, 5.49)	26.85 (11.76, 61.34)	0.70 (0.43, 1.15)	45.05 (21.71, 93.45)	13.6 (4.16, 44.54)
Breastfeeding duration (month)	0.91 (0.77, 1.08)	0.81 (0.78, 0.85)	0.60 (0.53, 0.68)	0.87 (0.82, 0.92)	1.10 (0.91, 1.32)	0.74 (0.65, 0.84)
Birth weight (100 g)	1.15 (1.01, 1.31)	0.98 (0.84, 1.10)	1.96 (1.88, 3.08)	0.99 (0.95, 1.04)	1.07 (0.92, 1.23)	0.94 (0.80, 1.09)
	p value	*p* value	*p* value	*p* value	*p* value	*p* value
Breastfeeding duration*Country	0.504	<0.001	<0.017	<0.001	0.187	<0.001
Birth weight*Country	0.211	0.578	<0.001	0.213	0.605	0.743

Notes: HDL-C, high-density lipoprotein cholesterol; MetS, metabolic syndrome. Data are presented as prevalence odds ratio (OR) with 95% confidence intervals (CI) using logistic regression model. Bold type indicates $p < 0.05$. All the shown risk factors in this model were included in the model at the same time.

4. Discussion

The results obtained showed that there were significant differences in the Chinese and Spanish samples in regard to most of the clinical features analyzed, whether anthropometric or metabolic. More specifically, Spanish adolescents were found to have considerably higher levels of TG and SBP in comparison to Chinese adolescents. In contrast, the children in the Chinese sample had lower BMI, WHR, and WC values. Generally speaking, these results suggest that the Chinese subjects were healthier than their Spanish counterparts, who had higher values for most of the clinical features [17,18]. This may be partially explained by the ethnic difference and different living environments. This evidently placed their health at risk and made them more vulnerable to cardiometabolic disorders [19]. These results indicate the need for an in-depth study of the lifestyle, and environmental factors affecting the population in China and Spain. Any or all of these could be factors that would explain the differences found between adolescents in the two countries.

Our results also showed differences between the Chinese and Spanish samples regarding MetS components. As in previous studies of the Spanish population [20] and based on the definition of MetS used, Spanish children and adolescents had higher levels of abdominal obesity, hyperglycemia, as well as a higher rate of hypertension when compared to the Chinese group. Nevertheless, the prevalence of MetS was still lower than that reported by Holst-Schumacher et al. [21] for adolescents in Costa Rica (5.6%) or that described by Alvarez et al. [22] for adolescents in Brazil (6%). The only variable that was higher in Chinese cohort was the value for hypertriglyceridemia, which was in agreement with Liang et al. [23] who studied another population of 976 Chinese adolescents.

Breastfeeding duration and birth weight correlated closely with the components of MetS. In this regard, Spanish schoolchildren had been breastfed for a longer time. This correlated positively with HDL-C levels and negatively with other variables such as FG, TG, and MetS. These findings suggest the potentially positive effect of breastfeeding as a way to prevent the development of metabolic disorders in young subjects. These results contrasted with Yakubov et al. [24], who found no association between breastfeeding duration and the development of MetS and/or impairments of its components. However, this lack of association could be explained by factors such as the small size of the sample, a possible selection bias of the subjects or the range of breastfeeding duration.

In contrast, other studies did find a correlation between breastfeeding duration and a reduced incidence of MetS later in life [25,26]. Yet, it could be argued that since in the present study Spanish adolescents were breastfed for a longer time and had a higher prevalence of MetS compared to the Chinese group, breastfeeding would increase, rather than decrease, the risk of developing MetS. However, this assumption can not be made directly, due to the multifactorial nature of the metabolic syndrome. The inverse association between breastfeeding duration and MetS in childhood and adolescence has been observed elsewhere [12,27]. Indeed, in a previous study, we found a higher prevalence of MetS in young subjects that had not been breastfed as babies [6]. Moreover, Ekelund et al. [28] stated that the most important benefits of maternal breastfeeding in terms of MetS prevention were for those subjects who had been breastfed for more than 6 months.

In the present study, breastfeeding duration was the main factor affecting the differences observed in the risk of MetS features between Chinese and Spanish adolescents. In fact, the interaction between breastfeeding duration and country for MetS and its components resulted strongly significant. Chinese mother breastfed their infants for less than half of the time than did Spanish mothers but no differences were on served for the range (0–13 months). A survey carried out in the city of Guangzhou (the same city of origin of our study), revealed that Chinese mothers tend to stop breastfeeding early before the six months. The reasons given for breastfeeding cessation were, among others, insufficient milk supply, medical reasons, lactational factors, and return to work [29]. Regardless of their antenatal intention, women with higher BMI have a higher risk of early cessation of exclusive breastfeeding [30], which has been associated to anatomical and physiological issues, medical conditions, and sociocultural and psychological factors [31]. Unfortunately, we do not have data on the prevalence of overweight mothers at the time of pregnancy. In our study, birth weight correlated positively with FG, TG, and MetS in

Spanish subjects, as well as with WC in Chinese subjects. These findings do not coincide with those in Dos Santos et al. [32], who studied a population of 172 adolescents in Brazil and found that birth weight was not a risk factor in the development of MetS during adolescence. This result was probably conditioned by the small size of the Brazilian cohort, a possible bias in the selection of participants, or methodological differences in the evaluation of adiposity. Nonetheless, Yuan et al. [33] did find an association between birth weight and disorders such as adolescent obesity and MetS. Their population sample was much larger and was composed of 16,580 Chinese children and adolescents, 7–17 years of age, which is consistent with the Chinese sample in our study. Strikingly, the results obtained by Yuan et al. [33] were more in consonance with the Spanish results in our study than with the Chinese ones.

The results of the multivariable analysis of early MetS predictors with MetS and MetS components showed that girls had a higher risk of abdominal obesity, which agrees with previous research [34,35]. The high prevalence of central obesity in Spanish and Chinese girls is a matter of concern, since according to Lee et al. [36], it increases the risk of morbidity and mortality at early ages. Additionally, MetS and its components showed a strong association with the participants' country of origin. In other words, Spanish adolescents had a greater risk of MetS or the alteration of any of its components (e.g., hypertension or hyperglycemia) than the Chinese adolescents.

These results also contrast with those of Haldar et al. [37], who reported that Asian adults who emigrated and lived in European countries were more apt to become obese than Caucasians, regardless of the degree of adiposity. However, this may very well be due to changes in their dietary habits. To explain the discrepancies between the Chinese and Spanish populations, it could be argued that Spaniards are not typical Caucasians in regard to metabolic disorders. In comparison to young people in other European countries, children and adolescents in Spain are more prone to be overweight, which means greater metabolic risk. Accordingly, the prevalence of MetS in Spanish adolescents is higher than the MetS prevalence in other European countries, such as Finland (2.1%), Greece (0.7%) [38], Denmark, Estonia, and Portugal (1.4%) [28]. Other studies also highlight differences between ethnic groups in the distribution of body fat, which signifies that they are at greater risk of developing cardiovascular and metabolic pathologies [39,40].

Interestingly, our study found that hypertriglyceridemia was strongly affected by the duration of breastfeeding (OR 0.87), regardless of the participants' gender or country of origin. The association between breastfeeding in infancy and triglyceride concentrations later in life is still a matter of debate. The absence of an association was reported by Victoria et al. [41] in a Brazilian population of 18-year-old boys and by Lawlor et al. [42] in Estonian and Danish children and adolescents. In Lawlor et al. [42], BMI and TG values were similar to those obtained for the Chinese sample in our study, but lower than those for the Spanish group. More recently, Ramirez-Silva et al. [43] observed that children who had not been breastfed had higher TG levels at the age of 4, compared with those who had been partially or exclusively breastfed. There is a lack of consensus regarding the influence of birth weight on hyperglycemia.

This research has a number of strengths as well as certain limitations. Without a doubt, one of its strengths is its pioneering nature. Our study focused on two populations of adolescents with very different cultural backgrounds and analyzed not only the prevalence of MetS, but also the association between MetS and early predictors such as breastfeeding duration (first year of life) and birth weight. Yet another strength is the size of the sample, which enhances the validity of the results and assures comparability in future studies. Nonetheless, an evident limitation of the study is its cross-sectional nature and the lack of information about the eating habits and physical activity of both populations. Finally, no data regarding pubertal status were collected or taken into account but two subjects were excluded as outliers with extremely high triglyceride levels. This may have been a factor in the differences between the two countries. The results should thus be interpreted with caution.

5. Conclusions

In conclusion, our initial hypothesis was confirmed since Spanish adolescents showed a higher number of altered MetS components, and consequently a higher prevalence of MetS than Chinese adolescents. In addition, in the Spanish sample, breastfeeding duration and birth weight strongly correlated with MetS components in comparison to the Chinese group, where this was not the case. The Spanish adolescents also had a higher risk for hyperglycemia, hypertension, hypertriglyceridemia, and abdominal obesity.

The results of this study should have an impact on clinical practice. It is advisable for healthcare professionals to have an in-depth understanding of all of the factors associated with MetS. This knowledge and awareness are crucial to the prevention of this disease in adolescents. Likewise, as reflected in our results, it is important for healthcare professionals to encourage pregnant women to breastfeed their babies. This would improve the metabolic status of the mothers and at the same time make their children less vulnerable to obesity, diabetes mellitus type 2, and MetS. This is especially true for Spain, as we found important differences in the prevalence of MetS and its components between Chinese and Spanish adolescents, which were importantly affected by differences in breastfeeding duration in both countries. For this reason, a clear priority for health professionals should be to encourage breastfeeding.

Author Contributions: J.W. and E.G.-J. had full access to all the data in the study and takes responsibility for the integrity of the data and the accuracy of the data analysis. E.G.-J., J.S.P., and J.S.-R. drafted the manuscript, critically revised the manuscript, and agreed to be accountable for all aspects of work ensuring integrity and accuracy. E.G.J., J.S.P., Y.C., and J.J. contributed to conception and whole study design. All authors have read and approved the final manuscript.

Acknowledgments: In China, the authors gratefully acknowledge the contribution of Yuexiu, Haizhu, Liwan and Luogang Education Bureau and ten schools. In Spain, we would like to thank the schools, parents, and guardians as well as the students for participating in this study.

References

1. Weiss, R.; Bremer, A.A.; Lustig, R.H. What is metabolic syndrome, and why are children getting it? *Ann. N. Y. Acad. Sci.* **2013**, *1281*, 123–140. [CrossRef] [PubMed]
2. Schubert, C.M.; Sun, S.S.; Burns, T.L.; Morrison, J.A.; Huang, T.T. Predictive ability of childhood metabolic components for adult metabolic syndrome and type 2 diabetes. *J. Pediatr.* **2009**, *155*, S1–S6. [CrossRef] [PubMed]
3. Huang, T.T.; Sun, S.S.; Daniels, S.R. Understanding the nature of metabolic syndrome components in children and what they can and cannot do to predict adult disease. *J. Pediatr.* **2009**, *155*, e13–e14. [CrossRef] [PubMed]
4. Chen, F.; Wang, Y.; Shan, X.; Cheng, H.; Hou, D.; Zhao, X.; Wang, T.; Zhao, D.; Mi, J. Association between childhood obesity and metabolic syndrome: Evidence from a large sample of Chinese children and adolescents. *PLoS ONE* **2012**, *7*, e47380. [CrossRef] [PubMed]
5. Miller, J.M.; Kaylor, M.B.; Johannsson, M.; Bay, C.; Churilla, J.R. Prevalence of metabolic syndrome and individual criterion in US adolescents: 2001–2010 national health and nutrition examination survey. *Metab. Syndr. Relat. Disord.* **2014**, *12*, 527–532. [CrossRef] [PubMed]
6. Gonzalez-Jimenez, E.; Montero-Alonso, M.A.; Schmidt-RioValle, J.; Garcia-Garcia, C.J.; Padez, C. Metabolic syndrome in Spanish adolescents and its association with birth weight, breastfeeding duration, maternal smoking, and maternal obesity: A cross-sectional study. *Eur. J. Nutr.* **2015**, *54*, 589–597. [CrossRef] [PubMed]

7. Xu, H.; Li, Y.; Liu, A.; Zhang, Q.; Hu, X.; Fang, H.; Li, T.; Guo, H.; Li, Y.; Xu, G.; et al. Prevalence of the metabolic syndrome among children from six cities of China. *BMC Public Health* **2012**, *12*, 13. [CrossRef] [PubMed]
8. Wang, J.; Zhu, Y.; Cai, L.; Jing, J.; Chen, Y.; Mai, J.; Ma, L.; Ma, Y.; Ma, J. Metabolic syndrome and its associated early-life factors in children and adolescents: A cross-sectional study in Guangzhou, China. *Public Health Nutr.* **2016**, *19*, 1147–1154. [CrossRef]
9. Ahmadi, A.; Gharipour, M.; Nouri, F.; Sarrafzadegan, N. Metabolic syndrome in Iranian youths: A population-based study on junior and high schools students in rural and urban areas. *J. Diabetes Res.* **2012**, *2013*, 738485. [CrossRef]
10. Agius, R.; Savona-Ventura, C.; Vassallo, J. Transgenerational metabolic determinants of fetal birth weight. *Exp. Clin. Endocrinol. Diabetes.* **2013**, *121*, 431–435. [CrossRef]
11. Stuebe, A. The risks of not breastfeeding for mothers and infants. *Rev. Obstet. Gynecol.* **2009**, *2*, 222–231. [PubMed]
12. Yang, Z.; Huffman, S.L. Nutrition in pregnancy and early childhood and associations with obesity in developing countries. *Matern. Child. Nutr.* **2013**, *9*, 105–119. [CrossRef] [PubMed]
13. Wang, X.; Liang, L.; Junfen, F.U.; Lizhong, D.U. Metabolic syndrome in obese children born large for gestational age. *Indian J. Pediatr.* **2007**, *74*, 561–565. [CrossRef] [PubMed]
14. Marfell-Jones, M.; Olds, T.; Stewart, A. *International Standards for Anthropometric Assessment*; ISAK: Potchefstroom, South Africa, 2006.
15. Pickering, T.G.; Hall, J.E.; Appel, L.J.; Falkner, B.; Graves, J.; Hill, M.; Jones, D.W.; Kurtz, T.; Sheps, S.G.; Roccella, E.J. Subcommittee of professional and public education of the American heart association council on high blood pressure research. Recommendations for blood pressure measurement in humans and experimental animals, part 1: Blood pressure measurement in humans: A statement for professionals from the subcommittee of professional and public education of the American heart association council on high blood pressure research. *Hypertension* **2005**, *45*, 142–161. [PubMed]
16. Zimmet, P.; Alberti, K.G.; Kaufman, F.; Tajima, N.; Silink, M.; Arslanian, S.; Wong, G.; Bennett, P.; Shaw, J.; Caprio, S.; et al. The metabolic syndrome in children and adolescents—An IDF consensus report. *Pediatr. Diabetes* **2007**, *8*, 299–306. [CrossRef]
17. Kelishadi, R. Childhood overweight, obesity, and the metabolic syndrome in developing countries. *Epidemiol. Rev.* **2007**, *29*, 62–76. [CrossRef] [PubMed]
18. Gupta, N.; Shah, P.; Nayyar, S.; Misra, A. Childhood obesity and the metabolic syndrome in developing countries. *Indian J. Pediatr.* **2013**, *80*, S28–S37. [CrossRef]
19. Faienza, M.F.; Wang, D.Q.; Fruhbeck, G.; Garruti, G.; Portincasa, P. The dangerous link between childhood and adulthood predictors of obesity and metabolic syndrome. *Intern. Emerg. Med.* **2016**, *11*, 175–182. [CrossRef]
20. Alvarez, L.E.; Ribas, B.L.; Serra, M.L. Prevalence of the metabolic syndrome in the population of Canary Islands, Spain. *Med. Clin.* **2003**, *120*, 172–174.
21. Holst-Schumacher, I.; Nunez-Rivas, H.; Monge-Rojas, R.; Barrantes-Santamaria, M. Components of the metabolic syndrome among a sample of overweight and obese Costa Rican schoolchildren. *Food Nutr. Bull.* **2009**, *30*, 161–170. [CrossRef]
22. Alvarez, M.M.; Vieira, A.C.; Sichieri, R.; Veiga, G.V. Prevalence of metabolic syndrome and of its specific components among adolescents from Niteroi city, Rio de Janeiro state, Brazil. *Arq. Bras. Endocrinol. Metab.* **2011**, *55*, 164–170. [CrossRef] [PubMed]
23. Liang, J.; Fu, J.; Jiang, Y.; Dong, G.; Wang, X.; Wu, W. TriGlycerides and high-density lipoprotein cholesterol ratio compared with homeostasis model assessment insulin resistance indexes in screening for metabolic syndrome in the chinese obese children: A cross section study. *BMC Pediatr.* **2015**, *15*, 138. [CrossRef] [PubMed]
24. Yakubov, R.; Nadir, E.; Stein, R.; Klein-Kremer, A. The duration of breastfeeding and its association with metabolic syndrome among obese children. *Sci. World J.* **2015**, *2015*, 731319. [CrossRef] [PubMed]
25. Owen, C.G.; Martin, R.M.; Whincup, P.H.; Smith, G.D.; Cook, D.G. Effect of infant feeding on the risk of obesity across the life course: A quantitative review of published evidence. *Pediatrics* **2005**, *115*, 1367–1377. [CrossRef] [PubMed]

26. Harder, T.; Bergmann, R.; Kallischnigg, G.; Plagemann, A. Duration of breastfeeding and risk of overweight: A meta-analysis. *Am. J. Epidemiol.* **2005**, *162*, 397–403. [CrossRef]
27. De Armas, M.G.; Megías, S.M.; Modino, S.C.; Bolaños, P.I.; Guardiola, P.D.; Alvarez, T.M. Importance of breastfeeding in the prevalence of metabolic syndrome and degree of childhood obesity. *Endocrinol. Nutr.* **2009**, *56*, 400–403. [CrossRef]
28. Ekelund, U.; Anderssen, S.; Andersen, L.B.; Riddoch, C.J.; Sardinha, L.B.; Luan, J.; Froberg, K.; Brage, S. Prevalence and correlates of the metabolic syndrome in a population-based sample of European youth. *Am. J. Clin. Nutr.* **2009**, *89*, 90–96. [CrossRef]
29. Sun, K.; Chen, M.; Yin, Y.; Wu, L.; Gao, L. Why Chinese mothers stop breastfeeding: Mothers' self-reported reasons for stopping during the first six months. *J. Child Health Care* **2017**, *21*, 353–363. [CrossRef]
30. De Jersey, S.J.; Mallan, K.; Forster, J.; Daniels, L.A. A prospective study of breastfeeding intentions of healthy weight and overweight women as predictors of breastfeeding outcomes. *Midwifery* **2017**, *53*, 20–27. [CrossRef]
31. Amir, L.H.; Donath, S. A systematic review of maternal obesity and breastfeeding intention, initiation and duration. *BMC Pregnancy Childbirth* **2007**, *7*, 9. [CrossRef]
32. Dos Santos Alves, P.J.; Henriques, A.C.; Pinto, L.R.; Mota, R.M.; Alencar, C.H.; Alves, R.S.; Carvalho, F.H. Endothelial and metabolic disorders in adolescence: Low birth weight is not an isolated risk factor. *J. Pediatr. Endocrinol. Metab.* **2015**, *28*, 407–413. [CrossRef] [PubMed]
33. Yuan, Z.P.; Yang, M.; Liang, L.; Fu, J.F.; Xiong, F.; Liu, G.L.; Gong, C.X.; Luo, F.H.; Chen, S.K.; Zhang, D.D.; et al. Possible role of birth weight on general and central obesity in Chinese children and adolescents: A cross-sectional study. *Ann. Epidemiol.* **2015**, *25*, 748–752. [CrossRef] [PubMed]
34. Zabeen, B.; Tayyeb, S.; Naz, F.; Ahmed, F.; Rahman, M.; Nahar, J.; Nahar, N.; Azad, K. Prevalence of obesity and central obesity among adolescent girls in a district school in Bangladesh. *Indian J. Endocrinol. Metab.* **2015**, *19*, 649–652. [CrossRef] [PubMed]
35. Schroder, H.; Ribas, L.; Koebnick, C.; Funtikova, A.; Gomez, S.F.; Fíto, M.; Perez-Rodrigo, C.; Serra-Majem, L. Prevalence of abdominal obesity in Spanish children and adolescents. Do we need waist circumference measurements in pediatric practice? *PLoS ONE* **2014**, *9*, e87549. [CrossRef] [PubMed]
36. Lee, C.M.; Huxley, R.R.; Wildman, R.P.; Woodward, M. Indices of abdominal obesity are better discriminators of cardiovascular risk factors than BMI: A meta-analysis. *J. Clin. Epidemiol.* **2008**, *61*, 646–653. [CrossRef]
37. Haldar, S.; Chia, S.C.; Henry, C.J. Body composition in Asians and caucasians: Comparative analyses and influences on cardiometabolic outcomes. *Adv. Food Nutr. Res.* **2015**, *75*, 97–154. [PubMed]
38. Papoutsakis, C.; Yannakoulia, M.; Ntalla, I.; Dedoussis, G.V. Metabolic syndrome in a Mediterranean pediatric cohort: Prevalence using international diabetes federation-derived criteria and associations with adiponectin and leptin. *Metabolism* **2012**, *61*, 140–145. [CrossRef] [PubMed]
39. Tai, E.S.; Lau, T.N.; Ho, S.C.; Fok, A.C.; Tan, C.E. Body fat distribution and cardiovascular risk in normal weight women. Associations with insulin resistance, lipids and plasma leptin. *Int. J. Obes. Relat. Metab. Disord.* **2000**, *24*, 751–757. [CrossRef]
40. Park, Y.W.; Allison, D.B.; Heymsfield, S.B.; Gallagher, D. Larger amounts of visceral adipose tissue in Asian Americans. *Obes. Res.* **2001**, *9*, 381–387. [CrossRef]
41. Victora, C.G.; Horta, B.L.; Post, P.; Lima, R.C.; De Leon Elizalde, J.W.; Gerson, B.M.; Barros, F.C. Breast feeding and blood lipid concentrations in male Brazilian adolescents. *J. Epidemiol. Community Health* **2006**, *60*, 621–625. [CrossRef]
42. Lawlor, D.A.; Riddoch, C.J.; Page, A.S.; Andersen, L.B.; Wedderkopp, N.; Harro, M.; Stansbie, D.; Smith, G.D. Infant feeding and components of the metabolic syndrome: Findings from the European youth heart study. *Arch. Dis. Child.* **2005**, *90*, 582–588. [CrossRef] [PubMed]
43. Ramirez-Silva, I.; Rivera, J.A.; Trejo-Valdivia, B.; Martorell, R.; Stein, A.D.; Romieu, I.; Ramakrishnan, U. Breastfeeding status at age 3 months is associated with adiposity and cardiometabolic markers at age 4 years in Mexican children. *J. Nutr.* **2015**, *145*, 1295–1302. [CrossRef] [PubMed]

11

Negative Energy Balance Induced by Exercise or Diet: Effects on Visceral Adipose Tissue and Liver Fat

Robert Ross *, Simrat Soni and Sarah Houle

School of Kinesiology and Health Studies, Department of Endocrinology and Metabolism, Queen's University, Kingston, ON K7L 3N6, Canada; s.soni@queensu.ca (S.S.); sarah.houle@queensu.ca (S.H.)

* Correspondence: rossr@queensu.ca

Abstract: The indisputable association between visceral adipose tissue (VAT) and cardiometabolic risk makes it a primary target for lifestyle-based strategies designed to prevent or manage health risk. Substantive evidence also confirms that liver fat (LF) is positively associated with increased health risk and that reduction is associated with an improved metabolic profile. The independent associations between reductions in VAT, LF, and cardiometabolic risk is less clear. In this narrative review, we summarize the evidence indicating whether a negative energy balance induced by either an increase in energy expenditure (aerobic exercise) or a decrease in energy intake (hypocaloric diet) are effective strategies for reducing both VAT and LF. Consideration will be given to whether a dose-response relationship exists between the negative energy balance induced by exercise or diet and reduction in either VAT or LF. We conclude with recommendations that will help fill gaps in knowledge with respect to lifestyle-based strategies designed to reduce VAT and LF.

Keywords: exercise; abdominal obesity; energy balance; caloric restriction; non-alcoholic fatty liver disease; physical activity

1. Introduction

Decades of evidence have firmly established that VAT is associated with cardiometabolic risk factors beyond obesity per se [1]. There is no dispute that VAT represents a primary treatment target for strategies designed to prevent or manage the health risks associated with abdominal obesity. The findings from systematic reviews confirm that a negative energy balance induced by exercise or diet is associated with significant reductions in VAT and associated cardiometabolic risk factors [2,3]. Routine exercise consistent with current guidelines, in combination with a balanced diet, is associated with significant reductions in VAT. Whether exercise or a hypocaloric diet is associated with VAT reduction in a dose-response manner remains unclear. It is also unclear whether exercise intensity is positively associated with VAT reduction. What is clear, however, is that exercise or diet is associated with a reduction in VAT and associated cardiometabolic risk factors with minimal or no weight loss [4]. This is good news for practitioners who seek treatment options for their patients/clients.

Non-alcoholic fatty liver disease (NAFLD), an umbrella term that encompasses the deposition of lipid in the liver to more progressive steatosis and associated hepatitis, fibrosis, and cirrhosis, is recognized as an ectopic site of fat deposition that has serious health consequences [5]. Although LF accumulation is positively associated with VAT, there is evidence to suggest that LF is associated with cardiometabolic risk factors independent of VAT [6]. Thus, LF represents another target for strategies designed to reduce obesity-related health risk. In adults with or without NAFLD, exercise induced-negative energy balance consistent with current guidelines is associated with a marked reduction in LF.

In this narrative review, we summarize the evidence indicating whether a negative energy balance induced by either an increase in energy expenditure (aerobic exercise), or a decrease in energy intake (hypocaloric diet), are effective strategies for reducing both VAT and LF. The primary focus of this review was to report on findings from randomized trials with supervised aerobic exercise and monitoredhypocaloric diet interventions. Consideration was given to whether a dose-response relationship exists between the negative energy balance induced by exercise or diet and reduction in either VAT or LF. We conclude with recommendations that will help fill gaps in knowledge with respect to lifestyle-based strategies designed to reduce VAT and LF.

2. Visceral Adipose Tissue (VAT)

2.1. *Measurement of VAT*

Several methodologies for assessing VAT volume and distribution have been established. The criterion methods, which provide direct measurement of partial or total volumes, include magnetic resonance imaging (MRI) and computed tomography (CT) [4]. More recently, dual energy X-ray absorptiometry (DXA) has been identified as a reference method for assessing body composition [7]. However, due to high cost and feasibility issues, indirect estimates of VAT are often performed using anthropometric measures, including waist circumference, sagittal diameter, and bioelectrical impedance analysis [4]. When using MRI or CT to determine the effects of exercise or diet on VAT, it is important to note that change in VAT determined using a single image (e.g., a single image obtained at the level of the L4-L5 intervertebral space) is not materially different from the corresponding reduction in VAT derived using a multiple-image protocol [8]. Thus, when accessible, a single MRI or CT image can be used to accurately determine VAT distribution and/or reduction throughout the abdomen.

2.2. *Is VAT Reduced in Response to Chronic Exercise or Hypocaloric Diets?*

Evidence from a systematic review and meta-analysis clearly established that an increase in energy expenditure (aerobic exercise), or a decrease in energy intake (hypocaloric diet), are both associated with significant reductions in VAT, measured using gold standard methods [2]. Ross and colleagues were the first to investigate whether differences in VAT reduction were observed in response to equivalent diet-versus exercise-induced weight loss in either men [9] or women [10]. These RCTs were characterized by control of both energy expenditure (supervised exercise) and energy intake (self-reported intake every day). VAT was quantified using MRI. In these trials, participants in the exercise group did not increase or decrease their energy intake throughout the intervention, whereas those in the hypocaloric diet group did not increase physical activity levels. The primary finding from these trials revealed that when the diet- and exercise-induced weight loss was carefully matched, reductions in abdominal obesity and VAT in response to 12–14 weeks of exercise or diet were similar. Regardless of biological sex, a ~7% weight loss was associated with a ~25% reduction in VAT in response to diet or exercise[1]. These observations are consistent with the recent systematic review of Verheggen et al., wherein the results from eight studies in adults revealed that diet or exercise is associated with similar reductions in VAT when the negative energy balance and duration of intervention is matched [2]. Additionally, in response to an 18-month diet and exercise-based intervention among 278 sedentary adults with abdominal obesity, Gepner and colleagues reported that diet combined with exercise results in greater reductions in VAT than diet alone, assessed using MRI [11]. In summary, regardless of age or biological sex, a negative energy balance induced by diet or exercise is associated with marked reductions in VAT that are not materially different.

2.2.1. Exercise Amount and VAT

While the evidence reviewed clearly establishes that regular exercise combined with a healthful diet is associated with a marked reduction in VAT, independent of age and biological sex, the separate effects of exercise amount and intensity on VAT are less clear. The findings from a systematic review suggest that a dose-response relationship exists between exercise amount, defined by the metabolic equivalent of task (MET-hours/week), and reductions in VAT in individuals without metabolic disorder [12]. All 16 studies included in the review measured VAT using CT or MRI.

The findings from the few randomized trials specifically designed to examine the independent contributions of exercise amount on VAT suggested that increasing exercise amount (caloric expenditure) is not positively associated with VAT reduction. Keating et al. randomized inactive, obese adults to eight weeks of either; (i) low to moderate intensity, high amount aerobic exercise (50% VO_2 peak, 60 min); (ii) high intensity, low amount aerobic exercise (70% VO_2 peak, 45 min); (iii) low to moderate intensity, low amount aerobic exercise (50% VO_2 peak, 45 min); or iv) control [13]. The authors' primary observation was that exercise conditions varying in amount (minutes) resulted in MRI-measured VAT reductions of a similar magnitude. Similarly, Slentz et al. randomized 175 sedentary, overweight adults to a control group, or for eight months, to one of three exercise groups: (i) low amount, moderate intensity, equivalent to walking 12 miles/week (19.2 km/week) at 40%–55% of VO_2 peak; (ii) low amount, vigorous intensity, equivalent to jogging 12 miles/week at 65%–80% of VO_2 peak; or (iii) high amount, vigorous intensity, equivalent to jogging 20 miles/week (32.0 km) [14]. Despite substantial differences in the amount (caloric expenditure) of exercise performed between groups, the primary finding was that there was no difference in CT-measured VAT reduction [12]. More recently, Cowan et al. randomized 103 previously sedentary, abdominally obese adults to one of four groups: (i) control; (ii) low amount, low-intensity exercise (180 kcal/session (women) and 300 kcal/session (men) at 50% VO_2 peak); (iii) high-amount, low-intensity exercise (HALI; 360 kcal/session (women) and 600 kcal/session (men) at 50% VO_2 peak); or (iv) high-amount, high-intensity exercise (HAHI; 360 kcal/session (women) and 600 kcal/session (men) at 75% VO_2 peak) for 24 weeks [15]. Consistent with prior findings, MRI-measured VAT was reduced by 15% to 20% by comparison to controls across exercise groups, despite substantial differences in exercise-induced energy expenditure between groups. Analysis of daily self-reported diet records suggested that change in dietary intake did not differ between groups. Similarly, reduction in body weight did not differ between exercise groups. Thus, increasing exercise amount (kilocalories) without changes in energy intake for six months was not associated with greater VAT reduction in adults with abdominal obesity.

2.2.2. Exercise Intensity and VAT

Whether exercise intensity is associated with VAT reduction independent of exercise amount is unclear. A systematic review that compared exercise groups that varied in exercise intensity from 14 studies suggests that exercise intensity should be at least moderate to vigorous if VAT reduction is the objective [16]. It is important to note, however, that this observation did not account for possible variation in exercise amount performed between studies. Indeed, with few exceptions, preliminary findings from randomized trials specifically designed to determine the effect of exercise intensity on VAT reduction suggest that the intensity of exercise performed is not a primary determinant of change in VAT [13–15,17]. Irving et al. reported that while VAT reduction was not significantly different between high intensity and low intensity exercise groups, significant within-group VAT changes by comparison to control were only observed in the high intensity group [17]. Similar to the observations for exercise amount described above, Keating et al. [13] and Slentz et al. [14] reported no effect of increasing exercise intensity on VAT reduction when measured using criterion methods. These observations were confirmed by Cowan et al. who reported that the reduction in VAT was not different independent of exercise intensity ranging from 50% to 70% of VO_2 peak performed for 24 weeks (Figure 1) [15].

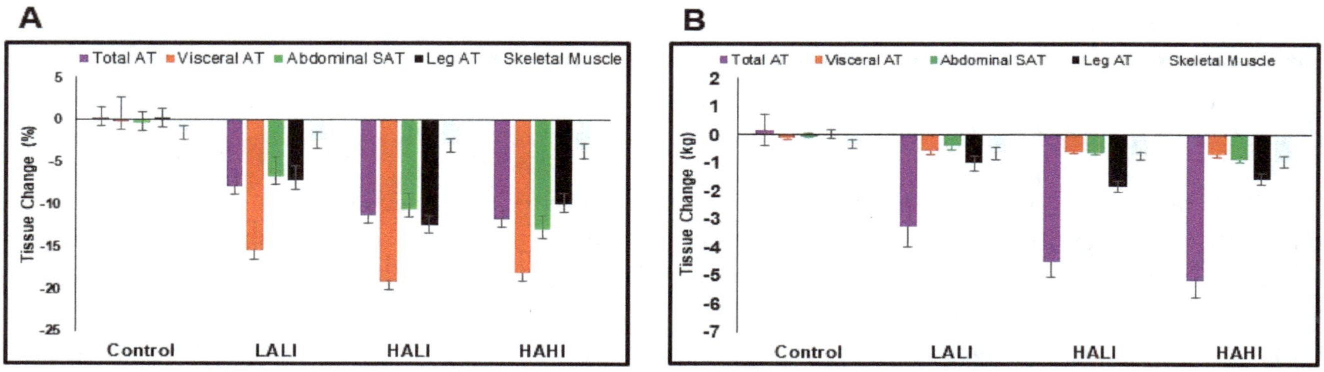

LALI = low amount, low intensity
HALI = high amount, low intensity
HAHI = high amount, high intensity

Figure 1. Illustration of relative (%, Panel **A**) and absolute (kg, Panel **B**) response of adipose and skeletal muscle tissues to variations in exercise dose. Taken from Reference [14]. Used with permission from Obesity. Absolute (left) and relative (right) changes in AT and skeletal muscle depots. With the exception of skeletal muscle, all AT depot changes (absolute and relative) were significantly different from control ($p < 0.008$; both panels). Relative change in VAT was greater than all other AT and skeletal muscle depots ($p < 0.01$; right panel). AT, adipose tissue; HAHI, high amount, high intensity; HALI, high amount, low intensity; LALI, low amount, low intensity.

These observations regarding the effects of exercise intensity on CT-measured VAT differ from a recently completed trial wherein 220 abdominally obese Chinese adults were randomized to either a high- or moderate-intensity exercise group for 12 months [18]. The primary finding was that vigorous-moderate exercise is associated with greater reductions in VAT compared to moderate exercise. However, it is important to note that in this trial, the vigorous exercise group performed supervised exercise for the entire 12 months, whereas the moderate exercise group self-reported their exercise behaviour. Self-reported physical activity behaviour is notoriously unreliable, thus confounds interpretation [19]. Self-reported physical activity can be under- or overestimated [19].

Emerging evidence has considered whether high intensity interval training (HITT) is associated with change in VAT. HITT is characterized by brief, intermittent bursts of exercise completed at a high intensity. High intensity exercise bouts are separated by brief recovery periods of inactivity or low-intensity exercise. Although there is no consensus established for the optimal durations of exercise and rest periods for HITT protocols, active bouts may be performed from 10 s to 5 min at 70–90% of VO_2 peak or 85%–95% of peak heart rate. Recovery periods range from 30 s to 3 min. Zhang et al. randomized 47 participants to a 12-week HIIT or moderate-intensity continuous training (MICT) intervention using a cycle ergometer three times a week [20]. Participants in the HIIT group performed cycles of 4-min high intensity bouts at 90% $VO_{2\,max}$, followed by 3 min of recovery until the targeted energy expenditure (300 kJ) was achieved. The MICT group performed continuous exercise until the matched energy expenditure target was reached (300 kJ). Similar reductions in VAT were observed regardless of exercise intervention. Winding et al. randomized 29 participants to an 11-week HIIT or MICT cycling intervention involving 10 1-min intervals (95% peak workload) with 1-min recovery or 40 min (50% peak workload), respectively [21]. Despite a lower exercise-induced energy expenditure, HIIT showed similar reductions in DXA-measured VAT compared to MICT. In both studies, participants were instructed to maintain their dietary intake throughout the intervention.

In summary, aerobic exercise combined with a balanced diet, wherein the participant does not increase energy intake, is associated with a robust reduction in VAT independent of amount or intensity. A 7% weight loss resulting from a lifestyle-based strategy consistent with current recommendations is likely to result in a 25% reduction in VAT. These observations provide treatment options for practitioners who target VAT reduction as part of a comprehensive lifestyle-based strategy designed to reduce health risk.

2.2.3. Individual Variability in VAT Response to Standardized Exercise

Since all adults acquire and inherit characteristics that vary substantially, their response to a treatment designed to change a given trait will vary substantially. Although increasing exercise is a primary determinant of improvement in numerous traits (e.g., cardiorespiratory fitness) at the group level, there is a growing body of evidence that the response to regular exercise varies substantially among individuals [22]. The extent to which individual variability in VAT response to a standard dose of exercise has only recently been considered. Brennan et al. performed a study to determine the effect of exercise amount and intensity on the proportion of individuals for whom the MRI-measured VAT response was above the minimal clinically important difference, defined as a reduction in VAT greater than 0.28 kg or 9%, and whether clinically meaningful changes in waist circumference, defined as greater than 2 cm, reflect individual VAT responses that are above the minimal clinically important difference [23]. Abdominally obese men and women were randomized to (i) control ($n = 20$); (ii) low amount, low intensity ($n = 24$); (iii) high amount, low intensity ($n = 30$); or (iv) high amount, high intensity ($n = 29$) treadmill exercise for 24 weeks.

Inspection of the individual responses to standardized exercise illustrated in Figure 2 clearly document the extraordinary variability in VAT response to exercise independent of exercise amount or intensity. The observation that most adults reduce VAT regardless of exercise strategy and that clinically important reductions in VAT can be determined by corresponding reductions in waist circumference that exceed 2 cm is encouraging (Figure 2). These observations underscore the value of routinely measuring waist circumference to determine the efficacy of treatment designed to reduce VAT and that, for some adults, substantial reduction in VAT may require altering the exercise dose by increasing either the amount and/or intensity of exercise. Whether some adults are resistant to reduction in VAT regardless of exercise dose is unknown and should be the subject of future investigations.

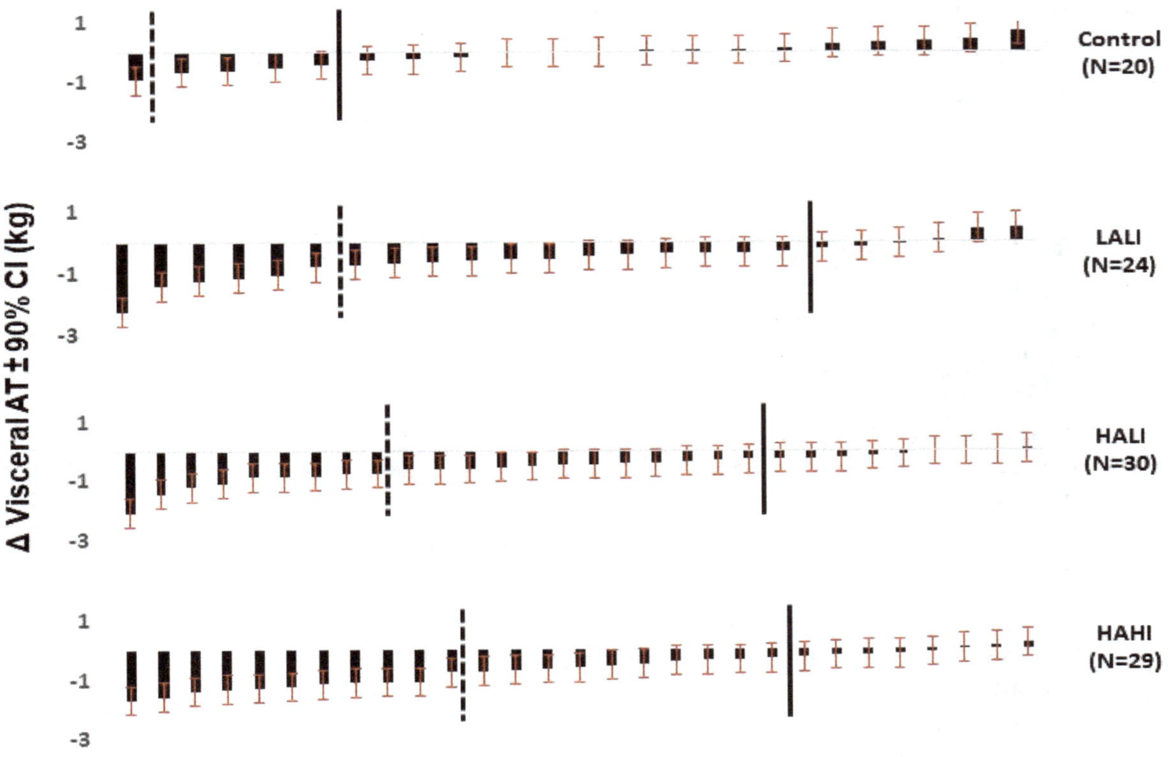

Figure 2. Variability of visceral adipose tissue (VAT) response to standardized exercise. Taken from Reference [19]. Used with permission from MSSE. Distribution of individual responses for change in VAT (kg) ± 90% CI in the control and intervention groups. The solid black line distinguishes participants whose observed response exceeds the MCID (e.g., those participants to the left of the solid line reduced visceral AT by < 0.28 kg). The dashed black line distinguishes participants whose observed response ± 90% CI exceeds the MCID (e.g., those participants to the left of the dashed line have CI where the top range is < 0.28 kg). LALI (low amount (~30 min), low intensity (50% VO_2 peak)), HALI (high amount (~60 min), low intensity (50% VO_2 peak)), HAHI (High amount (~40 min), high intensity (75% VO_2 peak)).

3. Liver Fat (LF)

3.1. Measurements of LF

Liver biopsy is an established method to assess liver fat and diagnose the severity of NAFLD with precision [6]. However, the invasive nature, cost, sampling error, and morbidity associated with the procedure are acknowledged limitations [6]. CT is a technique that estimates steatosis by quantitatively measuring liver density. However, the sensitivity and specificity of CT are clinically unacceptable at mild steatosis levels [6,16]. MRI is a technique that uses quantitative and qualitative information to assess intrahepatic fat content. The heterogeneity of the magnetic field, time demanding nature, low sensitivity, and poor image quality when disturbed are limitations of this technique [6]. Ultrasound is a common technique that is used to assess LF because of the low cost, vast availability and noninvasive nature [6]. Ultrasonography is limited as a single diagnostic tool because of the lack of sufficient sensitivity [6,24,25]. Accuracy of an ultrasound decreases with increasing body mass index [26–28]. Magnetic resonance spectroscopy (MRS) is cited as the gold standard MR technique to quantify LF. There is a high level of accuracy and reproducibility with this method, however, it is limited in availability because of the high degree of skill and specialized software required. Similar to liver biopsies, only a portion of the liver is analyzed, and so, sampling errors may occur [26].

3.2. Is Liver Fat Reduced in Response to Chronic Exercise or a Hypocaloric Diet?

As with VAT, evidence from systematic reviews and meta-analyses confirm that exercise or a hypocaloric diet is associated with a reduction in LF in previously sedentary, overweight and obese men and women [3,29].

3.3. Exercise and Liver Fat

Evidence from observational studies have established that adults with elevated levels of LF or NAFLD are physically inactive by comparison to those without NAFLD. Kistler and colleagues performed a retrospective analysis on 813 adults with biopsy-proven NAFLD, enrolled in the Nonalcoholic Steatohepatitis Clinical Research Network (NASH CRN) [30]. Physical activity levels were derived from self-reported responses to a questionnaire. The principle finding of this cross-sectional study was that neither moderate-intensity exercise nor total exercise per week was associated with NASH. However, vigorous exercise was associated with a decreased risk of having NASH (odds ratio (OR): 0.65 (0.43–0.98)). Thus, exercise intensity may be an important consideration when prescribing exercise to reduce LF. A limitation of this study was that exercise behaviour was assessed by self-report, which is notably unreliable [19].

Based on data derived from the National Health and Nutrition Examination Survey (NHANES) 2003–2006, Gerber and colleagues evaluated the associations between levels of physical activity and NAFLD in a large subsample of adults from this database [31]. NAFLD was defined as a fatty liver index >60 in the absence of other chronic liver diseases. The fatty liver index of hepatic steatosis is calculated based on measures of triglycerides, body mass index, waist circumference, and gamma-glutamyl transpeptidase. Physical activity levels were measured objectively over seven days using accelerometry.

Counter to the findings of Kistler et al. [30], Gerber and colleagues observed that adults with NAFLD (n = 1263), who were older and had a higher body mass index, perform less physical activity at any intensity level compared to adults without NAFLD (n = 1793) [31]. Thus, from initial epidemiological evidence, adults with NAFLD were physically inactive by comparison to adults without NAFLD, suggesting that exercise may be an important strategy for reducing LF. Physical activity was reported using accelerometers, which objectivity measure physical activity frequency and duration in a minimally invasive manner. However, accelerometers are limited in detecting non-ambulatory activities [19].

Evidence from controlled trials confirm the potential of exercise as a strategy to manage LF. Keating and colleagues reported that, in pooled data from six studies (156 overweight and abdominally obese adults), aerobic type exercise alone (no hypocaloric diet) ranging from two to 24 weeks at intensities between 45% and 85%, resulted in modest, yet significant reductions in LF (effect size 0.37) [29].

Keating et al. randomized 48 inactive overweight or obese adults to one of four groups varying in exercise amounts and intensities that are generally consistent with current exercise guidelines for 8 weeks [13]. LF was measured by MRS. The major finding was that LF was reduced by 1% to 3% compared to controls independent of exercise amount or intensity. The authors noted that, while the reductions in LF were modest, they were observed in association with minimal or no change in body weight.

In a much larger trial, Zhang et al. randomized 220 adults with NAFLD to 150 min per week for 12 months of either brisk walking (moderate intensity exercise) or jogging (moderate-vigorous intensity exercise) [18]. In this study, LF was assessed using MRS. All participants were asked not to change their diet during the trial. The principle finding was a decrease in LF that approximated 6% compared to controls, with no difference between exercise groups—thus, exercise intensity was not associated with LF reduction. In this trial, after controlling for the exercise-induced weight loss (3%–6%), the net changes in LF content were reduced and became nonsignificant between the exercise and control groups. Thus, the benefit of exercise was explained in large measure by the ability to induce weight loss.

Few studies have evaluated the association between cardiorespiratory fitness and LF. Pälve and colleagues found that in 463 adults, participants with fatty liver had lower cardiorespiratory fitness levels compared to participants without fatty liver ($VO_{2\,peak}$ 27.2 $mL\cdot kg^{-1}\cdot min^{-1}$ and 31.6 $mL\cdot kg^{-1}\cdot min^{-1}$, $p < 0.0001$) [32]. LF was assessed using ultrasound. This relationship remained significant when adjusted for physical activity, adiposity, smoking, alcohol consumption, serum lipids, insulin, glucose, and C-reactive protein. Participants with abdominal obesity (waist circumference > 80 cm in women and >94 cm in men) with higher fitness levels (higher than age- and sex-specific median of $VO_{2\,Peak}$) had lower prevalence of fatty liver than participants who were obese and unfit (below median), (11.7% vs. 34.8%, $p = 0.0003$). In a longitudinal study (nine months of follow up), Kantartzis et al. found that cardiorespiratory fitness (VO_2 peak) at baseline was a strong predictor of change in MRS-measured LF in response to an exercise intervention. Independent of total fat, visceral fat, subcutaneous fat or exercise intensity, cardiorespiratory fitness was negatively associated with LF at baseline [33].

Exercise-induced reductions in intrahepatic fat are observed independent of weight change [34]. A systematic review by Hashida and colleagues showed a 20-30% relative risk reduction in LF with exercise in the absence of weight loss [35]. Sullivan and colleagues found that the effect of MRS-measured LF following an exercise intervention, according to the physical activity guidelines (150–300 min of moderate intensity exercise), were independent of weight loss [36]. In previously sedentary adults, body weight, body fat mass, and fat-free mass did not change after the intervention. However, there was a decrease (10.3% ± 4.6%) in LF in the exercise group compared with the control group ($p = 0.04$). Interestingly, obese individuals who consumed moderate to excessive amounts of alcohol underwent a 12-week exercise intervention. In this randomized trial, exercise induced reductions in both subcutaneous and visceral fat, however, there was no reduction of MRI-measured LF. This finding suggests that moderate to excessive amounts of alcohol consumption may attenuate the beneficial effects of exercise on NAFLD [37].

Qiu and colleagues conducted a meta-analysis and observed that the amount of physical activity in men was inversely associated with the risk of NAFLD in a dose-dependent manner [38]. The authors report that 500 MET-minutes/week (approximately 150 minutes/week) of physical activity was associated with an 18% risk reduction of NALFD (RR = 0.82, 95% CI 0.73–0.91). Further increases in physical activity (1000 MET-minutes/week) were associated with a 33% risk reduction in NAFLD (RR = 0.67, 95% CI 0.54–0.83). These findings are consistent with those of Li and colleagues who reported that moderate- and vigorous-intensity physical activity effectively reduced the risk of NAFLD independent of energy intake and sedentary time (>684 MET-minutes/week compared to none: OR 0.58, 95% CI 0.40 to 0.86, vigorous-intensity physical activity: >960 MET-min/week compared to none: OR 0.63, 95% CI 0.41 to 0.95) [39]. Li et al. used ultrasound measurements to assess LF. Kwak et al. also found an inverse dose-response relationship between the amount of self-reported physical activity and the prevalence of NAFLD, independent of insulin resistance and VAT in 3718 adult men and women [40]. However, self-reported physical activity behaviour is notoriously unreliable, thus confounding interpretation [19].

Emerging evidence has also considered whether HITT is associated with change inLF. Hallworth and colleagues randomized participants to 12 weeks of HITT on a cycle ergometer three times a week. Participants were instructed to perform 5 intervals of cycling at 16–17 on the Borg scale for 3 min followed by 3 min of recovery [39]. Abdelbasset et al. randomized participants to an eight-week cycling protocol. Participants completed three sets of 4-min cycling at 80 to 85% of VO_2 max with 2-min recovery, three days a week [40]. In both studies, participants were instructed to make no modifications to their diets. Several authors have observed reductions in LF after HIIT compared to controls [41,42]. The change in LF was measured using MRI and/or ultrasonography. When HITT and moderate intensity exercise were matched for energy expenditure, there were no differences in LF reduction [41–43].

3.4. *Hypocaloric Diet and LF*

It is well established that diet-induced weight loss is a cornerstone of treatment for persons with NAFLD. In 2003, Tiikkainen and colleagues reported that LF, as measured by MRS, was reduced by about 39% in premenopausal women consequent to an 8% weight loss achieved within three to six months [43]. Of note, the authors reported that the reduction in LF was directly related to baseline levels. Larson-Meyer et al. reported results from the CALERIE study wherein a loss of body weight approximating 10% via hypocaloric diet or diet and exercise combined, was associated with a 29% to 40% reduction in MRS-measured LF in overweight adults. As with exercise-induced weight loss, diet-induced weight loss is associated with a marked reduction in MRI-measured LF [11]. Very low-calorie diets also resulted in significant reductions of LF, however, very low-calorie diets cannot be maintained long term [44–46].

Thoma and colleagues performed a systematic review of the literature to evaluate the effects of various lifestyle-based interventions on LF [3]. For diet only interventions, the authors uncovered 10 studies wherein 11 groups totaling 322 participants were prescribed a hypocaloric diet varying in composition and negative energy balance. Only two studies included control groups. The duration of the diet interventions ranged from one to six months. The mean weight loss across the studies ranged from 4% to 14% and the relative reduction in LF, as measured by MRS, ranged from 42% to 81%. No clear relationship between diet composition and LF reduction was reported. However, consistent with the evidence cited above, the reduction in LF was strongly associated with weight loss.

3.5. *Exercise and Hypocaloric Diet Combined*

Lifestyle interventions that include a hypocaloric diet and an exercise intervention have been considered in several systematic reviews. The reviews investigate if a combination of diet and exercise is more effective than exercise or diet alone to decrease LF [3,29,47–49]. Keating and colleagues did not find a significant pooled effect of combined interventions of diet and exercise; however, the authors discuss being limited by a low sample size and statistical power [29]. Thoma et al. reported on seven studies that conducted lifestyle modification interventions to decrease energy intake and increase physical activity or exercise over 3–12 months [3].The authors concluded that lifestyle modifications consistently resulted in LF reduction. Similarly, other systematic reviews conducted by Hens and colleagues, as well as Whitsett and colleagues, found that lifestyle modification can reduce LF [48,49]. Golabi et al. found that exercise alone and a combination of diet and exercise both significantly decrease LF [47].

4. Anthropometric Markers of VAT and LF

Criterion measurement of both VAT and LF requires sophisticated radiological techniques (e.g., magnetic resonance imaging or computed tomography) that are not readily accessible in most clinical settings. LF can also be determined using biopsy methods, but this too is invasive and presents a burden to the patient. Accordingly, the validity of simple anthropometric methods has been considered as an alternative, pragmatic option. There is general agreement that waist circumference represents the single best anthropometric marker of VAT [1,50]. However, due in large measure to the inter-individual variability between the quantity of abdominal subcutaneous and VAT [51], the variance explained in VAT change by waist circumference is modest, ranging from 25% to 75%[1]. At present, there is no universally accepted method for the measurement of waist circumference. The two most often used protocols are at the level of the iliac crest and the mid-point between the iliac crest and last rib [52]. Whether the associations between these two WC methods provide different values for VAT across sex, age, and ethnicity is unclear.

In 2006, Bedogni et al. derived a simple index (Fatty Liver Index) of hepatic steatosis that was calculated based on the measures of triglycerides, body mass index, waist circumference and gamma-glutamyl transpeptidase (GGT) [53]. Fatty liver index has a very good discriminative ability to predict fatty liver in both Asian and Western adult populations [54,55]. Motamed et al. recently validated the discriminative ability of the Fatty Liver Index to predict fatty liver in a sample of 5052 adults [56]. Fatty liver or NAFLD was determined by ultrasound. Interestingly, although the Fatty Liver Index showed good discriminative ability for the diagnosis of NAFLD (AUC = 0.87 (95%CI: 0.85–0.88), there was no significant difference in the discriminative ability determined by waist circumference alone (AUC = 0.85, 95%CI: 0.84–0.86). Thus, on a population basis, waist circumference alone may be a useful measure of both VAT and LF. However, the utility of either waist circumference or Fatty Liver Index to predict VAT and LF, respectively, on an individual basis is unknown.

5. Summary

It is now firmly established that both regular aerobic exercise and the consumption of a hypocaloric diet are associated with a substantial reduction in VAT and LF independent of age, biological sex, or ethnicity. Whereas exercise is associated with VAT reduction with or without weight loss, reductions in LF are positively associated with weight, independent of the strategy to induce weight loss. Despite decades of research into the associations between lifestyle-based interventions and VAT reduction, the threshold of VAT reduction that is required for health benefit remains unclear. Similarly, while it is clear that weight loss is associated with LF reduction, optimal levels of weight loss for attenuating LF are unclear. Nevertheless, it is extremely encouraging that regular exercise (4–6 months) consistent with consensus recommendations (30–60 min per day at moderate-to-vigorous intensity; e.g., brisk walking or jogging) combined with a balanced, healthful diet is associated with substantial reductions in VAT (15%–20%). Similarly, weight loss of 5% to 10% can be achieved by 4–6 months with reasonable reductions in caloric intake with or without exercise. Thus, practitioners in health care settings have options when counselling adults regarding the utility of lifestyle-based interventions designed to reduce both VAT and LF. The objective of this review was assessing strategies for reducing VAT and LF. The focus was on a negative energy balance induced aerobic exercise and a decrease in energy intake. Future research is required to determine if some adults are resistant to reductions in VAT and LF regardless of exercise dose.

Direct measurement of VAT or LF in most health care settings is not feasible. Waist circumference remains the single best anthropometric marker of change in VAT. While precise measurement of change in VAT using waist circumference on an individual basis is unlikely, it is extremely likely that reductions in waist circumference (e.g., greater than 2 cm) are associated with a corresponding reduction in VAT. While initial results suggest that waist circumference may be as useful as the LF Index to follow change in LF, additional evidence from large scale studies in diverse populations is required. Nevertheless, these observations are encouraging and reinforce the importance of measuring waist circumference in all health care settings.

Author Contributions: R.R. conceptualized the manuscript. S.H. and S.S. reviewed and assisted in writing the manuscript. All authors have read and agreed to the published version of the manuscript.

References

1. Neeland, I.J.; Ross, R.; Després, J.-P.; Matsuzawa, Y.; Yamashita, S.; Shai, I.; Seidell, J.; Magni, P.; Santos, R.D.; Arsenault, B.; et al. International Atherosclerosis Society; International Chair on Cardiometabolic Risk Working Group on Visceral Obesity. Visceral and Ectopic Fat, Atherosclerosis, and Cardiometabolic Disease: A Position Statement. *Lancet Diabetes Endocrinol.* **2019**, *7*, 715–725. [CrossRef]
2. Verheggen, R.J.H.M.; Maessen, M.F.H.; Green, D.J.; Hermus, A.R.M.M.; Hopman, M.T.E.; Thijssen, D.H.T. A Systematic Review and Meta-Analysis on the Effects of Exercise Training versus Hypocaloric Diet: Distinct Effects on Body Weight and Visceral Adipose Tissue. *Obes. Rev.* **2016**, *17*, 664–690. [CrossRef]
3. Thoma, C.; Day, C.P.; Trenell, M.I. Lifestyle Interventions for the Treatment of Non-Alcoholic Fatty Liver Disease in Adults: A Systematic Review. *J. Hepatol.* **2012**, *56*, 255–266. [CrossRef]
4. Shuster, A.; Patlas, M.; Pinthus, J.H.; Mourtzakis, M. The Clinical Importance of Visceral Adiposity: A Critical Review of Methods for Visceral Adipose Tissue Analysis. *Br. J. Radiol.* **2012**, *85*, 1–10. [CrossRef]
5. Targher, G.; Day, C.P.; Bonora, E. Risk of Cardiovascular Disease in Patients with Nonalcoholic Fatty Liver Disease. *N. Engl. J. Med.* **2010**, *363*, 1341–1350. [CrossRef]
6. Fabbrini, E.; Magkos, F.; Mohammed, B.S.; Pietka, T.; Abumrad, N.A.; Patterson, B.W.; Okunade, A.; Klein, S. Intrahepatic Fat, not Visceral Fat, Is Linked with Metabolic Complications of Obesity. *Proc. Natl. Acad. Sci. USA* **2009**, *106*, 15430–15435. [CrossRef]
7. Heymsfield, S.B.; Wang, Z.; Baumgartner, R.N.; Ross, R. Human Body Composition: Advances in Models and Methods. *Annu. Rev. Nutr.* **1997**, *17*, 527–558. [CrossRef]
8. Ross, R.; Rissanen, J.; Pedwell, H.; Clifford, J.; Shragge, P. Influence of Diet and Exercise on Skeletal Muscle and Visceral Adipose Tissue in Men. *J. Appl. Physiol.* **1996**, *81*, 2445–2455. [CrossRef]
9. Ross, R.; Dagnone, D.; Jones, P.J.; Smith, H.; Paddags, A.; Hudson, R.; Janssen, I. Reduction in Obesity and Related Comorbid Conditions after Diet-Induced Weight Loss or Exercise-Induced Weight Loss in Men. A Randomized, Controlled Trial. *Ann. Intern. Med.* **2000**, *133*, 92–103. [CrossRef]
10. Ross, R.; Janssen, I.; Dawson, J.; Kungl, A.-M.; Kuk, J.L.; Wong, S.L.; Nguyen-Duy, T.-B.; Lee, S.; Kilpatrick, K.; Hudson, R. Exercise-Induced Reduction in Obesity and Insulin Resistance in Women: A Randomized Controlled Trial. *Obes. Res.* **2004**, *12*, 789–798. [CrossRef]
11. Gepner, Y.; Shelef, I.; Schwarzfuchs, D.; Zelicha, H.; Tene, L.; Yaskolka Meir, A.; Tsaban, G.; Cohen, N.; Bril, N.; Rein, M.; et al. Effect of Distinct Lifestyle Interventions on Mobilization of Fat Storage Pools: Central Magnetic Resonance Imaging Randomized Controlled Trial. *Circulation* **2018**, *137*, 1143–1157. [CrossRef]
12. Ohkawara, K.; Tanaka, S.; Miyachi, M.; Ishikawa-Takata, K.; Tabata, I. A Dose-Response Relation between Aerobic Exercise and Visceral Fat Reduction: Systematic Review of Clinical Trials. *Int. J. Obes. (Lond.)* **2007**, *31*, 1786–1797. [CrossRef]

13. Keating, S.E.; Hackett, D.A.; Parker, H.M.; O'Connor, H.T.; Gerofi, J.A.; Sainsbury, A.; Baker, M.K.; Chuter, V.H.; Caterson, I.D.; George, J.; et al. Effect of Aerobic Exercise Training Dose on Liver Fat and Visceral Adiposity. *J. Hepatol.* **2015**, *63*, 174–182. [CrossRef]
14. Slentz, C.A.; Aiken, L.B.; Houmard, J.A.; Bales, C.W.; Johnson, J.L.; Tanner, C.J.; Duscha, B.D.; Kraus, W.E. Inactivity, Exercise, and Visceral Fat. STRRIDE: A Randomized, Controlled Study of Exercise Intensity and Amount. *J. Appl. Physiol.* **2005**, *99*, 1613–1618. [CrossRef]
15. Cowan, T.E.; Brennan, A.M.; Stotz, P.J.; Clarke, J.; Lamarche, B.; Ross, R. Separate Effects of Exercise Amount and Intensity on Adipose Tissue and Skeletal Muscle Mass in Adults with Abdominal Obesity. *Obesity (Silver Spring)* **2018**, *26*, 1696–1703. [CrossRef]
16. Vissers, D.; Hens, W.; Taeymans, J.; Baeyens, J.-P.; Poortmans, J.; Van Gaal, L. The Effect of Exercise on Visceral Adipose Tissue in Overweight Adults: A Systematic Review and Meta-Analysis. *PLoS ONE* **2013**, *8*, e56415. [CrossRef]
17. Irving, B.A.; Davis, C.K.; Brock, D.W.; Weltman, J.Y.; Swift, D.; Barrett, E.J.; Gaesser, G.A.; Weltman, A. Effect of Exercise Training Intensity on Abdominal Visceral Fat and Body Composition. *Med. Sci. Sports Exerc.* **2008**, *40*, 1863–1872. [CrossRef]
18. Zhang, H.-J.; He, J.; Pan, L.-L.; Ma, Z.-M.; Han, C.-K.; Chen, C.-S.; Chen, Z.; Han, H.-W.; Chen, S.; Sun, Q.; et al. Effects of Moderate and Vigorous Exercise on Nonalcoholic Fatty Liver Disease: A Randomized Clinical Trial. *JAMA Intern. Med.* **2016**, *176*, 1074–1082. [CrossRef]
19. Ainsworth, B.; Cahalin, L.; Buman, M.; Ross, R. The Current State of Physical Activity Assessment Tools. *Prog. Cardiovasc. Dis.* **2015**, *57*, 387–395. [CrossRef]
20. Zhang, H.; Tong, T.K.; Qiu, W.; Zhang, X.; Zhou, S.; Liu, Y.; He, Y. Comparable Effects of High-Intensity Interval Training and Prolonged Continuous Exercise Training on Abdominal Visceral Fat Reduction in Obese Young Women. Available online: https://www.hindawi.com/journals/jdr/2017/5071740/ (accessed on 14 March 2020).
21. Winding, K.M.; Munch, G.W.; Iepsen, U.W.; Van Hall, G.; Pedersen, B.K.; Mortensen, S.P. The Effect on Glycaemic Control of Low-Volume High-Intensity Interval Training versus Endurance Training in Individuals with Type 2 Diabetes. *Diabetes Obes. Metab.* **2018**, *20*, 1131–1139. [CrossRef]
22. Ross, R.; Goodpaster, B.H.; Koch, L.G.; Sarzynski, M.A.; Kohrt, W.M.; Johannsen, N.M.; Skinner, J.S.; Castro, A.; Irving, B.A.; Noland, R.C.; et al. Precision Exercise Medicine: Understanding Exercise Response Variability. *Br. J. Sports Med.* **2019**, *53*, 1141–1153. [CrossRef]
23. Brennan, A.M.; Day, A.G.; Cowan, T.E.; Clarke, G.J.; Lamarche, B.; Ross, R. Individual Response to Standardized Exercise: Total and Abdominal Adipose Tissue. *Med. Sci. Sports Exerc.* **2019**. [CrossRef]
24. Lv, S.; Jiang, S.; Liu, S.; Dong, Q.; Xin, Y.; Xuan, S. Noninvasive Quantitative Detection Methods of Liver Fat Content in Nonalcoholic Fatty Liver Disease. *J. Clin. Transl. Hepatol.* **2018**, *6*, 217–221. [CrossRef]
25. Kramer, H.; Pickhardt, P.J.; Kliewer, M.A.; Hernando, D.; Chen, G.-H.; Zagzebski, J.A.; Reeder, S.B. Accuracy of Liver Fat Quantification with Advanced CT, MRI, and Ultrasound Techniques: Prospective Comparison with MR Spectroscopy. *AJR Am. J. Roentgenol.* **2017**, *208*, 92–100. [CrossRef] [PubMed]
26. Chartampilas, E. Imaging of Nonalcoholic Fatty Liver Disease and Its Clinical Utility. *Hormones* **2018**, *17*, 69–81. [CrossRef]
27. Bohte, A.E.; van Werven, J.R.; Bipat, S.; Stoker, J. The Diagnostic Accuracy of US, CT, MRI and 1H-MRS for the Evaluation of Hepatic Steatosis Compared with Liver Biopsy: A Meta-Analysis. *Eur. Radiol.* **2011**, *21*, 87–97. [CrossRef]
28. Fitzpatrick, E.; Dhawan, A. Noninvasive Biomarkers in Non-Alcoholic Fatty Liver Disease: Current Status and a Glimpse of the Future. *World J. Gastroenterol.* **2014**, *20*, 10851–10863. [CrossRef]
29. Keating, S.E.; Hackett, D.A.; George, J.; Johnson, N.A. Exercise and Non-Alcoholic Fatty Liver Disease: A Systematic Review and Meta-Analysis. *J. Hepatol.* **2012**, *57*, 157–166. [CrossRef]
30. Kistler, K.D.; Brunt, E.M.; Clark, J.M.; Diehl, A.M.; Sallis, J.F.; Schwimmer, J.B.; NASH CRN Research Group. Physical Activity Recommendations, Exercise Intensity, and Histological Severity of Nonalcoholic Fatty Liver Disease. *Am. J. Gastroenterol.* **2011**, *106*, 460–468. [CrossRef]
31. Gerber, L.; Otgonsuren, M.; Mishra, A.; Escheik, C.; Birerdinc, A.; Stepanova, M.; Younossi, Z.M. Non-Alcoholic Fatty Liver Disease (NAFLD) Is Associated with Low Level of Physical Activity: A Population-Based Study. *Aliment. Pharmacol. Ther.* **2012**, *36*, 772–781. [CrossRef]

32. Pälve, K.S.; Pahkala, K.; Suomela, E.; Aatola, H.; Hulkkonen, J.; Juonala, M.; Lehtimäki, T.; Rönnemaa, T.; Viikari, J.S.A.; Kähönen, M.; et al. Cardiorespiratory Fitness and Risk of Fatty Liver: The Young Finns Study. *Med. Sci. Sports Exerc.* **2017**, *49*, 1834–1841. [CrossRef]
33. Kantartzis, K.; Thamer, C.; Peter, A.; Machann, J.; Schick, F.; Schraml, C.; Königsrainer, A.; Königsrainer, I.; Kröber, S.; Niess, A.; et al. High Cardiorespiratory Fitness Is an Independent Predictor of the Reduction in Liver Fat during a Lifestyle Intervention in Non-Alcoholic Fatty Liver Disease. *Gut* **2009**, *58*, 1281–1288. [CrossRef]
34. Katsagoni, C.N.; Georgoulis, M.; Papatheodoridis, G.V.; Panagiotakos, D.B.; Kontogianni, M.D. Effects of Lifestyle Interventions on Clinical Characteristics of Patients with Non-Alcoholic Fatty Liver Disease: A Meta-Analysis. *Metab. Clin. Exp.* **2017**, *68*, 119–132. [CrossRef]
35. Hashida, R.; Kawaguchi, T.; Bekki, M.; Omoto, M.; Matsuse, H.; Nago, T.; Takano, Y.; Ueno, T.; Koga, H.; George, J.; et al. Aerobic vs. Resistance Exercise in Non-Alcoholic Fatty Liver Disease: A Systematic Review. *J. Hepatol.* **2017**, *66*, 142–152. [CrossRef]
36. Sullivan, S.; Kirk, E.P.; Mittendorfer, B.; Patterson, B.W.; Klein, S. Randomized Trial of Exercise Effect on Intrahepatic Triglyceride Content and Lipid Kinetics in Nonalcoholic Fatty Liver Disease. *Hepatology* **2012**, *55*, 1738–1745. [CrossRef]
37. Houghton, D.; Hallsworth, K.; Thoma, C.; Cassidy, S.; Hardy, T.; Heaps, S.; Hollingsworth, K.G.; Taylor, R.; Day, C.P.; Masson, S.; et al. Effects of Exercise on Liver Fat and Metabolism in Alcohol Drinkers. *Clin. Gastroenterol. Hepatol.* **2017**, *15*, 1596–1603.e3. [CrossRef]
38. Qiu, S.; Cai, X.; Sun, Z.; Li, L.; Zügel, M.; Steinacker, J.M.; Schumann, U. Association between Physical Activity and Risk of Nonalcoholic Fatty Liver Disease: A Meta-Analysis. *Therap. Adv. Gastroenterol.* **2017**, *10*, 701–713. [CrossRef]
39. Li, Y.; He, F.; He, Y.; Pan, X.; Wu, Y.; Hu, Z.; Lin, X.; Xu, S.; Peng, X.-E. Dose-Response Association between Physical Activity and Non-Alcoholic Fatty Liver Disease: A Case-Control Study in a Chinese Population. *BMJ Open* **2019**, *9*, e026854. [CrossRef]
40. Kwak, M.-S.; Kim, D.; Chung, G.E.; Kim, W.; Kim, Y.J.; Yoon, J.-H. Role of Physical Activity in Nonalcoholic Fatty Liver Disease in Terms of Visceral Obesity and Insulin Resistance. *Liver Int.* **2015**, *35*, 944–952. [CrossRef]
41. Hallsworth, K.; Thoma, C.; Hollingsworth, K.G.; Cassidy, S.; Anstee, Q.M.; Day, C.P.; Trenell, M.I. Modified High-Intensity Interval Training Reduces Liver Fat and Improves Cardiac Function in Non-Alcoholic Fatty Liver Disease: A Randomized Controlled Trial. *Clin. Sci.* **2015**, *129*, 1097–1105. [CrossRef]
42. Abdelbasset, W.K.; Tantawy, S.A.; Kamel, D.M.; Alqahtani, B.A.; Soliman, G.S. A Randomized Controlled Trial on the Effectiveness of 8-Week High-Intensity Interval Exercise on Intrahepatic Triglycerides, Visceral Lipids, and Health-Related Quality of Life in Diabetic Obese Patients with Nonalcoholic Fatty Liver Disease. *Medicine (Baltim.)* **2019**, *98*, e14918. [CrossRef]
43. Tiikkainen, M.; Bergholm, R.; Vehkavaara, S.; Rissanen, A.; Häkkinen, A.-M.; Tamminen, M.; Teramo, K.; Yki-Järvinen, H. Effects of Identical Weight Loss on Body Composition and Features of Insulin Resistance in Obese Women with High and Low Liver Fat Content. *Diabetes* **2003**, *52*, 701–707. [CrossRef]
44. Lewis, M.C.; Phillips, M.L.; Slavotinek, J.P.; Kow, L.; Thompson, C.H.; Toouli, J. Change in Liver Size and Fat Content after Treatment with Optifast Very Low Calorie Diet. *Obes. Surg.* **2006**, *16*, 697–701. [CrossRef]
45. Gu, Y.; Yu, H.; Li, Y.; Ma, X.; Lu, J.; Yu, W.; Xiao, Y.; Bao, Y.; Jia, W. Beneficial Effects of an 8-Week, Very Low Carbohydrate Diet Intervention on Obese Subjects. *Evid. Based Complement Altern. Med.* **2013**, *2013*. [CrossRef]
46. Lim, E.L.; Hollingsworth, K.G.; Aribisala, B.S.; Chen, M.J.; Mathers, J.C.; Taylor, R. Reversal of Type 2 Diabetes: Normalisation of Beta Cell Function in Association with Decreased Pancreas and Liver Triacylglycerol. *Diabetologia* **2011**, *54*, 2506–2514. [CrossRef]
47. Golabi, P.; Locklear, C.T.; Austin, P.; Afdhal, S.; Byrns, M.; Gerber, L.; Younossi, Z.M. Effectiveness of Exercise in Hepatic Fat Mobilization in Non-Alcoholic Fatty Liver Disease: Systematic Review. *World J. Gastroenterol.* **2016**, *22*, 6318–6327. [CrossRef]
48. Hens, W.; Taeymans, J.; Cornelis, J.; Gielen, J.; Gaal, L.V.; Vissers, D. The Effect of Lifestyle Interventions on Excess Ectopic Fat Deposition Measured by Noninvasive Techniques in Overweight and Obese Adults: A Systematic Review and Meta-Analysis. *J. Phys. Act. Health* **2016**, *13*, 671–694. [CrossRef]

49. Whitsett, M.; VanWagner, L.B. Physical Activity as a Treatment of Non-Alcoholic Fatty Liver Disease: A Systematic Review. *World J. Hepatol.* **2015**, *7*, 2041–2052. [CrossRef]
50. Ross, R.; Neeland, I.J.; Yamashita, S.; Shai, I.; Seidell, J.; Magni, P.; Santos, R.D.; Arsenault, B.; Cuevas, A.; Hu, F.B.; et al. Waist Circumference as a Vital Sign in Clinical Practice: A Consensus Statement from the IAS and ICCR Working Group on Visceral Obesity. *Nat. Rev. Endocrinol.* **2020**, *16*, 177–189. [CrossRef]
51. Lee, S.; Janssen, I.; Ross, R. Interindividual Variation in Abdominal Subcutaneous and Visceral Adipose Tissue: Influence of Measurement Site. *J. Appl. Physiol.* **2004**, *97*, 948–954. [CrossRef]
52. Ross, R.; Berentzen, T.; Bradshaw, A.J.; Janssen, I.; Kahn, H.S.; Katzmarzyk, P.T.; Kuk, J.L.; Seidell, J.C.; Snijder, M.B.; Sørensen, T.I.A.; et al. Does the Relationship between Waist Circumference, Morbidity and Mortality Depend on Measurement Protocol for Waist Circumference? *Obes. Rev.* **2008**, *9*, 312–325. [CrossRef]
53. Bedogni, G.; Bellentani, S.; Miglioli, L.; Masutti, F.; Passalacqua, M.; Castiglione, A.; Tiribelli, C. The Fatty Liver Index: A Simple and Accurate Predictor of Hepatic Steatosis in the General Population. *BMC Gastroenterol.* **2006**, *6*, 33. [CrossRef]
54. Yang, B.-L.; Wu, W.-C.; Fang, K.-C.; Wang, Y.-C.; Huo, T.-I.; Huang, Y.-H.; Yang, H.-I.; Su, C.-W.; Lin, H.-C.; Lee, F.-Y.; et al. External Validation of Fatty Liver Index for Identifying Ultrasonographic Fatty Liver in a Large-Scale Cross-Sectional Study in Taiwan. *PLoS ONE* **2015**, *10*, e0120443. [CrossRef]
55. Koehler, E.M.; Schouten, J.N.L.; Hansen, B.E.; Hofman, A.; Stricker, B.H.; Janssen, H.L.A. External Validation of the Fatty Liver Index for Identifying Nonalcoholic Fatty Liver Disease in a Population-Based Study. *Clin. Gastroenterol. Hepatol.* **2013**, *11*, 1201–1204. [CrossRef]
56. Motamed, N.; Sohrabi, M.; Ajdarkosh, H.; Hemmasi, G.; Maadi, M.; Sayeedian, F.S.; Pirzad, R.; Abedi, K.; Aghapour, S.; Fallahnezhad, M.; et al. Fatty Liver Index vs. Waist Circumference for Predicting Non-Alcoholic Fatty Liver Disease. *World J. Gastroenterol.* **2016**, *22*, 3023–3030. [CrossRef]

12

Lifestyle and Metabolic Syndrome: Contribution of the Endocannabinoidome

Vincenzo Di Marzo [1,2,3,4,5,6] and Cristoforo Silvestri [3,4,5,*]

1 École de nutrition, Université Laval, Québec, QC G1V 0A6, Canada
2 Institut sur la nutrition et les aliments fonctionnels, Université Laval, Québec, QC G1V 0A6, Canada
3 Canada Excellence Research Chair on the Microbiome-Endocannabinoidome Axis in Metabolic Health, Université Laval, Québec, QC G1V 0A6, Canada
4 Centre de recherche de l'Institut universitaire de cardiologie et de pneumologie de Québec, Québec, QC G1V 4G5, Canada
5 Department de médecine, Université Laval, Québec, QC G1V 0A6, Canada
6 Institute of Biomolecular Chemistry, Consiglio Nazionale delle Ricerche, 80078 Pozzuoli, Italy
* Correspondence: cristoforo.silvestri@criucpq.ulaval.ca

Abstract: Lifestyle is a well-known environmental factor that plays a major role in facilitating the development of metabolic syndrome or eventually exacerbating its consequences. Various lifestyle factors, especially changes in dietary habits, extreme temperatures, unusual light–dark cycles, substance abuse, and other stressful factors, are also established modifiers of the endocannabinoid system and its extended version, the endocannabinoidome. The endocannabinoidome is a complex lipid signaling system composed of a plethora (>100) of fatty acid-derived mediators and their receptors and anabolic and catabolic enzymes (>50 proteins) which are deeply involved in the control of energy metabolism and its pathological deviations. A strong link between the endocannabinoidome and another major player in metabolism and dysmetabolism, the gut microbiome, is also emerging. Here, we review several examples of how lifestyle modifications (westernized diets, lack or presence of certain nutritional factors, physical exercise, and the use of cannabis) can modulate the propensity to develop metabolic syndrome by modifying the crosstalk between the endocannabinoidome and the gut microbiome and, hence, how lifestyle interventions can provide new therapies against cardiometabolic risk by ensuring correct functioning of both these systems.

Keywords: endocannabinoids; endocannabinoidome; metabolic syndrome; microbiome

---

1. Introduction

Diets poor in essential nutritional factors (e.g., dietary fibers or vitamins) and rich in high-calorie nutrients, lack of exercise, and uncontrolled use of recreational substances or certain therapeutic drugs, together with other environmental challenges such as recently changed lifestyle habits in populations living at extreme temperatures or regarding night–day cycles, are all known to negatively affect the body's ability to regulate energy metabolism and, hence, contribute to the development of metabolic syndrome [1]. A plethora of epidemiological studies point to these aspects as major predictors of various forms of dysmetabolism, including obesity and visceral adipose tissue accumulation [2], glucose intolerance, pre-diabetes and type 2 diabetes [3], dyslipidemia [4], hypertension [5] and, eventually, the development of atherogenic inflammation [6] and the ensuing cardiovascular disorders [7]. By contrast, several other studies show how fighting bad dietary habits and the introduction of some dietary supplements and vitamins, as well as the increase of physical exercise, can successfully counteract many features of metabolic syndrome [1,8,9].

At the same time, multifaceted lifestyle aspects are emerging as having a strong impact on an endogenous system of lipid signals known as the endocannabinoid system and its more recent expansion to the endocannabinoidome (see below), which play an important role in several physiological and pathological conditions and, particularly, in the control of energy metabolism and its dysfunctions [10,11]. Endocannabinoids and endocannabinoidome mediators are ultimately derived from long-chain fatty acids, and it is therefore predictable that prolonged diets rich in some fatty acids rather than others can affect the tissue concentrations of these molecules in as much as they can change the fatty acid composition of phospholipids acting as biosynthetic precursors [12,13]. Additionally, there is evidence that pre- and probiotics can produce beneficial effects partly mediated by endocannabinoidome mediators, pointing to the possibility that at least some of the numerous physiological and pathological actions respectively displayed by a healthy or disrupted gut microbiota (known as dysbiosis) may be due to changes in this complex system of lipid chemical signals, both at the central nervous system and peripheral tissue level. This seems to be particularly true in the context of metabolic control in which the intestinal flora, like the endocannabinoidome, is known to play a major role [14–16]. This evidence is reinforced by the recent finding that some commensal bacteria produce endocannabinoid-like compounds able to activate the same receptors as their host cell counterparts [17]. Conversely, in mice, pharmacological or tissue-selective genetic manipulation of the tissue concentrations and receptor-mediated activity of endocannabinoids and endocannabinoid-like molecules was found to affect, at the same time, the relative composition in phyla, orders, genera, and species of microorganisms that populate the intestinal tract as well as the metabolic response to high-fat diets [18–21]. If one considers that gut microbiota composition is altered by the same dietary and environmental factors and unhealthy behaviors that affect the endocannabinoid system [20,22–24], then it is perhaps not so farfetched to suggest that the lifestyle–gut microbiome–endocannabinoidome triangle plays a crucial role in the development of metabolic syndrome.

In this article, we shall discuss several ways through which lifestyle-induced alterations of the endocannabinoidome—very often through direct or indirect effects on the gut microbiome (μB; that is the ensemble of genes, proteins, and metabolites provided by intestinal microorganisms)—can either worsen or ameliorate energy metabolism in mammals and, hence, influence the development of the metabolic syndrome.

2. The Endocannabinoidome

The very popular drug of abuse, marijuana, is prepared from the flowers of *Cannabis sativa* varieties containing relatively high contents of the non-psychotropic precursor of Δ^9-tetrahydrocannabinol (THC), i.e., Δ^9-tetrahydrocannabinolic acid, wherefrom the better known THC is obtained following desiccation and/or heating. However, *Cannabis sativa*—including those varieties that have been used for centuries for their fibers and employed to make ropes and paper—contains more than one hundred other THC and THC acid-like compounds in the inflorescence. These compounds have little or no psychotropic action and, together with THC and THC-acid, are known as *cannabinoids*. The euphoric, appetite-stimulating, and many other "central" actions of THC, are due to its unique capability to bind and activate a G-protein-coupled receptor (GPCR), the cannabinoid receptor type-1 (CB1), whereas another GPCR, the cannabinoid receptor type-2 (CB2), with little more than 50% homology with CB1 [1,2], is responsible for the immune-modulatory effects of this compound. So far, THC is the only plant-derived cannabinoid known to be capable of potently and efficaciously activating these receptors (which is why they should, in our opinion, be renamed "THC receptors"), although a THC congener, Δ^9-tetrahydrocannabivarine (THCV), was more recently shown to antagonize CB1 [25]. The discovery of cannabinoid receptors suggested the existence of endogenous ligands for such receptors. Two small lipids ultimately derived from arachidonic acid, *N*-arachidonoylethanolamine (AEA or anandamide) and 2-arachidonoylglycerol (2-AG), were indeed identified and shown to be capable of high-affinity binding to both CB1 and CB2 receptors, stimulating their activity with good efficacy [26,27]. These molecules were named *endocannabinoids* (eCBs) [28].

The eCBs come with their own anabolic and catabolic routes and enzymes, biosynthetic precursors, and hydrolysis products, which are inactive at cannabinoid receptors. By the turn of the last century, it was established that AEA is biosynthesized from the hydrolysis of *N*-arachidonoyl-phosphatidylethanolamines catalyzed by an *N*-acyl-phosphatidylethanolamine-specific phospholipase D-like enzyme (NAPE-PLD), whereas 2-AG is produced from the hydrolysis of 1-acyl-*sn*-2-arachidonoyl-glycerols (AcArGs), catalyzed by either *sn*-1 selective diacylglycerol lipase-α or -β (DAGLα or DAGLβ). AEA is hydrolyzed to arachidonic acid (AA) and ethanolamine by fatty acid amide hydrolase (FAAH), and 2-AG to AA and glycerol by monoacylglycerol lipase (MAGL) [29–32]. This ensemble of lipids, enzymes, and CB1 and CB2 receptors is known as the "endocannabinoid system". While the enzymes mentioned above are historically considered to be the canonical ones that regulate endocannabinoid levels, it must be noted that other pathways have also been identified (see Figure 1B, recently reviewed in [33]). For example, AEA may be synthesized by the combined action of ABDH4 and GDE1 [34] or PTPN22 [35].

It was soon realized that AEA and 2-AG, like several other lipid mediators, are quite promiscuous in their pharmacological activity in as much as they were suggested to modulate the activity of other proteins at concentrations often, but not necessarily, higher than those required to activate CB1 and CB2. These receptors were later found to often be even better targets for some of the congeners of AEA and 2-AG, i.e., the long-chain *N*-acylethanolamines (NAEs) and 2-monoacylglycerols (2-MAGs), respectively, and include (1) thermosensitive transient receptor potential (TRP) channels, such as the "capsaicin receptor", or TRP of vanilloid type-1 (TRPV1), the "menthol receptor", or TRP of melastatin type-8 (TRPM8), and the TRP of vanilloid type-2 (TRPV2) channels, as well as the T-type Ca^{2+} channel ($Ca_{v.3.1}$); (2) some orphan GPCRs, such as GPR55, GPR110, or GPR119; and (3) peroxisome proliferator-activated receptor-α and -γ (PPARα and PPARγ) (Figure 1A; recently reviewed in [33]. The eCB congeners, which are biosynthesized using NAPE-PLD or DAGLs from precursors similar to those of the two eCBs, and inactivated to the respective fatty acids and ethanolamine or glycerol by FAAH and MAGL, can also be produced and degraded via alternative pathways and enzymes, and, as mentioned above, this also applies to AEA and 2-AG (Figure 1B). Finally, several other long-chain fatty acid derivatives have also been identified during the last 15 years, including primary fatty acid amides and several *N*-acylated amino acids and neurotransmitters that often share molecular targets and/or inactivating enzymes with eCBs (Figure 1A,B). These findings led to the definition of the "expanded eCB system" or *endocannabinoidome* (eCBome), which includes a plethora of lipid mediators (including some enzymatic oxidation products of AEA and 2-AG) and tens of proteins acting as biosynthetic and inactivating enzymes, or molecular targets, for these mediators (recently reviewed in [33]).

The existence of the eCBome complicates the development of selective pharmacological and genetic tools to be used for the understanding of the several tissue-specific local functions of the eCBs, and for the exploitation of this knowledge for the development of new therapies against pathological conditions in which AEA and 2-AG are involved. On the other hand, if one looks at the eCBome as a whole and as the potential target of several physiopathological and environmental clues, and at eCBome profiles as possible personalized fingerprints of disease and responses to lifestyle, this complex signaling *hypersystem*, no matter how challenging, may open new therapeutic and diagnostic avenues. Indeed, as will be discussed below, diet and dietary components, habits, exercise, and the environment strongly impact on the eCBome—to an extent of which we have had perhaps, so far, only a partial view.

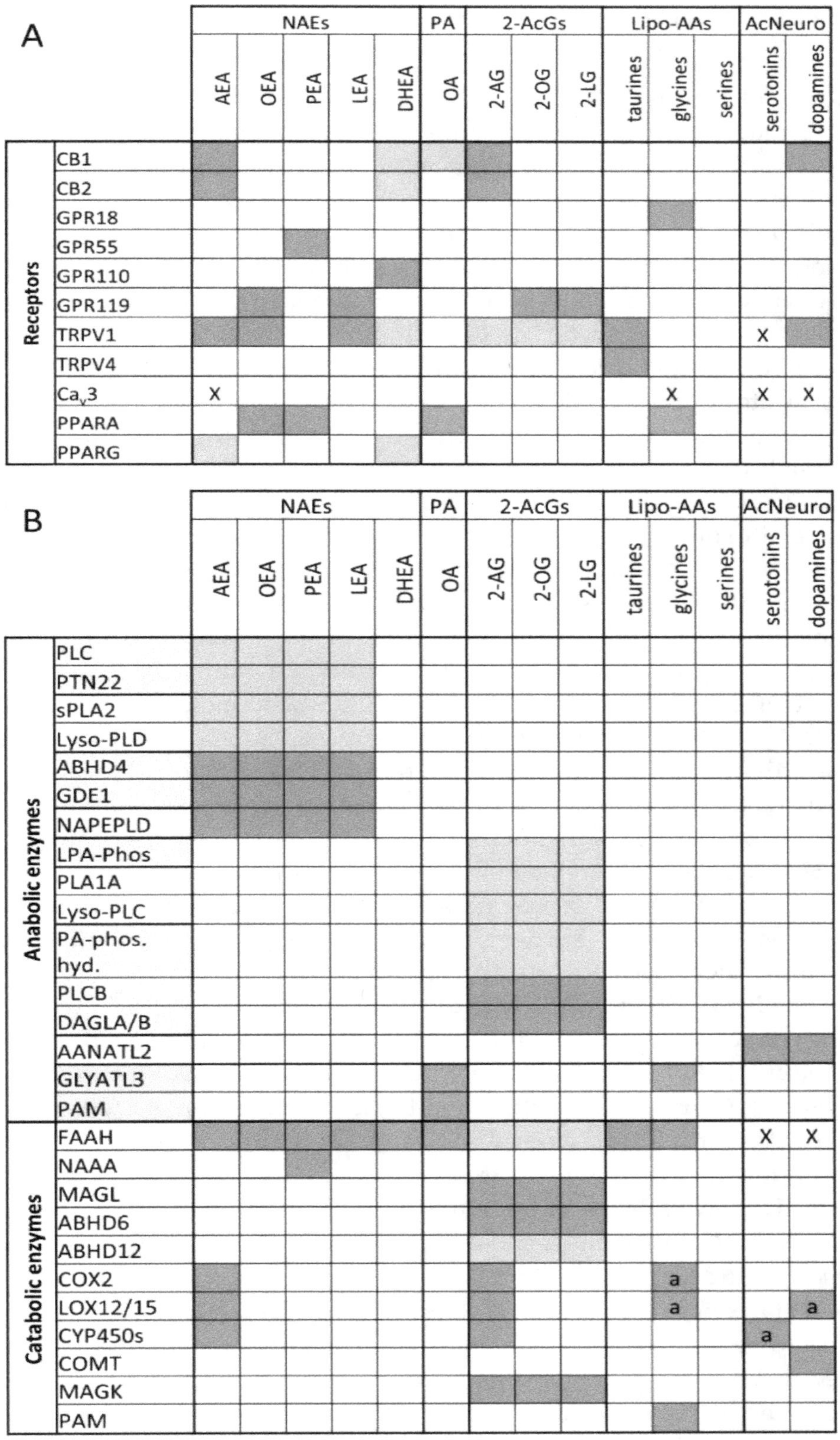

Figure 1. Endocannabinoidome mediators and their receptors (**A**) and anabolic and catabolic enzymes (**B**). Interactions are indicated by dark shaded boxes, and anabolic enzymes that function in concert are grouped together; "X" indicates inhibitory interactions; "a" indicates that enzymes only function with arachidonoyl homologs. A lighter shade of gray indicates a lower interaction with the receptors or a lesser role of the enzymes in biosynthesis or degradation.

3. Dietary Fats and the Endocannabinoidome

In the obese state, the eCB system is modulated at the level of anabolic and catabolic enzyme activity, endocannabinoid levels, and CB1 receptor expression, resulting in a generally increased eCB tone "in the wrong place and at the wrong time" [36]. BMI positively correlates with circulating AEA and 2-AG levels, especially when fat distribution is partitioned more towards intra-abdominal stores [37–39]. However, the levels of AEA are dysregulated in obesity with respect to responses to feeding or the time of day as viscerally obese men were found to have significantly lower levels of AEA in the morning than normoweights [38]. The observed increases in AEA and 2-AG levels appear to be due to changes in expression of adipose tissue-metabolizing enzymes, as the AEA-catabolizing enzyme FAAH was decreased and the 2-AG-anabolizing enzyme DAGLα was increased in the adipose tissue from obese individuals in conjunction with decreased CB1 expression, perhaps as a homeostatic compensatory response [37,39,40]. Changes in eCBome gene expression within adipose tissue appear to be depot-specific, however, since gluteal subcutaneous adipose tissue from obese subjects had decreased eCBome gene expression (including FAAH, DAGLα, and CB1) while abdominal subcutaneous adipose tissue showed the opposite trend, with visceral adipose tissue similarly having increased CB1 expression [41].

Obesogenic diets characterized by high fat content are increasingly prevalent in westernized societies. High-fat diets increase AEA and/or 2-AG levels [12,13]. While *N*-oleoylethanolamine (OEA), *N*-palmitoylethanolamine (PEA), and *N*-linoleoylethanolamine (LEA) levels are reduced in the jejunum and/or stomach in response to 1 week [42] or up to 8 weeks [43] of high-fat feeding, prolonged feeding (14 weeks) increased OEA levels in the stomach concomitant with increased NAPE-PLD and decreased FAAH expression [43]. In the liver, a high-fat diet increased AEA levels and CB1 signaling, which contributed to the activation of genetic programs that increase fatty acid production [13]. In a very recent study in which circulating eCBome levels were tracked over time in mice on a high-fat diet, AEA, PEA, and *N*-docosahexanoylethanolamine (DHEA) levels increased rapidly over the course of a week, while SEA and 2-AG increases became significant only after 4 weeks and, finally, OEA increased after 10 weeks [44]. While gene expression changes in eCBome enzymes were observed in muscle and liver tissues, they were transient; however, the expression of the 2-AG anabolic enzyme DAGLβ was constantly increased in white and brown adipose tissue (BAT) from 4 weeks, while the NAE anabolic enzyme NAPE-PLD was constantly increased only in the BAT from 3 days on [44]. This study supports the conclusions inferred from human studies, that adipose tissue is one of the main regulators of circulating 2-AG in obesity. The potential contribution of BAT (at least in mice) to the regulation of NAEs was a surprising result, though at least in the case of OEA, it cannot be ruled out that the intestinal tract is one of the major sources [43].

Changes in eCBome mediator levels in response to high-fat feeding occur very quickly in mice. Recently, Everard et al. showed that after just 4 h of initial high-fat-diet feeding, jejunal AEA and 2-AG levels decreased while OEA, 2-OG, 2-LG, and 2-PG levels increased [18], but after 5 weeks of exposure AEA, LEA increased, as did 2-OG and 2-PG.

In utero or neonatal exposure to dietary perturbations can have long-lasting effects on an individual and, indeed, the eCBome is significantly impacted by exposure to high-fat diets early on in life with long-lasting consequences. Maternal high-fat feeding resulted in sustained elevation of CB1/2, FAAH, and MAGL levels in the livers of adult male rats, with changes in redox homeostasis [45]. Maternal exposure to high-fat diet also increased CB1 in the male, and CB2 in the female hypothalamus at birth, while CB1 and FAAH expression were increased, and CB2 and MGLL were decreased in the BAT of males and females, respectively. Both sexes developed an increased adiposity and preference for high-fat diets [46].

Dietary linoleic acid (LA) is a major *n*-6 fatty acid component of Western diets, making up over 80% of the polyunsaturated fatty acid (PUFA) consumed in the United States [47], resulting in an imbalance the ratio of *n*-6/*n*-3 fatty acids consumed greatly in favor of the former. LA is linked to obesity and is efficiently converted to the AEA and 2-AG constituent arachidonic acid (AA), thus explaining its ability to increase AEA and 2-AG levels and to produce obesogenic effects [48,49]. Indeed, even within the context of a low-fat diet, high levels of LA increased liver AEA and 2-AG levels, promoting obesity and associated adipose tissue inflammation [50]. Inclusion of n-3 fatty acids to an LA-rich diet reverses the latter's effects on AEA and 2-AG levels [48]. Similar results have been obtained with EPA/DHA n-3 fatty acid-rich krill and, to a lesser extent, fish oil [12,51–53]. Additionally, supplementing young mice on a lard diet with flax seed oil rich in the n-3 fatty acid α-linolenic acid significantly decreased liver AEA levels and improved glucose homeostasis after a subsequent 10 weeks on a high-lard diet [54]. These effects are believed to largely be the result of decreasing the n-6/n-3 PUFA ratio, which results in AA displacement from phospholipid membranes, thus reducing the amounts of the biosynthetic precursors of AEA and 2-AG. In support of this, n-3 PUFAs provided as phospholipids, rather than free fatty acids, result in more significant decreases in eCB levels [12,52]. Correspondingly, decreasing n-3 PUFA phospholipid content increased 2-AG liver levels and promoted hepatosteatosis and insulin resistance [55].

These data suggest that some of the therapeutic properties against metabolic disorders (such as against high triglycerides) of n-3 fatty PUFA may be ascribed to a reduction of eCB overactivity, and this has also been suggested to be the case in obese humans [53]. However, the metabolic benefits of dietary n-3 PUFAs may also result from the elevation of n-3 PUFA-derived NAEs (DHEA, *N*-eicosapentaenoylethanolamine (EPEA)), which has been observed in several tissues and blood [52,56,57], as well as of the corresponding monoacylglycerols [58] and other monoacylamides [59], which possess anti-inflammatory and anticancer actions and potential cardiometabolic- and neuroprotective effects independent of cannabinoid receptors [60–63]. A recent study comparing DHA and EPA supplementation in diet-induced obese mice and type 2 diabetic patients found significantly increased levels of DHEA and EPEA in both circulation and adipose tissue, but decreases in AEA and 2-AG were only observed in mice [64]. Of note, this study by Rossmeisl et al. utilized n-3 PUFAs as triglycerides; however, when provided mostly as phospholipids (from krill powder) to obese men, circulating AEA levels were reduced along with triglycerides [53].

Gut microbes (collectively termed the microbiome (μB)), are not a group of commensalist microorganisms living within animals but, rather, many are mutualists, benefiting the host in a variety of ways such as aiding in energy harvesting and digestion, modulating the immune system, and influencing many aspects of metabolic health, including weight, adiposity, and lipid and glucose metabolism [65]. The μB responds quickly to dietary interventions [66], and westernized diets are linked to dysbiosis (an imbalance of microbial communities) and associated with obesity, which is generally characterized by decreased bacterial diversity with an increase in the Firmicutes/Bacteroidetes phyla ratio [67,68]. Alterations in the μB are associated with other aspects of metabolic syndrome, including dyslipidemia, hypertension, and insulin resistance (reviewed extensively in [69–72]), and their consideration for the development of targeted therapies for "precision health" plans has recently been suggested for diabetes [73,74]. Like the eCBome, the gut μB is modified by dietary fatty acids, including supplementation with n-3 fatty acids from fish oil and krill oil [22,75,76]. Although few studies have assessed the effects of α-linolenic acid, at least one clinical trial has indicated that α-linolenic acid-rich oils can modify the μB at the genera level [77].

In the study by Everard et al. discussed above, the chronic high-fat-diet-induced changes in the jejunum eCBome lipid levels were associated with significant alterations in the gut μB, with the proportions of 19 bacterial genera identified as being significantly modified [18]. The same group had previously shown that 4 weeks of high-fat-diet feeding increased 2-AG levels in the ileum which was also associated with an altered μB [78]. High-fat-diet-induced μB changes were associated with increased CB1 expression in the colon whereas FAAH was increased in the jejunum [79]. Thus, it appears that μB alterations in response to high-fat diets impacts upon the intestinal eCBome directly which, under obesity-inducing conditions, increases gut barrier permeability, subsequently resulting in increased circulating bacterially derived lipopolysaccharide (LPS) that subsequently modulates adipose tissue eCBome and functionality (reviewed in [80]).

4. Dietary Fiber and Prebiotics: Improving Gut Barrier Function through the Endocannabinoidome

The health benefits of dietary fiber have been extensively studied and reviewed, and there is little doubt that higher fiber is beneficial for cardiovascular disease, supporting prevalent recommendations that fiber intake be increased in order to maintain a healthy diet [81]. The positive effects of fiber on obesity and metabolic syndrome are believed to be intimately linked to alterations of the gut μB [23,82]. Increasing attention is being paid to "prebiotic" fiber, which is non-digestible by the host but is metabolized by gut microbiota, resulting in an alteration of the composition and/or activity of the μB, producing bioactive metabolites (such as short-chain fatty acids) that provide physiological benefits to the host [83].

One of the main positive effects of prebiotics is in regulating intestinal epithelial barrier permeability, in which short-chain fatty acids play a crucial role. The term "leaky gut" has been used to describe the phenomenon in which the tight junctions within the intestinal epithelial lining are compromised, leading to the movement of bacterially derived LPS into circulation, resulting in metabolic endotoxemia-induced inflammation that is associated with obesity [84,85]. Supplementing the diets of genetically (*ob/ob*) or diet-induced obese mice with the prebiotic oligofructose increases *Bifidobacterium* species and *Akkermansia muciniphila* in association with improved gut barrier function and decreased inflammation [79,86,87]. Similarly, women with type 2 diabetes who were given oligofructose-enriched inulin (10 g/day) for 8 weeks had significantly lower circulating levels of LPS and other inflammatory markers, along with decreased fasting glucose and glycosylated hemoglobin [88]. Finally, administration of pasteurized *A. muciniphila* improved insulin sensitivity and reduced total plasma cholesterol levels [89].

The eCBome has been found to regulate intestinal permeability. Using the same genetic model discussed above (*ob/ob* mice), Muccioli et al. showed that CB1 antagonism partially rescued tight junction integrity within the intestinal epithelium and reduced plasma LPS levels, while CB1 agonism in wild type mice increased gut permeability [79]. Further, blocking CB1 activity in mice on an obesity-inducing diet not only inhibited the development of obesity and improved glucose homeostasis, as expected, but also decreased intestinal permeability as evidenced by reduced circulating LPS levels in association with decreased adipose tissue inflammation and circulating inflammatory cytokine profile, indicating a decrease in systemic inflammation [21]. Importantly, these changes were observed in conjunction with an increase in the relative amounts of intestinal *A. muciniphila* and decreased *Lachnospiraceae*. The reduction in metabolic endotoxemia induced in *ob/ob* mice fed oligofructose correlated with decreased colonic CB1 expression and AEA levels, with the latter presumably due to increased expression of the AEA catabolic enzyme FAAH [79]. Thus, CB1 regulation of gut permeability, under the influence of the μB, is another mechanism by which CB1 regulates inflammation in addition to direct proinflammatory effects such as, for example, the stimulation of proinflammatory cytokine release from macrophages, which has developmental consequences for type 2 diabetes [90,91]. These results collectively support the notion that the cardiometabolic health effects of dietary prebiotic fiber is associated with alteration of the gut microbiota and intestinal eCBome, resulting in decreased intestinal permeability and the ensuing metabolic endotoxemia/systemic inflammation.

5. TRPV1: Linking the Endocannabinoidome to the Metabolic Benefits Attributed to Spicy Food

The consumption of spicy food has been associated with overall decreased mortality and significant reduction in hazard ratios for deaths caused by ischemic heart diseases and, in the case of the consumption of fresh chili peppers, reduced diabetes [92]. Capsaicin is the active component endowing chili peppers with their spiciness, due to activation of transient receptor potential vanilloid-1 (TRPV1) cation channels. TRPV1 channels primarily respond to noxious heat (>42 °C), but are also modulated by several eCBome members (including long-chain-saturated NAEs, monoacylglycerols, *N*-acyldopamines, and *N*-acyltaurines) [33]. Several human studies have indicated the various metabolic benefits of dietary capsaicin, which improved postprandial glucose handling in both healthy individuals and overweight individuals and women with gestational diabetes [93–95]. While a meta-analysis of capsaicin studies supported the positive effects of this dietary component on energy expenditure and appetite regulation, the overall effects were very small and more evident at high doses [96]. In rodent models, oral capsaicin is able to combat diet-induced obesity, insulin resistance, and hepatosteatosis [97]. The positive metabolic effects of capsaicin appear to be mediated by both TRPV1 and PPARα [97,98]. However, the role of TRPV1 in obesity and associated side effects—especially dysregulation of glucose homeostasis—is complex, as indicated by contrasting results from *Trpv1*$^{-/-}$ mice in diet-induced obesity, in which both beneficial [99] and detrimental [100] effects have been observed. These differences may be due to variations in the diets used between studies or the ages of the mice, as *Trpv1*$^{-/-}$ mice have been shown to have increased activity at young ages, but decreased activity at older ages, in association with increased weight gain [100,101].

Capsaicin and TRP channels have also been linked to the gut μB. The antiobesity effects of capsaicin have been associated with changes in the gut μB, including also increases in *A. muciniphila* [20,102,103]. The gut μB appears to have a causative role in mediating capsaicin antiobesity effects as gut μB transplantation from capsaicin-treated to germ-free mice replicated the capsaicin-dependent antimetabolic endotoxemia effects, which were mitigated by antibiotics in capsaicin-treated mice [104]. These changes were defined by decreases in lipopolysaccharide (LPS)-producing, gram-negative bacteria and LPS biosynthetic genes, and increases in short-chain fatty acid (SCFA)-producing bacteria, such as *Lachnospiraceae*, *Ruminococcaceae*, and *Roseburia*, as well as decreased colonic CB1 expression [104]. Accordingly, TRPV1 has been suggested to counteract increased intestinal permeability in vitro [105]. Most interestingly, in a human study, different μB enterotypes (different gut μB ecosystems) of participants were associated with the extent of capsaicin-mediated positive metabolic effects. Capsaicin increased the Firmicutes/Bacteroidetes ratio and *Faecalibacterium* abundance more prevalently in participants with the *Bacteroides* enterotype than the *Prevotella* enterotype, in combination with increased serum incretin (GIP and GLP-1) levels, which stimulate insulin production, and decreased LBP, which was assessed as a marker of inflammation [106]. As in the case of eCBs and CB1 receptors, also the communication between TRPV1 and the gut μB seems to be bi-directional. In fact, the visceral antinociceptive effects of the probiotic *Lactobacillus reuteri* has been attributed to inhibition of TRPV1 activity in mesenteric neurons [107], indicating also that the eCBome may play a significant role in mediating the activity of microbial influences on the gut–brain axis, at least with respect to pain.

6. Sunlight Effects on the Endocannabinoidome: A Role for Vitamin D?

Vitamin D deficiency represents a global health issue, with over a billion people being deficient [108], largely due to inadequate sun exposure. Yet, significant levels of deficiency still occur in populations living in areas of abundant sunlight [109]. Vitamin D is found only in a few foods and is thus a common dietary supplement recommended by health authorities, especially in winter months [110]. Several aspects of the metabolic syndrome are associated with vitamin D deficiency, including obesity, dyslipidemia, insulin resistance, hepatosteatosis, and hypertension [111]. The causal role of vitamin D in the pathophysiology of these aspects of the metabolic syndrome is not known, but the gut μB also appears to play a significant role. In a mouse model of diet-induced obesity, vitamin D deficiency aggravated high-fat-diet-induced insulin resistance and hepatosteatosis along with inflammation. These results occurred in conjunction with mucosal breakdown within the ileum, endotoxemia and dysbiosis with increased levels of pathogenic *Helicobacter hepaticus*, and decreased levels of the metabolically beneficial *A. muciniphila* [112]. Vitamin D receptor knockout mice also develop dysbiosis, exemplified by an alteration in the ratio of Bacteroidetes/Firmicutes phyla with increases in Lactobacillaceae and Lachnospiraceae families [113]. However, while the mechanisms remain to be determined, UVR has recently been found to alter the mouse gut μB independently of vitamin D [114].

Endogenous vitamin D is produced upon UV irradiation of 7-hehydrocholesterol in skin, which is then further metabolized, mostly in the liver and kidney, to produce bioactive 1,25-dihydroxyvitamin D_3 [115]. The skin contains not only 2-AG and AEA, but also several other NAEs in both the dermis and epidermis [116]. Whether the skin provides a significant source of circulating eCBome mediators remains to be determined. However, in vitro exposure of melanocytes to low doses of UVB upregulates CB1 mRNA expression and increases the levels of AEA, PEA, and 2-AG in keratinocytes [117]. Further, 6 weeks of cutaneous UV exposure increased circulating 2-AG levels in both light- and dark-skinned people, without significantly altering NAEs [118]. This finding was in apparent contrast to results obtained earlier by Magina et al., who found that in psoriasis patients, whole-body narrowband UVB therapy resulted in a decrease in AEA plasma levels without affecting 2-AG [119]. The differences in these results may have been due to a variety of factors, including the fact that the employed UV radiation regimens differed between the studies and that Madina et al. studied effects only in psoriasis patients.

Vitamin D deficiency in mice increased pain sensitization and decreased CB1, but increased CB2 and PPARα in the spinal cord along with increased AEA and DHEA [120]. In the colon, 2-AG was significantly decreased together with microbial diversity, leading to an increased Firmicutes/Bacteroidetes ratio and lower levels of *A. muciniphila*. Treatment of vitamin D-deficient mice with the PPARα agonist and AEA congener, PEA, reversed the observed pain sensitization in conjunction with an increase in the levels of several microbial genera, including *A. muciniphila* [120].

Taken together, these studies suggest that sunlight exposure, and the elevation in vitamin D levels that results from it, modify the eCBome as well as the μB. Whether there is a link between the two remains to be determined. For this reason, and given that these alterations are associated with μB changes that are believed to impact on metabolic health, such as increased Firmicutes/Bacteroidetes ratios and the presence of low *A. muciniphila* levels, it will be interesting to investigate if μB–eCBome crosstalk plays a significant role in regulating obesity and associated metabolic complications downstream of vitamin D.

7. Effects of Exercise on the Endocannabinoidome

Exercise is the second pillar, together with the diet, which maintains metabolic health. Viscerally obese men who underwent a lifestyle modification program that included the addition of regular exercise for one year had significant improvements in several metabolic parameters as well as reduced circulating 2-AG and, to a lesser extent, AEA levels [121]. These latter alterations were very likely associated with decreased adiposity. However, while physically active men have higher lymphocyte FAAH activity than sedentary controls, suggesting higher eCBome tone within these cells, basal circulating levels of AEA, PEA, and 2-AG were not found to be different from those of sedentary males [122]. By contrast, in a study of normoweight and obese women whose activity was tracked over 6 days, while 2-AG was associated with BMI, as expected, AEA and OEA levels were positively associated with moderate–vigorous physical activity [123].

In contrast to the scarcity of data on the effects of chronic physical activity on basal eCBome mediator levels, much more research has been conducted on their response to acute exercise. Many studies have shown that physical activity quickly increases circulating AEA, but not 2-AG, levels in humans ([124–126] and reviewed in [127]). However, a recent study found that 2-AG, and not AEA, increased after exercise [128], and this discrepancy with previous studies may be due to the fact that the participants fasted before exercising. Interestingly, AEA increases only appear in response to medium-intensity exercise [124]. Heyman et al. showed that similar to AEA, PEA and OEA also increase during and after exercise and, in fact, are more responsive to lower intensity exercise than AEA [126]. The source of these eCBome mediators remains to be determined. However, in rats, exercise alters the levels of many NAE metabolic enzymes within the adipose tissue [129]. It has been suggested that AEA and related NAEs exert positive metabolic effects in muscle, such as improving glucose uptake and mitochondrial activity by acting at the PPARγ and TRPV1 eCBome receptors [127]. Further, exercise may modulate AEA levels directly in muscle, as has been found in the extensor digitorum longus muscles of rats [129].

Several physiological mechanisms by which exercise affects mood have been proposed, including increasing endorphins, altered mitochondrial function, and thermogenesis, as well as modulation of the endocannabinoid system [130]. The notion that increased AEA levels may be, in part, responsible for feelings of euphoria associated with exercise is supported by the finding in mice that exercise increased AEA and OEA, but not 2-AG or PEA, levels in association with decreased GABAergic neuron CB1-dependent anxiety [131]. In fact, exercise also increases eCB tone in the brain. Mice with free access to a running wheel for 8 days had increased AEA levels and CB1 binding site density in the hippocampus [132]. Furthermore, wheel running in mice results in potentiated CB1 activity within the striatum, playing a protective role against stress [133], which does not appear to be simply due to increased CB1 expression, as chronic exercise does not alter the levels of this receptor in any part of the brain [134]. Similarly, a recent study showed that singing increased circulating AEA, PEA, and OEA levels in association with improved positive mood [135]. In the same study, the effects of 30 min of cycling were also examined, and significantly increased OEA levels were observed, while AEA and PEA only showed trends towards increases. The lack of statistical increases in AEA, commonly observed in other studies, may have been due to the intensity of the cycling or the relatively small sample size. Further, exercise addicts, which have increased negative mood in response to exercise deprivation, also have lower basal circulating AEA levels than non-addicted regular runners, and exercise withdrawal and reintroduction only decreases and increases AEA levels, respectively, in non-addicts [136]. The lack of response of AEA in exercise addicts suggests that perhaps their increased amount of exercise is a homeostatic attempt to increase eCB tone.

Recent evidence indicates that exercise and the μB interact with each other (reviewed in [24]). Germ-free mice have decreased exercise performance as compared to conventional controls, and reintroduction of a single bacterial species (*Bacteroides fragilis*) partially reversed this [137]. While the sample sizes were small, Petriz et al. found that moderate exercise differentially changes the μB in wild type Wistar, obese Zucker, and spontaneously hypertensive rats, suggesting that exercise-induced changes in the μB may be dependent on the metabolic state of the host organism [138]. Similarly, high-intensity interval training of high-fat-diet-fed mice altered the μB differentially along the gastrointestinal tract with the most significant changes found in the distal regions [139]. Interestingly, exercise reversed the high-fat-diet-induced decrease in microbial diversity and the Bacteroidetes/Firmicutes ratio, which are indicative of obesity [139]. Furthermore, fecal microbiota transplant from exercised mice to mice on a high-fat diet resulted in improved metabolic parameters, suggesting that that μB can confer, at least in part, the benefits of exercise [140]. However, a more recent study found that high- or medium-intensity training had no effect on the μB of obese Zucker rats [141]. In humans, studies on professional rugby players found that their μBs were more diverse than sedentary controls and produced more short-chain fatty acids, though these changes were also associated with dietary differences [142,143]. However, other studies have found that independent of diet or BMI, higher levels of cardiorespiratory fitness correlated with higher μB diversity and short-chain fatty acid production [144]. Similarly, independent of diet, six weeks of endurance exercise in overweight women significantly altered the μB of participants with an increase in *A. muciniphila* [145], which has been shown to increase the levels of eCBome monoacylglycerols, including 2-AG [87] and, as mentioned above, to be regulated by both CB1 and TRPV1 activity [21,103]. To date, no studies have examined the potential link between the eCBome, exercise, and the gut μB. However, given that activities of several eCBome receptors (CB1, TRPV1, PPARα) have been linked to μB changes [21,103,146], it is possible that their modulation through exercise-induced changes in eCBome mediator levels may play a role in exercise-induced changes in the μB, or vice versa.

8. Cannabis Use and Metabolic Health

The principal psychoactive component of marijuana/cannabis (THC), one of the most commonly used recreational drugs the world over, acts mainly through CB1 activation (reviewed in [25]). Given the strong association of CB1 and its ligands AEA and 2-AG with several aspects of metabolic syndrome and obesity in general [10], it is somewhat counterintuitive that cannabis use is generally associated with an improved metabolic phenotype. Analysis of the NHANES survey from 2005–2010 found that current and past cannabis use is generally associated with significantly lower odds of metabolic syndrome [147]. Combined examination of two large epidemiological studies (NESARC and NCS-R) concluded that chronic cannabis users had significantly decreased adjusted prevalence rates of obesity, from 22%–25% in non-users to 14%–17% in users [148]. A very recent prospective analysis of NESARC data supports the above, finding that cannabis use is inversely associated with BMI increases over 3 years [149]. Several large studies have also shown inverse associations between cannabis and diabetes [150–152], which were corroborated by a Swedish study involving 18,000 participants, though the observed protective effects on diabetes were attenuated when adjusted for age [153]. Interestingly, these associations, observed in large heterogeneous populations, are also observed in Inuit from the Canadian north, a relatively isolated ethnic group in which the decreased weight associated with cannabis use was found to account for an association with improved glucose metabolism [154]. Cannabis use is also associated with reduced prevalence of both alcoholic and non-alcoholic fatty liver disease [155,156]. It should be noted that cannabis use is not always associated with positive metabolic outcomes; among individuals with type 1 diabetes, it is correlated with an increased risk in ketoacidosis [157], subclinical atherosclerosis (but only among cigarette smokers) [158], and mortality in patients with myocardial infarction, despite having lower rates of diabetes and hyperlipidemia [159].

The positive metabolic effects of cannabis have been attributed to the downregulation of CB1 in response to chronic cannabis use/THC exposure. Post-mortem analysis of chronic cannabis users' brains found decreased CB1 (*CNR1*) mRNA and ligand-binding in several brain regions [160], and in vivo positron emission tomography (PET) imaging similarly showed globally decreased CB1 availability compared to controls [161]. Chronic THC administration to rats decreases 2-AG and AEA levels in the striatum, but increases AEA levels in the limbic forebrain [162], and in chronic cannabis users, AEA levels are decreased in cerebrospinal fluid while 2-AG levels are increased in the serum as compared to infrequent users [163]. The mechanism by which eCB levels were altered in these studies are unknown; however, ex vivo treatment of placental explants with THC for long (72 h) but not short (24 h) periods of time increased AEA levels, concomitant with a counterintuitive decrease in NAPE-PLD levels and a trend for increased FAAH levels [164]. In hepatocytes, THC increased both AEA and 2-AG levels, presumably by blocking the activity of fatty acid binding protein 1 (FABP1), which can act as an eCB "chaperone", allowing eCB enzymatic degradation [165]. While THC does not appear to be able to inhibit eCBome catabolic or anabolic enzymes, several other phytocannabinoids do, though at relatively high concentrations [166], suggesting that their combination within cannabis may contribute to its ability to alter eCBome mediator levels.

In agreement with epidemiological studies, chronic THC administration to mice inhibited the development of obesity in response to a high-fat diet [167]. However, other cannabis-produced phytocannabinoids are also able to elicit positive metabolic effects. Delta-9-tetrahydrocannabivarin (THCV) is a CB1 antagonist and cannabidiol (CBD) is a CB1 negative allosteric modulator,) and both are TRPV1 agonists as well as acting on other receptors (reviewed in [25]). THCV markedly improved glucose metabolism in genetically, and diet-induced obese mice [168] and as did CBD in a genetic model of type 1 diabetes [169] Similarly, a clinical study found decreased fasting glucose levels in participants treated twice per day with 5 mg of THCV [170], whereas both THCV and CBD reduced hepatic triglyceride content in genetically obese mice [168,171].

More than 25% of non-antibiotic drugs induce dysbiosis of the μB [172]. There is limited evidence that cannabis use can modulate the gut μB. To date, only two studies have investigated the effects of cannabis use on the human gut μB. Panee et al. assayed the stools of 19 lifetime cannabis users and 20 non-users for the relative abundance of only two specific genera, *Prevotella* and *Bacteroides*, given that they are main determinants of human enterotypes [173]. They found that non-users had an average 13-fold higher *Prevotella/Bacteroides* ratio than cannabis users, which has been associated with plant-based as compared to animal-based diets [174]. This raised the possibility that the observed changes were attributed to alterations in the diets of users vs non-users, consistent with observations that cannabis users consume fewer fruits and more animal products and have higher caloric intake but, paradoxically, have similar nutrient serum status and lower BMIs than non-users [175]. In a second study, archived anal swabs were used to assess the μBs of HIV-positive individuals [176]. Cannabis use in these individuals was also associated with alterations in bacterial populations, including a decreased abundance of *Prevotella* as well as *Acidaminococcus* and *Dorea*, the latter two of which have been associated with obesity [177,178], along with increased abundances of other genera. The role of the *Prevotella* genus in metabolic health is complicated, due likely to the genetic diversity between individual species and, thus, several conflicting studies exist on its association with obesity, diabetes, and NAFLD, while others report positive correlations with improvements in various metabolic parameters (recently reviewed in [179]).

Chronic treatment with THC reduced weight and fat mass gain as well as energy intake in diet-induced obese but not lean mice, in association with alterations in the gut μB, which included increased levels of *A. muciniphila* and inhibition of the obesity-induced shift in the Firmicutes/Bacteroidetes ratio [167]. In an experimental autoimmune encephalomyelitis mouse model meant to mimic multiple sclerosis, a combination of the phytocannabinoids THC and CBD attenuated the induced inflammation and disease scores and significantly modulated the μB, decreasing the levels of *A. muciniphila* [180]. Fecal material transplantation confirmed that the protective effects were mediated by changes in the μB. Further unpublished data suggest that THC-mediated effects on the μB may be due, in part, to alterations in the host immune system, which has a complex interaction with the μB throughout a host's lifespan [181].

It is still unclear if the modulation of the μB by THC is dependent on CB1 activity. However, inhibition of CB1 with the inverse agonist rimonabant alters the μB composition of diet-induced obese mice, including increasing *A. muciniphila* in conjunction with metabolic parameter improvements [21]. Further, an adipose tissue-specific knockout of a major NAE anabolic enzyme, NAPE-PLD, which reduced local OEA, PEA and SEA, but not AEA levels, inhibited adipose tissue browning, and led to increased weight gain, glucose intolerance, and dyslipidemia in addition to exacerbating diet-induced obesity [19]. These effects were associated with an alteration in the gut μB which when transferred to germ-free mice, partially reproduced the phenotype, and are therefore likely to be CB1-independent, as the affected NAEs are ligands for other eCBome receptors, including TRPV1, which, as indicated above, impacts upon metabolic health, at least in part through alteration of the μB. Taken together, the above studies indicate that cannabis use—through its psychoactive constituent, THC, and non-psychoactive phytocannabinoids—potentially impacts upon metabolic health, in part by modulating μB constituents.

9. Conclusions

In summary, we have reviewed several examples of how the lifestyle–eCBome–μB triangle, with its multifaceted aspects, is likely to play a fundamental role in both metabolic health and metabolic syndrome (Figure 2). It is likely that several healthy and "bad" lifestyle habits, in synergy with other environmental factors, independently affect both eCBome signaling and the μB, and hence help in determining their correct or defective control of energy metabolism, respectively. It is also possible, however, that eCBome and μB crosstalk—which has not yet been fully explored—directs the manner in which lifestyle cues result in virtuous or vicious circles that can respectively counteract or accelerate the development of metabolic syndrome. The molecular aspects of the lifestyle–eCBome–μB triangle, therefore, need now to be fully elucidated in order to exploit this knowledge for new lifestyle (e.g., nutritional, physical activity, etc.) and pharmacological interventions aimed at combating the appearance of one or more of the metabolic syndrome features that together contribute to the development of type 2 diabetes and cardiovascular risk factors.

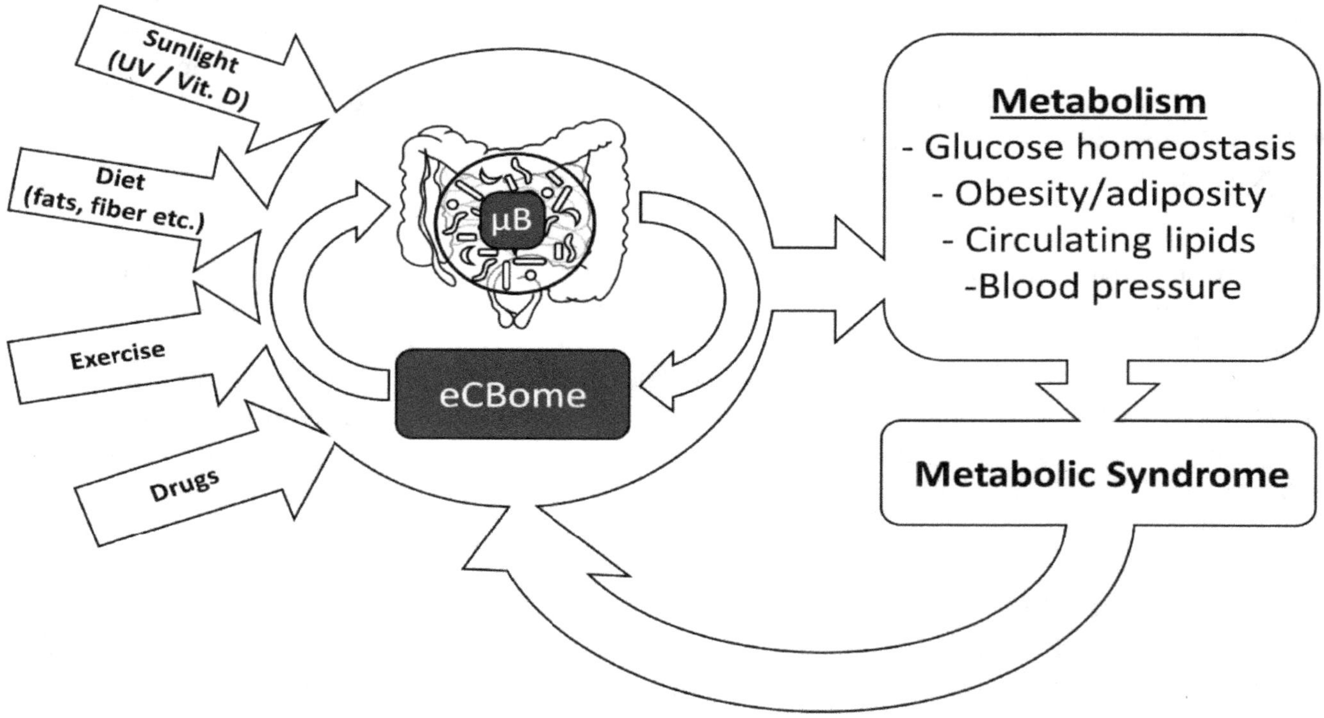

Figure 2. The endocannabinoidome–microbiome axis as a mechanism through which lifestyle choices affect various aspects of metabolism, which in turn may lead to the metabolic syndrome when dysregulated. This can, in turn, impact on both endocannabinoidome and microbiome-mediated signaling and, ultimately, also on lifestyle, thus creating potential vicious circles.

Author Contributions: C.S. and V.D.M. wrote the manuscript.

Abbreviations

Mediators	
2-AcGs	2-acylglycerols
2-AG	2-arachidonoylglycerol
2-LG	2-linoleoyl glycerol
2-OG	2-oleoylglycerol
AcNeuro	acyl neurotransmitters
AEA	*N*-arachidonoylethanolamine
DHEA	*N*-docosahexanoylethanolamine
LEA	*N*-linoleoylethanolamine
Lipo-AAs	lipoamino acids
NAEs	*N*-acylethanolamines
OA	oleoylamide
OEA	*N*-oleoylethanolamine
PA	fatty acid primary amides
PEA	*N*-palmitoylethanolamine

Receptors	
Ca_v3	T-type Ca^{2+} channel
CB1	cannabinoid receptor 1
CB2	cannabinoid receptor 2
GPR110	G protein-coupled receptor 110
GPR119	G protein-coupled receptor 119
GPR18	G protein-coupled receptor 18
GPR55	G protein-coupled receptor 55
PPARA	peroxisome proliferator-activated receptor alpha
PPARG	peroxisome proliferator-activated receptor gamma
TRPV1	transient receptor potential cation channel sub-family V member 1
TRPV4	transient receptor potential cation channel subfamily V member 4
Anabolic enzymes	
AANATL2	arylalkylamine *N*-acyltransferase-like 2, isoform A
ABHD4	alpha/beta-hydrolase domain containing 4
DAGLA/B	diacylglycerol lipase alpha/beta
GDE1	glycerophosphodiester phosphodiesterase 1
GLYATL3	glycine *N*-acyltransferase-like protein 3
LPA-Phos	lysophosphatidic acid phosphatase
Lyso-PLC	lysophospholipase C Lyso-PLC, lysophospholipase D
NAPEPLD	*N*-acyl phosphatidylethanolamine-hydrolyzing phospholipase D
PA-phos. hyd.	phosphatidic acid phosphohydrolase
PLA1A	phospholipase A1 member A
PLC	phospholipase C
PLCB	phospholipase C beta
PTPN22	tyrosine protein phosphatase non-receptor type 22
sPLA2	soluble phospholipase A2.
Catabolic enzymes	
ABHD12	alpha/beta-hydrolase domain containing 12
ABHD6	alpha/beta hydrolase domain containing 6
COMT	catechol-*O*-methyltransferase
COX2	cyclooxygenase 2
CYP450	cytochrome P450
FAAH	fatty acid amide hydrolase
LOX12/15	arachidonate lipoxygenase 12/15
MAGK	monoacylglycerol kinase
MGLL	monoacylglycerol lipase
NAAA	*N*-acylethanolamine-hydrolyzing acid amidase
PAM	peptidyl-glycine α-amidating monooxygenase

References

1. Yamaoka, K.; Tango, T. Effects of lifestyle modification on metabolic syndrome: A systematic review and meta-analysis. *BMC Med.* **2012**, *10*, 138. [CrossRef]
2. Reilly, J.J.; El-Hamdouchi, A.; Diouf, A.; Monyeki, A.; Somda, S.A. Determining the worldwide prevalence of obesity. *Lancet* **2018**, *391*, 1773–1774. [CrossRef]
3. NCD Risk Factor Collaboration (NCD-RisC). Worldwide trends in diabetes since 1980: A pooled analysis of 751 population-based studies with 4·4 million participants. *Lancet* **2016**, *387*, 1513–1530. [CrossRef]
4. Liu, H.-H.; Li, J.-J. Aging and dyslipidemia: A review of potential mechanisms. *Ageing Res. Rev.* **2015**, *19*, 43–52. [CrossRef] [PubMed]
5. Blacher, J.; Levy, B.I.; Mourad, J.-J.; Safar, M.E.; Bakris, G. From epidemiological transition to modern cardiovascular epidemiology: Hypertension in the 21st century. *Lancet* **2016**, *388*, 530–532. [CrossRef]

6. Halcox, J.P.; Banegas, J.R.; Roy, C.; Dallongeville, J.; De Backer, G.; Guallar, E.; Perk, J.; Hajage, D.; Henriksson, K.M.; Borghi, C. Prevalence and treatment of atherogenic dyslipidemia in the primary prevention of cardiovascular disease in Europe: EURIKA, a cross-sectional observational study. *BMC Cardiovasc. Disord.* **2017**, *17*, 160. [CrossRef] [PubMed]
7. Barquera, S.; Pedroza-Tobías, A.; Medina, C.; Hernández-Barrera, L.; Bibbins-Domingo, K.; Lozano, R.; Moran, A.E. Global Overview of the Epidemiology of Atherosclerotic Cardiovascular Disease. *Arch. Med. Res.* **2015**, *46*, 328–338. [CrossRef] [PubMed]
8. Saboya, P.P.; Bodanese, L.C.; Zimmermann, P.R.; da Silva Gustavo, A.; Macagnan, F.E.; Feoli, A.P.; da Silva Oliveira, M. Lifestyle Intervention on Metabolic Syndrome and its Impact on Quality of Life: A Randomized Controlled Trial. *Arq. Bras. Cardiol.* **2017**, *108*, 60–69. [CrossRef] [PubMed]
9. VanWormer, J.J.; Boucher, J.L.; Sidebottom, A.C.; Sillah, A.; Knickelbine, T. Lifestyle changes and prevention of metabolic syndrome in the Heart of New Ulm Project. *Prev. Med. Rep.* **2017**, *6*, 242–245. [CrossRef]
10. Silvestri, C.; Di Marzo, V. The Endocannabinoid System in Energy Homeostasis and the Etiopathology of Metabolic Disorders. *Cell Metab.* **2013**, *17*, 475–490. [CrossRef]
11. Cristino, L.; Becker, T.; Di Marzo, V. Endocannabinoids and energy homeostasis: An update: Regolatory Role of Endocannabinoids in Obesity. *BioFactors* **2014**, *40*, 389–397. [CrossRef] [PubMed]
12. Piscitelli, F.; Carta, G.; Bisogno, T.; Murru, E.; Cordeddu, L.; Berge, K.; Tandy, S.; Cohn, J.S.; Griinari, M.; Banni, S.; et al. Effect of dietary krill oil supplementation on the endocannabinoidome of metabolically relevant tissues from high-fat-fed mice. *Nutr. Metab. (Lond.)* **2011**, *8*, 51. [CrossRef] [PubMed]
13. Osei-Hyiaman, D.; DePetrillo, M.; Pacher, P.; Liu, J.; Radaeva, S.; Bátkai, S.; Harvey-White, J.; Mackie, K.; Offertáler, L.; Wang, L.; et al. Endocannabinoid activation at hepatic CB1 receptors stimulates fatty acid synthesis and contributes to diet-induced obesity. *J. Clin. Invest.* **2005**, *115*, 1298–1305. [CrossRef] [PubMed]
14. Bäckhed, F.; Ding, H.; Wang, T.; Hooper, L.V.; Koh, G.Y.; Nagy, A.; Semenkovich, C.F.; Gordon, J.I. The gut microbiota as an environmental factor that regulates fat storage. *Proc. Natl. Acad. Sci. USA* **2004**, *101*, 15718–15723. [CrossRef] [PubMed]
15. Esteve, E.; Ricart, W.; Fernández-Real, J.-M. Gut microbiota interactions with obesity, insulin resistance and type 2 diabetes: Did gut microbiote co-evolve with insulin resistance? *Curr. Opin. Clin. Nutr. Metab. Care* **2011**, *14*, 483–490. [CrossRef]
16. Ridaura, V.K.; Faith, J.J.; Rey, F.E.; Cheng, J.; Duncan, A.E.; Kau, A.L.; Griffin, N.W.; Lombard, V.; Henrissat, B.; Bain, J.R.; et al. Gut Microbiota from Twins Discordant for Obesity Modulate Metabolism in Mice. *Science* **2013**, *341*, 1241214. [CrossRef] [PubMed]
17. Cohen, L.J.; Esterhazy, D.; Kim, S.-H.; Lemetre, C.; Aguilar, R.R.; Gordon, E.A.; Pickard, A.J.; Cross, J.R.; Emiliano, A.B.; Han, S.M.; et al. Commensal bacteria make GPCR ligands that mimic human signalling molecules. *Nature* **2017**, *549*, 48–53. [CrossRef]
18. Everard, A.; Plovier, H.; Rastelli, M.; Van Hul, M.; de Wouters d'Oplinter, A.; Geurts, L.; Druart, C.; Robine, S.; Delzenne, N.M.; Muccioli, G.G.; et al. Intestinal epithelial N-acylphosphatidylethanolamine phospholipase D links dietary fat to metabolic adaptations in obesity and steatosis. *Nat. Commun.* **2019**, *10*, 457. [CrossRef]
19. Geurts, L.; Everard, A.; Van Hul, M.; Essaghir, A.; Duparc, T.; Matamoros, S.; Plovier, H.; Castel, J.; Denis, R.G.P.; Bergiers, M.; et al. Adipose tissue NAPE-PLD controls fat mass development by altering the browning process and gut microbiota. *Nat. Commun.* **2015**, *6*, 6495. [CrossRef]
20. Song, J.-X.; Ren, H.; Gao, Y.-F.; Lee, C.-Y.; Li, S.-F.; Zhang, F.; Li, L.; Chen, H. Dietary Capsaicin Improves Glucose Homeostasis and Alters the Gut Microbiota in Obese Diabetic ob/ob Mice. *Front. Physiol.* **2017**, *8*, 602. [CrossRef]
21. Mehrpouya-Bahrami, P.; Chitrala, K.N.; Ganewatta, M.S.; Tang, C.; Murphy, E.A.; Enos, R.T.; Velazquez, K.T.; McCellan, J.; Nagarkatti, M.; Nagarkatti, P. Blockade of CB1 cannabinoid receptor alters gut microbiota and attenuates inflammation and diet-induced obesity. *Sci. Rep.* **2017**, *7*, 15645. [CrossRef] [PubMed]
22. Costantini, L.; Molinari, R.; Farinon, B.; Merendino, N. Impact of Omega-3 Fatty Acids on the Gut Microbiota. *Int. J. Mol. Sci.* **2017**, *18*, 2645. [CrossRef] [PubMed]
23. Dahiya, D.K.; Renuka; Puniya, M.; Shandilya, U.K.; Dhewa, T.; Kumar, N.; Kumar, S.; Puniya, A.K.; Shukla, P. Gut Microbiota Modulation and Its Relationship with Obesity Using Prebiotic Fibers and Probiotics: A Review. *Front. Microbiol.* **2017**, *8*, 563. [CrossRef] [PubMed]

24. Mailing, L.J.; Allen, J.M.; Buford, T.W.; Fields, C.J.; Woods, J.A. Exercise and the Gut Microbiome: A Review of the Evidence, Potential Mechanisms, and Implications for Human Health. *Exerc. Sport Sci. Rev.* **2019**, *47*, 75–85. [CrossRef] [PubMed]
25. Pertwee, R.; Cascio, M.G. Chapter 6: Known Pharmacological Actions of Delta-9-Tetrahydrocannabinol and of Four Other Chemical Constituents of Cannabis that Activate Cannabinoid Receptors. In *Handbook of Cannabis*; Pertwee, R., Ed.; Oxford University Press: Oxford, UK, 2014; pp. 115–136. ISBN 978-0-19-178756-0.
26. Devane, W.A.; Hanus, L.; Breuer, A.; Pertwee, R.G.; Stevenson, L.A.; Griffin, G.; Gibson, D.; Mandelbaum, A.; Etinger, A.; Mechoulam, R. Isolation and structure of a brain constituent that binds to the cannabinoid receptor. *Science* **1992**, *258*, 1946–1949. [CrossRef] [PubMed]
27. Mechoulam, R.; Ben-Shabat, S.; Hanus, L.; Ligumsky, M.; Kaminski, N.E.; Schatz, A.R.; Gopher, A.; Almog, S.; Martin, B.R.; Compton, D.R. Identification of an endogenous 2-monoglyceride, present in canine gut, that binds to cannabinoid receptors. *Biochem. Pharmacol.* **1995**, *50*, 83–90. [CrossRef]
28. Di Marzo, V.; De Petrocellis, L.; Bisogno, T. The biosynthesis, fate and pharmacological properties of endocannabinoids. *Handb. Exp. Pharmacol.* **2005**, 147–185.
29. Dinh, T.P.; Carpenter, D.; Leslie, F.M.; Freund, T.F.; Katona, I.; Sensi, S.L.; Kathuria, S.; Piomelli, D. Brain monoglyceride lipase participating in endocannabinoid inactivation. *Proc. Natl. Acad. Sci. USA* **2002**, *99*, 10819–10824. [CrossRef] [PubMed]
30. Cravatt, B.F.; Giang, D.K.; Mayfield, S.P.; Boger, D.L.; Lerner, R.A.; Gilula, N.B. Molecular characterization of an enzyme that degrades neuromodulatory fatty-acid amides. *Nature* **1996**, *384*, 83–87. [CrossRef]
31. Bisogno, T.; Howell, F.; Williams, G.; Minassi, A.; Cascio, M.G.; Ligresti, A.; Matias, I.; Schiano-Moriello, A.; Paul, P.; Williams, E.-J.; et al. Cloning of the first sn1-DAG lipases points to the spatial and temporal regulation of endocannabinoid signaling in the brain. *J. Cell Biol.* **2003**, *163*, 463–468. [CrossRef]
32. Okamoto, Y.; Morishita, J.; Tsuboi, K.; Tonai, T.; Ueda, N. Molecular Characterization of a Phospholipase D Generating Anandamide and Its Congeners. *J. Biol. Chem.* **2004**, *279*, 5298–5305. [CrossRef] [PubMed]
33. Di Marzo, V. New approaches and challenges to targeting the endocannabinoid system. *Nat. Rev. Drug Discov.* **2018**, *17*, 623–639. [CrossRef] [PubMed]
34. Simon, G.M.; Cravatt, B.F. Anandamide Biosynthesis Catalyzed by the Phosphodiesterase GDE1 and Detection of Glycerophospho-N-acyl Ethanolamine Precursors in Mouse Brain. *J. Biol. Chem.* **2008**, *283*, 9341–9349. [CrossRef] [PubMed]
35. Liu, J.; Wang, L.; Harvey-White, J.; Osei-Hyiaman, D.; Razdan, R.; Gong, Q.; Chan, A.C.; Zhou, Z.; Huang, B.X.; Kim, H.-Y.; et al. A biosynthetic pathway for anandamide. *Proc. Natl. Acad. Sci. USA* **2006**, *103*, 13345–13350. [CrossRef] [PubMed]
36. Naughton, S.S.; Mathai, M.L.; Hryciw, D.H.; McAinch, A.J. Fatty Acid modulation of the endocannabinoid system and the effect on food intake and metabolism. *Int. J. Endocrinol.* **2013**, *2013*, 361895. [CrossRef] [PubMed]
37. Bluher, M.; Engeli, S.; Kloting, N.; Berndt, J.; Fasshauer, M.; Batkai, S.; Pacher, P.; Schon, M.R.; Jordan, J.; Stumvoll, M. Dysregulation of the Peripheral and Adipose Tissue Endocannabinoid System in Human Abdominal Obesity. *Diabetes* **2006**, *55*, 3053–3060. [CrossRef] [PubMed]
38. Côté, M.; Matias, I.; Lemieux, I.; Petrosino, S.; Alméras, N.; Després, J.-P.; Di Marzo, V. Circulating endocannabinoid levels, abdominal adiposity and related cardiometabolic risk factors in obese men. *Int. J. Obes.* **2007**, *31*, 692–699. [CrossRef]
39. Engeli, S.; Böhnke, J.; Feldpausch, M.; Gorzelniak, K.; Janke, J.; Bátkai, S.; Pacher, P.; Harvey-White, J.; Luft, F.C.; Sharma, A.M.; et al. Activation of the Peripheral Endocannabinoid System in Human Obesity. *Diabetes* **2005**, *54*, 2838–2843. [CrossRef]
40. Karvela, A.; Rojas-Gil, A.P.; Samkinidou, E.; Papadaki, H.; Pappa, A.; Georgiou, G.; Spiliotis, B.E. Endocannabinoid (EC) receptor, CB1, and EC enzymes' expression in primary adipocyte cultures of lean and obese pre-pubertal children in relation to adiponectin and insulin. *J. Pediatr. Endocrinol. Metab.* **2010**, *23*, 1011–1024. [CrossRef]
41. Pagano, C.; Pilon, C.; Calcagno, A.; Urbanet, R.; Rossato, M.; Milan, G.; Bianchi, K.; Rizzuto, R.; Bernante, P.; Federspil, G.; et al. The Endogenous Cannabinoid System Stimulates Glucose Uptake in Human Fat Cells via Phosphatidylinositol 3-Kinase and Calcium-Dependent Mechanisms. *J. Clin. Endocrinol. Metab.* **2007**, *92*, 4810–4819. [CrossRef]

42. Diep, T.A.; Madsen, A.N.; Holst, B.; Kristiansen, M.M.; Wellner, N.; Hansen, S.H.; Hansen, H.S. Dietary fat decreases intestinal levels of the anorectic lipids through a fat sensor. *FASEB J.* **2011**, *25*, 765–774. [CrossRef] [PubMed]
43. Aviello, G.; Matias, I.; Capasso, R.; Petrosino, S.; Borrelli, F.; Orlando, P.; Romano, B.; Capasso, F.; Di Marzo, V.; Izzo, A.A. Inhibitory effect of the anorexic compound oleoylethanolamide on gastric emptying in control and overweight mice. *J. Mol. Med.* **2008**, *86*, 413–422. [CrossRef] [PubMed]
44. Kuipers, E.N.; Kantae, V.; Maarse, B.C.E.; van den Berg, S.M.; van Eenige, R.; Nahon, K.J.; Reifel-Miller, A.; Coskun, T.; de Winther, M.P.J.; Lutgens, E.; et al. High Fat Diet Increases Circulating Endocannabinoids Accompanied by Increased Synthesis Enzymes in Adipose Tissue. *Front. Physiol.* **2019**, *9*, 1913. [CrossRef] [PubMed]
45. Miranda, R.A.; De Almeida, M.M.; Rocha, C.P.D.D.; de Brito Fassarella, L.; De Souza, L.L.; Souza, A.F.P.D.; Andrade, C.B.V.D.; Fortunato, R.S.; Pazos-Moura, C.C.; Trevenzoli, I.H. Maternal high-fat diet consumption induces sex-dependent alterations of the endocannabinoid system and redox homeostasis in liver of adult rat offspring. *Sci. Rep.* **2018**, *8*, 14751. [CrossRef] [PubMed]
46. Dias-Rocha, C.P.; Almeida, M.M.; Santana, E.M.; Costa, J.C.B.; Franco, J.G.; Pazos-Moura, C.C.; Trevenzoli, I.H. Maternal high-fat diet induces sex-specific endocannabinoid system changes in newborn rats and programs adiposity, energy expenditure and food preference in adulthood. *J. Nutr. Biochem.* **2018**, *51*, 56–68. [CrossRef] [PubMed]
47. Kris-Etherton, P.M.; Taylor, D.S.; Yu-Poth, S.; Huth, P.; Moriarty, K.; Fishell, V.; Hargrove, R.L.; Zhao, G.; Etherton, T.D. Polyunsaturated fatty acids in the food chain in the United States. *Am. J. Clin. Nutr.* **2000**, *71*, 179S–188S. [CrossRef] [PubMed]
48. Alvheim, A.R.; Malde, M.K.; Osei-Hyiaman, D.; Lin, Y.H.; Pawlosky, R.J.; Madsen, L.; Kristiansen, K.; Frøyland, L.; Hibbeln, J.R. Dietary linoleic acid elevates endogenous 2-AG and anandamide and induces obesity. *Obesity (Silver Spring)* **2012**, *20*, 1984–1994. [CrossRef] [PubMed]
49. Matias, I.; Petrosino, S.; Racioppi, A.; Capasso, R.; Izzo, A.A.; Di Marzo, V. Dysregulation of peripheral endocannabinoid levels in hyperglycemia and obesity: Effect of high fat diets. *Mol. Cell. Endocrinol.* **2008**, *286*, S66–S78. [CrossRef]
50. Alvheim, A.R.; Torstensen, B.E.; Lin, Y.H.; Lillefosse, H.H.; Lock, E.-J.; Madsen, L.; Frøyland, L.; Hibbeln, J.R.; Malde, M.K. Dietary Linoleic Acid Elevates the Endocannabinoids 2-AG and Anandamide and Promotes Weight Gain in Mice Fed a Low Fat Diet. *Lipids* **2014**, *49*, 59–69. [CrossRef]
51. Batetta, B.; Griinari, M.; Carta, G.; Murru, E.; Ligresti, A.; Cordeddu, L.; Giordano, E.; Sanna, F.; Bisogno, T.; Uda, S.; et al. Endocannabinoids may mediate the ability of (n-3) fatty acids to reduce ectopic fat and inflammatory mediators in obese Zucker rats. *J. Nutr.* **2009**, *139*, 1495–1501. [CrossRef]
52. Rossmeisl, M.; Jilkova, Z.M.; Kuda, O.; Jelenik, T.; Medrikova, D.; Stankova, B.; Kristinsson, B.; Haraldsson, G.G.; Svensen, H.; Stoknes, I.; et al. Metabolic Effects of n-3 PUFA as Phospholipids Are Superior to Triglycerides in Mice Fed a High-Fat Diet: Possible Role of Endocannabinoids. *PLoS ONE* **2012**, *7*, e38834. [CrossRef] [PubMed]
53. Berge, K.; Piscitelli, F.; Hoem, N.; Silvestri, C.; Meyer, I.; Banni, S.; Di Marzo, V. Chronic treatment with krill powder reduces plasma triglyceride and anandamide levels in mildly obese men. *Lipids Health Dis.* **2013**, *12*, 78. [CrossRef] [PubMed]
54. Demizieux, L.; Piscitelli, F.; Troy-Fioramonti, S.; Iannotti, F.A.; Borrino, S.; Gresti, J.; Muller, T.; Bellenger, J.; Silvestri, C.; Di Marzo, V.; et al. Early Low-Fat Diet Enriched With Linolenic Acid Reduces Liver Endocannabinoid Tone and Improves Late Glycemic Control After a High-Fat Diet Challenge in Mice. *Diabetes* **2016**, *65*, 1824–1837. [CrossRef] [PubMed]
55. Pachikian, B.D.; Essaghir, A.; Demoulin, J.-B.; Neyrinck, A.M.; Catry, E.; De Backer, F.C.; Dejeans, N.; Dewulf, E.M.; Sohet, F.M.; Portois, L.; et al. Hepatic n-3 polyunsaturated fatty acid depletion promotes steatosis and insulin resistance in mice: Genomic analysis of cellular targets. *PLoS ONE* **2011**, *6*, e23365. [CrossRef] [PubMed]
56. Berger, A.; Crozier, G.; Bisogno, T.; Cavaliere, P.; Innis, S.; Marzo, V.D. Anandamide and diet: Inclusion of dietary arachidonate and docosahexaenoate leads to increased brain levels of the corresponding N-acylethanolamines in piglets. *Proc. Natl. Acad. Sci. USA* **2001**, *98*, 6402–6406. [CrossRef] [PubMed]

57. Artmann, A.; Petersen, G.; Hellgren, L.I.; Boberg, J.; Skonberg, C.; Nellemann, C.; Hansen, S.H.; Hansen, H.S. Influence of dietary fatty acids on endocannabinoid and N-acylethanolamine levels in rat brain, liver and small intestine. *Biochimica et Biophysica Acta (BBA) Mol. Cell Biol. Lipids* **2008**, *1781*, 200–212. [CrossRef] [PubMed]
58. Ramsden, C.E.; Zamora, D.; Makriyannis, A.; Wood, J.T.; Mann, J.D.; Faurot, K.R.; MacIntosh, B.A.; Majchrzak-Hong, S.F.; Gross, J.R.; Courville, A.B.; et al. Diet-Induced Changes in n-3- and n-6-Derived Endocannabinoids and Reductions in Headache Pain and Psychological Distress. *J. Pain* **2015**, *16*, 707–716. [CrossRef] [PubMed]
59. Verhoeckx, K.C.M.; Voortman, T.; Balvers, M.G.J.; Hendriks, H.F.J.; Wortelboer, H.M.; Witkamp, R.F. Presence, formation and putative biological activities of N-acyl serotonins, a novel class of fatty-acid derived mediators, in the intestinal tract. *Biochimica et Biophysica Acta (BBA) Mol. Cell Biol. Lipids* **2011**, *1811*, 578–586. [CrossRef] [PubMed]
60. Arshad, A.; Chung, W.Y.; Steward, W.; Metcalfe, M.S.; Dennison, A.R. Reduction in circulating pro-angiogenic and pro-inflammatory factors is related to improved outcomes in patients with advanced pancreatic cancer treated with gemcitabine and intravenous omega-3 fish oil. *HPB (Oxford)* **2013**, *15*, 428–432. [CrossRef]
61. Watson, J.E.; Kim, J.S.; Das, A. Emerging class of omega-3 fatty acid endocannabinoids & their derivatives. *Prostaglandins Other Lipid Mediat.* **2019**, *143*, 106337.
62. Wainwright, C.L.; Michel, L. Endocannabinoid system as a potential mechanism for n-3 long-chain polyunsaturated fatty acid mediated cardiovascular protection. *Proc. Nutr. Soc.* **2013**, *72*, 460–469. [CrossRef] [PubMed]
63. Meijerink, J.; Balvers, M.; Witkamp, R. N-Acyl amines of docosahexaenoic acid and other n-3 polyunsatured fatty acids—From fishy endocannabinoids to potential leads. *Br. J. Pharmacol.* **2013**, *169*, 772–783. [CrossRef] [PubMed]
64. Rossmeisl, M.; Pavlisova, J.; Janovska, P.; Kuda, O.; Bardova, K.; Hansikova, J.; Svobodova, M.; Oseeva, M.; Veleba, J.; Kopecky, J.; et al. Differential modulation of white adipose tissue endocannabinoid levels by n-3 fatty acids in obese mice and type 2 diabetic patients. *Biochimica et Biophysica Acta (BBA) Mol. Cell Biol. Lipids* **2018**, *1863*, 712–725. [CrossRef] [PubMed]
65. Moran, C.P.; Shanahan, F. Gut microbiota and obesity: Role in aetiology and potential therapeutic target. *Best Pract. Res. Clin. Gastroenterol.* **2014**, *28*, 585–597. [CrossRef] [PubMed]
66. David, L.A.; Maurice, C.F.; Carmody, R.N.; Gootenberg, D.B.; Button, J.E.; Wolfe, B.E.; Ling, A.V.; Devlin, A.S.; Varma, Y.; Fischbach, M.A.; et al. Diet rapidly and reproducibly alters the human gut microbiome. *Nature* **2014**, *505*, 559–563. [CrossRef]
67. Finucane, M.M.; Sharpton, T.J.; Laurent, T.J.; Pollard, K.S. A Taxonomic Signature of Obesity in the Microbiome? Getting to the Guts of the Matter. *PLoS ONE* **2014**, *9*, e84689. [CrossRef]
68. Turnbaugh, P.J.; Hamady, M.; Yatsunenko, T.; Cantarel, B.L.; Duncan, A.; Ley, R.E.; Sogin, M.L.; Jones, W.J.; Roe, B.A.; Affourtit, J.P.; et al. A core gut microbiome in obese and lean twins. *Nature* **2009**, *457*, 480–484. [CrossRef]
69. Kasselman, L.J.; Vernice, N.A.; DeLeon, J.; Reiss, A.B. The gut microbiome and elevated cardiovascular risk in obesity and autoimmunity. *Atherosclerosis* **2018**, *271*, 203–213. [CrossRef]
70. Ascher, S.; Reinhardt, C. The gut microbiota: An emerging risk factor for cardiovascular and cerebrovascular disease. *Eur. J. Immunol.* **2018**, *48*, 564–575. [CrossRef] [PubMed]
71. Ma, J.; Li, H. The Role of Gut Microbiota in Atherosclerosis and Hypertension. *Front. Pharmacol.* **2018**, *9*, 1082. [CrossRef]
72. van den Munckhof, I.C.L.; Kurilshikov, A.; ter Horst, R.; Riksen, N.P.; Joosten, L.A.B.; Zhernakova, A.; Fu, J.; Keating, S.T.; Netea, M.G.; de Graaf, J.; et al. Role of gut microbiota in chronic low-grade inflammation as potential driver for atherosclerotic cardiovascular disease: A systematic review of human studies: Impact of gut microbiota on low-grade inflammation. *Obes. Rev.* **2018**, *19*, 1719–1734. [CrossRef] [PubMed]
73. Zhou, W.; Sailani, M.R.; Contrepois, K.; Zhou, Y.; Ahadi, S.; Leopold, S.R.; Zhang, M.J.; Rao, V.; Avina, M.; Mishra, T.; et al. Longitudinal multi-omics of host–microbe dynamics in prediabetes. *Nature* **2019**, *569*, 663. [CrossRef] [PubMed]
74. Rose, S.M.S.-F.; Contrepois, K.; Moneghetti, K.J.; Zhou, W.; Mishra, T.; Mataraso, S.; Dagan-Rosenfeld, O.; Ganz, A.B.; Dunn, J.; Hornburg, D.; et al. A longitudinal big data approach for precision health. *Nat. Med.* **2019**, *25*, 792.

75. Cui, C.; Li, Y.; Gao, H.; Zhang, H.; Han, J.; Zhang, D.; Li, Y.; Zhou, J.; Lu, C.; Su, X. Modulation of the gut microbiota by the mixture of fish oil and krill oil in high-fat diet-induced obesity mice. *PLoS ONE* **2017**, *12*, e0186216. [CrossRef] [PubMed]
76. Shen, W.; Gaskins, H.R.; McIntosh, M.K. Influence of dietary fat on intestinal microbes, inflammation, barrier function and metabolic outcomes. *J. Nutr. Biochem.* **2014**, *25*, 270–280. [CrossRef]
77. Pu, S.; Khazanehei, H.; Jones, P.J.; Khafipour, E. Interactions between Obesity Status and Dietary Intake of Monounsaturated and Polyunsaturated Oils on Human Gut Microbiome Profiles in the Canola Oil Multicenter Intervention Trial (COMIT). *Front. Microbiol.* **2016**, *7*, 1612. [CrossRef] [PubMed]
78. Everard, A.; Cani, P.D. Diabetes, obesity and gut microbiota. *Best Pract. Res. Clin. Gastroenterol.* **2013**, *27*, 73–83. [CrossRef]
79. Muccioli, G.G.; Naslain, D.; Bäckhed, F.; Reigstad, C.S.; Lambert, D.M.; Delzenne, N.M.; Cani, P.D. The endocannabinoid system links gut microbiota to adipogenesis. *Mol. Syst. Biol.* **2010**, *6*, 392. [CrossRef]
80. Cani, P.D.; Plovier, H.; Van Hul, M.; Geurts, L.; Delzenne, N.M.; Druart, C.; Everard, A. Endocannabinoids—At the crossroads between the gut microbiota and host metabolism. *Nat. Rev. Endocrinol.* **2016**, *12*, 133–143. [CrossRef]
81. Veronese, N.; Solmi, M.; Caruso, M.G.; Giannelli, G.; Osella, A.R.; Evangelou, E.; Maggi, S.; Fontana, L.; Stubbs, B.; Tzoulaki, I. Dietary fiber and health outcomes: An umbrella review of systematic reviews and meta-analyses. *Am. J. Clin. Nutr.* **2018**, *107*, 436–444. [CrossRef]
82. Ahmadi, S.; Mainali, R.; Nagpal, R.; Sheikh-Zeinoddin, M.; Soleimanian-Zad, S.; Wang, S.; Deep, G.; Kumar Mishra, S.; Yadav, H. Dietary Polysaccharides in the Amelioration of Gut Microbiome Dysbiosis and Metabolic Diseases. *Obes. Control Ther.* **2017**, *4*. [CrossRef]
83. Bindels, L.B.; Delzenne, N.M.; Cani, P.D.; Walter, J. Towards a more comprehensive concept for prebiotics. *Nat. Rev. Gastroenterol. Hepatol.* **2015**, *12*, 303–310. [CrossRef] [PubMed]
84. Cani, P.D.; Amar, J.; Iglesias, M.A.; Poggi, M.; Knauf, C.; Bastelica, D.; Neyrinck, A.M.; Fava, F.; Tuohy, K.M.; Chabo, C.; et al. Metabolic endotoxemia initiates obesity and insulin resistance. *Diabetes* **2007**, *56*, 1761–1772. [CrossRef] [PubMed]
85. Cani, P.D.; Bibiloni, R.; Knauf, C.; Waget, A.; Neyrinck, A.M.; Delzenne, N.M.; Burcelin, R. Changes in gut microbiota control metabolic endotoxemia-induced inflammation in high-fat diet-induced obesity and diabetes in mice. *Diabetes* **2008**, *57*, 1470–1481. [CrossRef] [PubMed]
86. Cani, P.D.; Possemiers, S.; Van de Wiele, T.; Guiot, Y.; Everard, A.; Rottier, O.; Geurts, L.; Naslain, D.; Neyrinck, A.; Lambert, D.M.; et al. Changes in gut microbiota control inflammation in obese mice through a mechanism involving GLP-2-driven improvement of gut permeability. *Gut* **2009**, *58*, 1091–1103. [CrossRef]
87. Everard, A.; Belzer, C.; Geurts, L.; Ouwerkerk, J.P.; Druart, C.; Bindels, L.B.; Guiot, Y.; Derrien, M.; Muccioli, G.G.; Delzenne, N.M.; et al. Cross-talk between Akkermansia muciniphila and intestinal epithelium controls diet-induced obesity. *Proc. Natl. Acad. Sci. USA* **2013**, *110*, 9066–9071. [CrossRef]
88. Dehghan, P.; Pourghassem Gargari, B.; Asghari Jafar-abadi, M. Oligofructose-enriched inulin improves some inflammatory markers and metabolic endotoxemia in women with type 2 diabetes mellitus: A randomized controlled clinical trial. *Nutrition* **2014**, *30*, 418–423. [CrossRef]
89. Depommier, C.; Everard, A.; Druart, C.; Plovier, H.; Hul, M.V.; Vieira-Silva, S.; Falony, G.; Raes, J.; Maiter, D.; Delzenne, N.M.; et al. Supplementation with Akkermansia muciniphila in overweight and obese human volunteers: A proof-of-concept exploratory study. *Nat. Med.* **2019**, *25*, 1096. [CrossRef]
90. Jourdan, T.; Szanda, G.; Cinar, R.; Godlewski, G.; Holovac, D.J.; Park, J.K.; Nicoloro, S.; Shen, Y.; Liu, J.; Rosenberg, A.Z.; et al. Developmental Role of Macrophage Cannabinoid-1 Receptor Signaling in Type 2 Diabetes. *Diabetes* **2017**, *66*, 994–1007. [CrossRef]
91. Jourdan, T.; Godlewski, G.; Cinar, R.; Bertola, A.; Szanda, G.; Liu, J.; Tarn, J.; Han, T.; Mukhopadhyay, B.; Skarulis, M.C.; et al. Activation of the Nlrp3 inflammasome in infiltrating macrophages by endocannabinoids mediates beta cell loss in type 2 diabetes. *Nat. Med.* **2013**, *19*, 1132–1140. [CrossRef]
92. Lv, J.; Qi, L.; Yu, C.; Yang, L.; Guo, Y.; Chen, Y.; Bian, Z.; Sun, D.; Du, J.; Ge, P.; et al. Consumption of spicy foods and total and cause specific mortality: Population based cohort study. *BMJ* **2015**, *351*, h3942. [CrossRef] [PubMed]

93. Yuan, L.-J.; Qin, Y.; Wang, L.; Zeng, Y.; Chang, H.; Wang, J.; Wang, B.; Wan, J.; Chen, S.-H.; Zhang, Q.-Y.; et al. Capsaicin-containing chili improved postprandial hyperglycemia, hyperinsulinemia, and fasting lipid disorders in women with gestational diabetes mellitus and lowered the incidence of large-for-gestational-age newborns. *Clin. Nutr.* **2016**, *35*, 388–393. [CrossRef] [PubMed]
94. Kroff, J.; Hume, D.J.; Pienaar, P.; Tucker, R.; Lambert, E.V.; Rae, D.E. The metabolic effects of a commercially available chicken peri-peri (African bird's eye chilli) meal in overweight individuals. *Br. J. Nutr.* **2017**, *117*, 635–644. [CrossRef] [PubMed]
95. Dömötör, A.; Szolcsányi, J.; Mózsik, G. Capsaicin and glucose absorption and utilization in healthy human subjects. *Eur. J. Pharmacol.* **2006**, *534*, 280–283. [CrossRef] [PubMed]
96. Ludy, M.-J.; Moore, G.E.; Mattes, R.D. The Effects of Capsaicin and Capsiate on Energy Balance: Critical Review and Meta-analyses of Studies in Humans. *Chem. Senses* **2012**, *37*, 103–121. [CrossRef] [PubMed]
97. Kang, J.-H.; Tsuyoshi, G.; Han, I.-S.; Kawada, T.; Kim, Y.M.; Yu, R. Dietary Capsaicin Reduces Obesity-induced Insulin Resistance and Hepatic Steatosis in Obese Mice Fed a High-fat Diet. *Obesity* **2010**, *18*, 780–787. [CrossRef]
98. Zhang, L.L.; Yan Liu, D.; Ma, L.Q.; Luo, Z.D.; Cao, T.B.; Zhong, J.; Yan, Z.C.; Wang, L.J.; Zhao, Z.G.; Zhu, S.J.; et al. Activation of Transient Receptor Potential Vanilloid Type-1 Channel Prevents Adipogenesis and Obesity. *Circ. Res.* **2007**, *100*, 1063–1070. [CrossRef] [PubMed]
99. Motter, A.L.; Ahern, G.P. TRPV1-null mice are protected from diet-induced obesity. *FEBS Lett.* **2008**, *582*, 2257–2262. [CrossRef]
100. Lee, E.; Jung, D.Y.; Kim, J.H.; Patel, P.R.; Hu, X.; Lee, Y.; Azuma, Y.; Wang, H.-F.; Tsitsilianos, N.; Shafiq, U.; et al. Transient receptor potential vanilloid type-1 channel regulates diet-induced obesity, insulin resistance, and leptin resistance. *FASEB J.* **2015**, *29*, 3182–3192. [CrossRef]
101. Wanner, S.P.; Garami, A.; Romanovsky, A.A. Hyperactive when young, hypoactive and overweight when aged: Connecting the dots in the story about locomotor activity, body mass, and aging in Trpv1 knockout mice. *Aging (Albany NY)* **2011**, *3*, 450–454. [CrossRef]
102. Baboota, R.K.; Murtaza, N.; Jagtap, S.; Singh, D.P.; Karmase, A.; Kaur, J.; Bhutani, K.K.; Boparai, R.K.; Premkumar, L.S.; Kondepudi, K.K.; et al. Capsaicin-induced transcriptional changes in hypothalamus and alterations in gut microbial count in high fat diet fed mice. *J. Nutr. Biochem.* **2014**, *25*, 893–902. [CrossRef] [PubMed]
103. Shen, W.; Shen, M.; Zhao, X.; Zhu, H.; Yang, Y.; Lu, S.; Tan, Y.; Li, G.; Li, M.; Wang, J.; et al. Anti-obesity Effect of Capsaicin in Mice Fed with High-Fat Diet Is Associated with an Increase in Population of the Gut Bacterium Akkermansia muciniphila. *Front. Microbiol.* **2017**, *8*, 272. [CrossRef] [PubMed]
104. Kang, C.; Wang, B.; Kaliannan, K.; Wang, X.; Lang, H.; Hui, S.; Huang, L.; Zhang, Y.; Zhou, M.; Chen, M.; et al. Gut Microbiota Mediates the Protective Effects of Dietary Capsaicin against Chronic Low-Grade Inflammation and Associated Obesity Induced by High-Fat Diet. *mBio* **2017**, *8*, e00470-17. [CrossRef] [PubMed]
105. Karwad, M.A.; Macpherson, T.; Wang, B.; Theophilidou, E.; Sarmad, S.; Barrett, D.A.; Larvin, M.; Wright, K.L.; Lund, J.N.; O'Sullivan, S.E. Oleoylethanolamine and palmitoylethanolamine modulate intestinal permeability in vitro via TRPV1 and PPARα. *FASEB J.* **2017**, *31*, 469–481. [CrossRef] [PubMed]
106. Kang, C.; Zhang, Y.; Zhu, X.; Liu, K.; Wang, X.; Chen, M.; Wang, J.; Chen, H.; Hui, S.; Huang, L.; et al. Healthy Subjects Differentially Respond to Dietary Capsaicin Correlating with Specific Gut Enterotypes. *J. Clin. Endocrinol. Metab.* **2016**, *101*, 4681–4689. [CrossRef]
107. Perez-Burgos, A.; Wang, L.; McVey Neufeld, K.-A.; Mao, Y.-K.; Ahmadzai, M.; Janssen, L.J.; Stanisz, A.M.; Bienenstock, J.; Kunze, W.A. The TRPV1 channel in rodents is a major target for antinociceptive effect of the probiotic Lactobacillus reuteri DSM 17938. *J. Physiol.* **2015**, *593*, 3943–3957. [CrossRef]
108. Holick, M.F.; Chen, T.C. Vitamin D deficiency: A worldwide problem with health consequences. *Am. J. Clin. Nutr.* **2008**, *87*, 1080S–1086S. [CrossRef]
109. Al-Dabhani, K.; Tsilidis, K.K.; Murphy, N.; Ward, H.A.; Elliott, P.; Riboli, E.; Gunter, M.; Tzoulaki, I. Prevalence of vitamin D deficiency and association with metabolic syndrome in a Qatari population. *Nutr. Diabetes* **2017**, *7*, e263. [CrossRef]
110. Moon, R.J.; Curtis, E.M.; Cooper, C.; Davies, J.H.; Harvey, N.C. Vitamin D supplementation: Are multivitamins sufficient? *Arch. Dis. Child.* **2019**. [CrossRef]

111. Strange, R.C.; Shipman, K.E.; Ramachandran, S. Metabolic syndrome: A review of the role of vitamin D in mediating susceptibility and outcome. *World J. Diabetes* **2015**, *6*, 896–911. [CrossRef]
112. Su, D.; Nie, Y.; Zhu, A.; Chen, Z.; Wu, P.; Zhang, L.; Luo, M.; Sun, Q.; Cai, L.; Lai, Y.; et al. Vitamin D Signaling through Induction of Paneth Cell Defensins Maintains Gut Microbiota and Improves Metabolic Disorders and Hepatic Steatosis in Animal Models. *Front. Physiol.* **2016**, *7*, 498. [CrossRef] [PubMed]
113. Ooi, J.H.; Li, Y.; Rogers, C.J.; Cantorna, M.T. Vitamin D regulates the gut microbiome and protects mice from dextran sodium sulfate-induced colitis. *J. Nutr.* **2013**, *143*, 1679–1686. [CrossRef] [PubMed]
114. Ghaly, S.; Kaakoush, N.O.; Lloyd, F.; Gordon, L.; Forest, C.; Lawrance, I.C.; Hart, P.H. Ultraviolet Irradiation of Skin Alters the Faecal Microbiome Independently of Vitamin D in Mice. *Nutrients* **2018**, *10*, 1069. [CrossRef] [PubMed]
115. Bikle, D. Vitamin D: Production, Metabolism, and Mechanisms of Action. In *Endotext*; Feingold, K.R., Anawalt, B., Boyce, A., Chrousos, G., Dungan, K., Grossman, A., Hershman, J.M., Kaltsas, G., Koch, C., et al., Eds.; MDText.com, Inc.: South Dartmouth, MA, USA, 2000.
116. Kendall, A.C.; Pilkington, S.M.; Massey, K.A.; Sassano, G.; Rhodes, L.E.; Nicolaou, A. Distribution of Bioactive Lipid Mediators in Human Skin. *J. Invest. Dermatol.* **2015**, *135*, 1510–1520. [CrossRef] [PubMed]
117. Magina, S.; Esteves-Pinto, C.; Moura, E.; Serrão, M.P.; Moura, D.; Petrosino, S.; Di Marzo, V.; Vieira-Coelho, M.A. Inhibition of basal and ultraviolet B-induced melanogenesis by cannabinoid CB1 receptors: A keratinocyte-dependent effect. *Arch. Dermatol. Res.* **2011**, *303*, 201–210. [CrossRef] [PubMed]
118. Felton, S.J.; Kendall, A.C.; Almaedani, A.F.M.; Urquhart, P.; Webb, A.R.; Kift, R.; Vail, A.; Nicolaou, A.; Rhodes, L.E. Serum endocannabinoids and N-acyl ethanolamines and the influence of simulated solar UVR exposure in humans in vivo. *Photochem. Photobiol. Sci.* **2017**, *16*, 564–574. [CrossRef] [PubMed]
119. Magina, S.; Vieira-Coelho, M.A.; Moura, E.; Serrão, M.P.; Piscitelli, F.; Moura, D.; Di Marzo, V. Effect of narrowband ultraviolet B treatment on endocannabinoid plasma levels in patients with psoriasis. *Br. J. Dermatol.* **2014**, *171*, 198–201. [CrossRef] [PubMed]
120. Guida, F.; Boccella, S.; Belardo, C.; Iannotta, M.; Piscitelli, F.; De Filippis, F.; Paino, S.; Ricciardi, F.; Siniscalco, D.; Marabese, I.; et al. Altered gut microbiota and endocannabinoid system tone in vitamin D deficiency-mediated chronic pain. *Brain Behav. Immunity* **2019**. [CrossRef]
121. Di Marzo, V.; Côté, M.; Matias, I.; Lemieux, I.; Arsenault, B.J.; Cartier, A.; Piscitelli, F.; Petrosino, S.; Alméras, N.; Després, J.-P. Changes in plasma endocannabinoid levels in viscerally obese men following a 1 year lifestyle modification programme and waist circumference reduction: Associations with changes in metabolic risk factors. *Diabetologia* **2009**, *52*, 213–217. [CrossRef]
122. Gasperi, V.; Ceci, R.; Tantimonaco, M.; Talamonti, E.; Battista, N.; Parisi, A.; Florio, R.; Sabatini, S.; Rossi, A.; Maccarrone, M. The Fatty Acid Amide Hydrolase in Lymphocytes from Sedentary and Active Subjects. *Med. Sci. Sports Exerc.* **2014**, *46*, 24–32. [CrossRef]
123. Fernández-Aranda, F.; Sauchelli, S.; Pastor, A.; Gonzalez, M.L.; de la Torre, R.; Granero, R.; Jiménez-Murcia, S.; Baños, R.; Botella, C.; Fernández-Real, J.M.; et al. Moderate-Vigorous Physical Activity across Body Mass Index in Females: Moderating Effect of Endocannabinoids and Temperament. *PLoS ONE* **2014**, *9*, e104534. [CrossRef] [PubMed]
124. Raichlen, D.A.; Foster, A.D.; Seillier, A.; Giuffrida, A.; Gerdeman, G.L. Exercise-induced endocannabinoid signaling is modulated by intensity. *Eur. J. Appl. Physiol.* **2013**, *113*, 869–875. [CrossRef] [PubMed]
125. Raichlen, D.A.; Foster, A.D.; Gerdeman, G.L.; Seillier, A.; Giuffrida, A. Wired to run: Exercise-induced endocannabinoid signaling in humans and cursorial mammals with implications for the "runner's high". *J. Exp. Biol.* **2012**, *215*, 1331–1336. [CrossRef] [PubMed]
126. Heyman, E.; Gamelin, F.-X.; Goekint, M.; Piscitelli, F.; Roelands, B.; Leclair, E.; Di Marzo, V.; Meeusen, R. Intense exercise increases circulating endocannabinoid and BDNF levels in humans—Possible implications for reward and depression. *Psychoneuroendocrinology* **2012**, *37*, 844–851. [CrossRef] [PubMed]
127. Heyman, E.; Gamelin, F.-X.; Aucouturier, J.; Marzo, V.D. The role of the endocannabinoid system in skeletal muscle and metabolic adaptations to exercise: Potential implications for the treatment of obesity. *Obes. Rev.* **2012**, *13*, 1110–1124. [CrossRef] [PubMed]
128. Cedernaes, J.; Fanelli, F.; Fazzini, A.; Pagotto, U.; Broman, J.-E.; Vogel, H.; Dickson, S.L.; Schiöth, H.B.; Benedict, C. Sleep restriction alters plasma endocannabinoids concentrations before but not after exercise in humans. *Psychoneuroendocrinology* **2016**, *74*, 258–268. [CrossRef] [PubMed]

129. Gamelin, F.-X.; Aucouturier, J.; Iannotti, F.A.; Piscitelli, F.; Mazzarella, E.; Aveta, T.; Leriche, M.; Dupont, E.; Cieniewski-Bernard, C.; Montel, V.; et al. Effects of chronic exercise on the endocannabinoid system in Wistar rats with high-fat diet-induced obesity. *J. Physiol. Biochem.* **2016**, *72*, 183–199. [CrossRef] [PubMed]
130. Mikkelsen, K.; Stojanovska, L.; Polenakovic, M.; Bosevski, M.; Apostolopoulos, V. Exercise and mental health. *Maturitas* **2017**, *106*, 48–56. [CrossRef] [PubMed]
131. Fuss, J.; Steinle, J.; Bindila, L.; Auer, M.K.; Kirchherr, H.; Lutz, B.; Gass, P. A runner's high depends on cannabinoid receptors in mice. *Proc. Natl. Acad. Sci. USA* **2015**, *112*, 13105–13108. [CrossRef]
132. Hill, M.N.; Titterness, A.K.; Morrish, A.C.; Carrier, E.J.; Lee, T.T.-Y.; Gil-Mohapel, J.; Gorzalka, B.B.; Hillard, C.J.; Christie, B.R. Endogenous cannabinoid signaling is required for voluntary exercise-induced enhancement of progenitor cell proliferation in the hippocampus. *Hippocampus* **2010**, *20*, 513–523. [CrossRef] [PubMed]
133. De Chiara, V.; Errico, F.; Musella, A.; Rossi, S.; Mataluni, G.; Sacchetti, L.; Siracusano, A.; Castelli, M.; Cavasinni, F.; Bernardi, G.; et al. Voluntary exercise and sucrose consumption enhance cannabinoid CB1 receptor sensitivity in the striatum. *Neuropsychopharmacology* **2010**, *35*, 374–387. [CrossRef] [PubMed]
134. Swenson, S.; Hamilton, J.; Robison, L.; Thanos, P.K. Chronic aerobic exercise: Lack of effect on brain CB1 receptor levels in adult rats. *Life Sci.* **2019**, *230*, 84–88. [CrossRef] [PubMed]
135. Stone, N.L.; Millar, S.A.; Herrod, P.J.J.; Barrett, D.A.; Ortori, C.A.; Mellon, V.A.; O'Sullivan, S.E. An Analysis of Endocannabinoid Concentrations and Mood Following Singing and Exercise in Healthy Volunteers. *Front. Behav. Neurosci.* **2018**, *12*, 269. [CrossRef] [PubMed]
136. Antunes, H.K.M.; Leite, G.S.F.; Lee, K.S.; Barreto, A.T.; dos Santos, R.V.T.; de Sá Souza, H.; Tufik, S.; de Mello, M.T. Exercise deprivation increases negative mood in exercise-addicted subjects and modifies their biochemical markers. *Physiol. Behav.* **2016**, *156*, 182–190. [CrossRef] [PubMed]
137. Hsu, Y.J.; Chiu, C.C.; Li, Y.P.; Huang, W.C.; Huang, Y.T.; Huang, C.C.; Chuang, H.L. Effect of Intestinal Microbiota on Exercise Performance in Mice. *J. Strength Cond. Res.* **2015**, *29*, 552–558. [CrossRef] [PubMed]
138. Petriz, B.A.; Castro, A.P.; Almeida, J.A.; Gomes, C.P.; Fernandes, G.R.; Kruger, R.H.; Pereira, R.W.; Franco, O.L. Exercise induction of gut microbiota modifications in obese, non-obese and hypertensive rats. *BMC Genom.* **2014**, *15*, 511. [CrossRef] [PubMed]
139. Denou, E.; Marcinko, K.; Surette, M.G.; Steinberg, G.R.; Schertzer, J.D. High-intensity exercise training increases the diversity and metabolic capacity of the mouse distal gut microbiota during diet-induced obesity. *Am. J. Physiol.-Endocrinol. Metab.* **2016**, *310*, E982–E993. [CrossRef]
140. Lai, Z.-L.; Tseng, C.-H.; Ho, H.J.; Cheung, C.K.Y.; Lin, J.-Y.; Chen, Y.-J.; Cheng, F.-C.; Hsu, Y.-C.; Lin, J.-T.; El-Omar, E.M.; et al. Fecal microbiota transplantation confers beneficial metabolic effects of diet and exercise on diet-induced obese mice. *Sci. Rep.* **2018**, *8*, 15625. [CrossRef]
141. Maillard, F.; Vazeille, E.; Sauvanet, P.; Sirvent, P.; Combaret, L.; Sourdrille, A.; Chavanelle, V.; Bonnet, R.; Otero, Y.F.; Delcros, G.; et al. High intensity interval training promotes total and visceral fat mass loss in obese Zucker rats without modulating gut microbiota. *PLoS ONE* **2019**, *14*, e0214660. [CrossRef]
142. Barton, W.; Penney, N.C.; Cronin, O.; Garcia-Perez, I.; Molloy, M.G.; Holmes, E.; Shanahan, F.; Cotter, P.D.; O'Sullivan, O. The microbiome of professional athletes differs from that of more sedentary subjects in composition and particularly at the functional metabolic level. *Gut* **2017**. [CrossRef]
143. Clarke, S.F.; Murphy, E.F.; O'Sullivan, O.; Lucey, A.J.; Humphreys, M.; Hogan, A.; Hayes, P.; O'Reilly, M.; Jeffery, I.B.; Wood-Martin, R.; et al. Exercise and associated dietary extremes impact on gut microbial diversity. *Gut* **2014**, *63*, 1913–1920. [CrossRef] [PubMed]
144. Estaki, M.; Pither, J.; Baumeister, P.; Little, J.P.; Gill, S.K.; Ghosh, S.; Ahmadi-Vand, Z.; Marsden, K.R.; Gibson, D.L. Cardiorespiratory fitness as a predictor of intestinal microbial diversity and distinct metagenomic functions. *Microbiome* **2016**, *4*, 42. [CrossRef] [PubMed]
145. Munukka, E.; Ahtiainen, J.P.; Puigbó, P.; Jalkanen, S.; Pahkala, K.; Keskitalo, A.; Kujala, U.M.; Pietilä, S.; Hollmén, M.; Elo, L.; et al. Six-Week Endurance Exercise Alters Gut Metagenome That Is not Reflected in Systemic Metabolism in Over-weight Women. *Front. Microbiol.* **2018**, *9*, 2323. [CrossRef] [PubMed]
146. Cristiano, C.; Pirozzi, C.; Coretti, L.; Cavaliere, G.; Lama, A.; Russo, R.; Lembo, F.; Mollica, M.P.; Meli, R.; Calignano, A.; et al. Palmitoylethanolamide counteracts autistic-like behaviours in BTBR T+tf/J mice: Contribution of central and peripheral mechanisms. *Brain Behav. Immunity* **2018**, *74*, 166–175. [CrossRef] [PubMed]

147. Vidot, D.C.; Prado, G.; Hlaing, W.M.; Florez, H.J.; Arheart, K.L.; Messiah, S.E. Metabolic Syndrome among Marijuana Users in the United States: An Analysis of National Health and Nutrition Examination Survey Data. *Am. J. Med.* **2016**, *129*, 173–179. [CrossRef] [PubMed]
148. Le Strat, Y.; Le Foll, B. Obesity and Cannabis Use: Results from 2 Representative National Surveys. *Am. J. Epidemiol.* **2011**, *174*, 929–933. [CrossRef] [PubMed]
149. Alshaarawy, O.; Anthony, J.C. Are cannabis users less likely to gain weight? Results from a national 3-year prospective study. *Int. J. Epidemiol.* **2019**. [CrossRef] [PubMed]
150. Penner, E.A.; Buettner, H.; Mittleman, M.A. The Impact of Marijuana Use on Glucose, Insulin, and Insulin Resistance among US Adults. *Am. J. Med.* **2013**, *126*, 583–589. [CrossRef]
151. Alshaarawy, O.; Anthony, J.C. Cannabis Smoking and Diabetes Mellitus: Results from Meta-Analysis with Eight Independent Replication Samples. *Epidemiology* **2015**, *26*, 597–600. [CrossRef]
152. Rajavashisth, T.B.; Shaheen, M.; Norris, K.C.; Pan, D.; Sinha, S.K.; Ortega, J.; Friedman, T.C. Decreased prevalence of diabetes in marijuana users: Cross-sectional data from the National Health and Nutrition Examination Survey (NHANES) III. *BMJ Open* **2012**, *2*, e000494. [CrossRef]
153. Danielsson, A.K.; Lundin, A.; Yaregal, A.; Östenson, C.G.; Allebeck, P.; Agardh, E.E. Cannabis Use as Risk or Protection for Type 2 Diabetes: A Longitudinal Study of 18 000 Swedish Men and Women. *J. Diabetes Res.* **2016**, *2016*, 1–6. [CrossRef] [PubMed]
154. Ngueta, G.; Bélanger, R.E.; Laouan-Sidi, E.A.; Lucas, M. Cannabis use in relation to obesity and insulin resistance in the inuit population. *Obesity* **2015**, *23*, 290–295. [CrossRef] [PubMed]
155. Adejumo, A.C.; Ajayi, T.O.; Adegbala, O.M.; Adejumo, K.L.; Alliu, S.; Akinjero, A.M.; Onyeakusi, N.E.; Ojelabi, O.; Bukong, T.N. Cannabis use is associated with reduced prevalence of progressive stages of alcoholic liver disease. *Liver Int.* **2018**, *38*, 1475–1486. [CrossRef] [PubMed]
156. Adejumo, A.C.; Alliu, S.; Ajayi, T.O.; Adejumo, K.L.; Adegbala, O.M.; Onyeakusi, N.E.; Akinjero, A.M.; Durojaiye, M.; Bukong, T.N. Cannabis use is associated with reduced prevalence of non-alcoholic fatty liver disease: A cross-sectional study. *PLoS ONE* **2017**, *12*, e0176416. [CrossRef] [PubMed]
157. Akturk, H.K.; Taylor, D.D.; Camsari, U.M.; Rewers, A.; Kinney, G.L.; Shah, V.N. Association Between Cannabis Use and Risk for Diabetic Ketoacidosis in Adults With Type 1 Diabetes. *JAMA Intern. Med.* **2019**, *179*, 115. [CrossRef] [PubMed]
158. Auer, R.; Sidney, S.; Goff, D.; Vittinghoff, E.; Pletcher, M.J.; Allen, N.B.; Reis, J.P.; Lewis, C.E.; Carr, J.; Rana, J.S. Lifetime marijuana use and subclinical atherosclerosis: The Coronary Artery Risk Development in Young Adults (CARDIA) study. *Addiction* **2018**, *113*, 845–856. [CrossRef]
159. DeFilippis, E.M.; Singh, A.; Divakaran, S.; Gupta, A.; Collins, B.L.; Biery, D.; Qamar, A.; Fatima, A.; Ramsis, M.; Pipilas, D.; et al. Cocaine and Marijuana Use Among Young Adults With Myocardial Infarction. *J. Am. Coll. Cardiol.* **2018**, *71*, 2540–2551. [CrossRef] [PubMed]
160. Villares, J. Chronic use of marijuana decreases cannabinoid receptor binding and mRNA expression in the human brain. *Neuroscience* **2007**, *145*, 323–334. [CrossRef]
161. Ceccarini, J.; Kuepper, R.; Kemels, D.; van Os, J.; Henquet, C.; Laere, K.V. [18F]MK-9470 PET measurement of cannabinoid CB1 receptor availability in chronic cannabis users. *Addict. Biol.* **2015**, *20*, 357–367. [CrossRef]
162. Marzo, V.D.; Berrendero, F.; Bisogno, T.; González, S.; Cavaliere, P.; Romero, J.; Cebeira, M.; Ramos, J.A.; Fernández-Ruiz, J.J. Enhancement of Anandamide Formation in the Limbic Forebrain and Reduction of Endocannabinoid Contents in the Striatum of Δ9-Tetrahydrocannabinol-Tolerant Rats. *J. Neurochem.* **2000**, *74*, 1627–1635. [CrossRef]
163. Morgan, C.J.A.; Page, E.; Schaefer, C.; Chatten, K.; Manocha, A.; Gulati, S.; Curran, H.V.; Brandner, B.; Leweke, F.M. Cerebrospinal fluid anandamide levels, cannabis use and psychotic-like symptoms. *Br. J. Psychiatry* **2013**, *202*, 381–382. [CrossRef] [PubMed]
164. Maia, J.; Midão, L.; Cunha, S.C.; Almada, M.; Fonseca, B.M.; Braga, J.; Gonçalves, D.; Teixeira, N.; Correia-da-Silva, G. Effects of cannabis tetrahydrocannabinol on endocannabinoid homeostasis in human placenta. *Arch. Toxicol.* **2019**, *93*, 649–658. [CrossRef] [PubMed]
165. McIntosh, A.L.; Martin, G.G.; Huang, H.; Landrock, D.; Kier, A.B.; Schroeder, F. Δ^9-Tetrahydrocannabinol induces endocannabinoid accumulation in mouse hepatocytes: Antagonism by *Fabp1* gene ablation. *J. Lipid Res.* **2018**, *59*, 646–657. [CrossRef] [PubMed]

166. De Petrocellis, L.; Ligresti, A.; Moriello, A.S.; Allarà, M.; Bisogno, T.; Petrosino, S.; Stott, C.G.; Di Marzo, V. Effects of cannabinoids and cannabinoid-enriched Cannabis extracts on TRP channels and endocannabinoid metabolic enzymes. *Br. J. Pharmacol.* **2011**, *163*, 1479–1494. [CrossRef] [PubMed]
167. Cluny, N.L.; Keenan, C.M.; Reimer, R.A.; Le Foll, B.; Sharkey, K.A. Prevention of Diet-Induced Obesity Effects on Body Weight and Gut Microbiota in Mice Treated Chronically with Δ9-Tetrahydrocannabinol. *PLoS ONE* **2015**, *10*, e0144270. [CrossRef] [PubMed]
168. Wargent, E.T.; Zaibi, M.S.; Silvestri, C.; Hislop, D.C.; Stocker, C.J.; Stott, C.G.; Guy, G.W.; Duncan, M.; Di Marzo, V.; Cawthorne, M.A. The cannabinoid Δ9-tetrahydrocannabivarin (THCV) ameliorates insulin sensitivity in two mouse models of obesity. *Nutr. Diabetes* **2013**, *3*, e68. [CrossRef] [PubMed]
169. Weiss, L.; Zeira, M.; Reich, S.; Har-Noy, M.; Mechoulam, R.; Slavin, S.; Gallily, R. Cannabidiol lowers incidence of diabetes in non-obese diabetic mice. *Autoimmunity* **2006**, *39*, 143–151. [CrossRef]
170. Jadoon, K.A.; Ratcliffe, S.H.; Barrett, D.A.; Thomas, E.L.; Stott, C.; Bell, J.D.; O'Sullivan, S.E.; Tan, G.D. Efficacy and Safety of Cannabidiol and Tetrahydrocannabivarin on Glycemic and Lipid Parameters in Patients With Type 2 Diabetes: A Randomized, Double-Blind, Placebo-Controlled, Parallel Group Pilot Study. *Diabetes Care* **2016**, *39*, 1777–1786. [CrossRef]
171. Silvestri, C.; Paris, D.; Martella, A.; Melck, D.; Guadagnino, I.; Cawthorne, M.; Motta, A.; Di Marzo, V. Two non-psychoactive cannabinoids reduce intracellular lipid levels and inhibit hepatosteatosis. *J. Hepatol.* **2015**, *62*, 1382–1390. [CrossRef]
172. Le Bastard, Q.; Al-Ghalith, G.A.; Grégoire, M.; Chapelet, G.; Javaudin, F.; Dailly, E.; Batard, E.; Knights, D.; Montassier, E. Systematic review: Human gut dysbiosis induced by non-antibiotic prescription medications. *Aliment. Pharmacol. Ther.* **2018**, *47*, 332–345. [CrossRef]
173. Panee, J.; Gerschenson, M.; Chang, L. Associations between Microbiota, Mitochondrial Function, and Cognition in Chronic Marijuana Users. *J. Neuroimmune Pharmacol.* **2018**, *13*, 113–122. [CrossRef] [PubMed]
174. Wu, G.D.; Chen, J.; Hoffmann, C.; Bittinger, K.; Chen, Y.-Y.; Keilbaugh, S.A.; Bewtra, M.; Knights, D.; Walters, W.A.; Knight, R.; et al. Linking Long-Term Dietary Patterns with Gut Microbial Enterotypes. *Science* **2011**, *334*, 105–108. [CrossRef] [PubMed]
175. Smit, E.; Crespo, C.J. Dietary intake and nutritional status of US adult marijuana users: Results from the Third National Health and Nutrition Examination Survey. *Public Health Nutr.* **2001**, *4*, 781–786. [CrossRef] [PubMed]
176. Fulcher, J.A.; Hussain, S.K.; Cook, R.; Li, F.; Tobin, N.H.; Ragsdale, A.; Shoptaw, S.; Gorbach, P.M.; Aldrovandi, G.M. Effects of Substance Use and Sex Practices on the Intestinal Microbiome During HIV-1 Infection. *J. Infect. Dis.* **2018**, *218*, 1560–1570. [CrossRef] [PubMed]
177. Yun, Y.; Kim, H.-N.; Kim, S.E.; Heo, S.G.; Chang, Y.; Ryu, S.; Shin, H.; Kim, H.-L. Comparative analysis of gut microbiota associated with body mass index in a large Korean cohort. *BMC Microbiol.* **2017**, *17*, 151. [CrossRef] [PubMed]
178. Ottosson, F.; Brunkwall, L.; Ericson, U.; Nilsson, P.M.; Almgren, P.; Fernandez, C.; Melander, O.; Orho-Melander, M. Connection Between BMI-Related Plasma Metabolite Profile and Gut Microbiota. *J. Clin. Endocrinol. Metab.* **2018**, *103*, 1491–1501. [CrossRef] [PubMed]
179. Precup, G.; Vodnar, D.-C. Gut Prevotella as a possible biomarker of diet and its eubiotic versus dysbiotic roles-A comprehensive literature review. *Br. J. Nutr.* **2019**, 1–24. [CrossRef]
180. Al-Ghezi, Z.Z.; Busbee, P.B.; Alghetaa, H.; Nagarkatti, P.S.; Nagarkatti, M. Combination of cannabinoids, delta-9-tetrahydrocannabinol (THC) and cannabidiol (CBD), mitigates experimental autoimmune encephalomyelitis (EAE) by altering the gut microbiome. *Brain Behav. Immun.* **2019**. [CrossRef]
181. Becker, W.J.; Nagarkatti, M.; Nagarkatti, P.S. Δ^9-tetrahydrocannabinol (THC) activation of cannabinoid receptors induces unique changes in the murine gut microbiome and associated induction of myeloid-derived suppressor cells and Th17 cells. *J. Immunol.* **2017**, *198*, 218.11.

13

Trimethylamine-N-Oxide (TMAO) as Novel Potential Biomarker of Early Predictors of Metabolic Syndrome

Luigi Barrea [1,*,†], Giuseppe Annunziata [2,†], Giovanna Muscogiuri [1], Carolina Di Somma [3], Daniela Laudisio [1], Maria Maisto [2], Giulia de Alteriis [1], Gian Carlo Tenore [2], Annamaria Colao [1] and Silvia Savastano [1]

1 Dipartimento di Medicina Clinica e Chirurgia, Unit of Endocrinology, Federico II University Medical School of Naples, Via Sergio Pansini 5, 80131 Naples, Italy; giovanna.muscogiuri@gmail.com (G.M.); daniela.laudisio@libero.it (D.L.); dealteriisgiulia@gmail.com (G.d.A.); colao@unina.it (A.C.); sisavast@unina.it (S.S.)

2 Department of Pharmacy, University of Naples "Federico II", Via Domenico Montesano 49, 80131 Naples, Italy; giuseppe.annunziata@unina.it (G.A.); maria.maisto@unina.it (M.M.); giancarlo.tenore@unina.it (G.C.T.)

3 IRCCS SDN, Napoli Via Gianturco 113, 80143 Naples, Italy; cdisomma@unina.it

* Correspondence: luigi.barrea@unina.it

† These Authors contributed equally to this work.

Abstract: There is a mechanistic link between the gut-derived metabolite trimethylamine-N-oxide (TMAO) and obesity-related diseases, suggesting that the TMAO pathway may also be linked to the pathogenesis of obesity. The Visceral Adiposity Index (VAI), a gender-specific indicator of adipose dysfunction, and the Fatty Liver Index (FLI), a predictor of non-alcoholic fatty liver disease (NAFLD), are early predictors of metabolic syndrome (MetS). In this cross-sectional observational study, we investigated TMAO levels in adults stratified according to Body Mass Index (BMI) and the association of TMAO with VAI and FLI. One hundred and thirty-seven adult subjects (59 males; 21–56 years) were enrolled. TMAO levels were detected using HPLC/MS analysis. Homeostatic Model Assessment of Insulin Resistance (HoMA-IR), VAI and FLI were included as cardio-metabolic indices. TMAO levels increased along with BMI and were positively associated with VAI and FLI, independently, on common potential covariates. The most sensitive and specific cut-offs for circulating levels of TMAO to predict the presence of NAFLD-FLI and MetS were $\geq$8.02 μM and $\geq$8.74 μM, respectively. These findings allow us to hypothesize a role of TMAO as an early biomarker of adipose dysfunction and NAFLD-FLI in all borderline conditions in which overt MetS is not present, and suggest that a specific cut-off of TMAO might help in identifying subjects at high risk of NAFLD.

Keywords: trimethylamine N-oxide (TMAO); obesity; visceral adiposity index (VAI); fatty liver index (FLI); metabolic syndrome (MetS)

1. Introduction

TMAO is a small, organic, gut microbiota-derived metabolite, which is emerging as a new potentially important cause of increased atherosclerosis and cardiovascular risk [1–3]. Circulating levels of TMAO increase after the gut microbial metabolism of dietary L-carnitine and phosphatidylcholine-rich foods, including red meat, eggs, dairy products, which are common nutrients of the Western diet. Very recently we reported a novel association between circulating levels of TMAO and the Mediterranean diet in healthy normal-weight adults, with a clear gender difference in this association [4]. The metabolic pathway of TMAO includes the digestion of these amines from gut microbiota with the production of trimethylamine (TMA), which is then converted to TMAO via flavin-monooxygenase-3 (FMO3) in the liver [5,6]. The interplay between dietary composition, gut microbiota and microbe-generated metabolites has been intensely investigated [7,8].

Several studies have shown a mechanistic link between TMAO, inflammatory pathways [9] atherosclerosis, type 2 diabetes mellitus (T2DM), and cardiovascular diseases (CVD) [1–3,6,10,11]. Namely, circulating levels of TMAO and its metabolites (choline and betaine) are associated with atherosclerosis risks in both humans and mice [1]. Among the pro-atherosclerotic mechanisms proposed for TMAO there are the inhibition of the reverse cholesterol transport, although this effect was reported in animal studies only [6], and the enhancement of human platelet hyperresponsiveness and thrombosis potential [10]. A systematic review and meta-analysis by Schiattarella et al. [2] demonstrated that in humans there is a positive dose-dependent association between circulating levels of TMAO and increased cardiovascular risk and mortality [2]. Nevertheless, in this metanalysis, the population samples were not divided according the BMI classes. More recently, Kanitsoraphan et al. [3] reported that in patients with T2DM higher circulating levels of TMAO were significantly associated with higher overall mortality by 2.07- to 2.7-fold, also after adjustment for BMI [3]. Recently, the strong association between gut microbiota and either obesity and obesity-related diseases in humans on the one hand, and the association between the TMAO pathway and cardio-metabolic diseases on the other, suggested that the TMAO pathway may be also mechanistically linked to the pathogenesis of obesity. Schugar et al. [11] reported that plasma TMAO levels were linked to with obesity traits in the different inbred strains of mice receiving a high-fat diet and suggested that the TMAO-generating pathway is linked to obesity and energy metabolism [11], although scientific evidence to support this association in humans has not yet been provided. Only Randrianarisoa et al. [12] reported that TMAO correlated positively with BMI, insulin resistance, visceral fat mass, and liver fat content [12]. In addition, Chen et al. [13] showed positive associations of the circulating TMAO levels and two of its nutrient precursors, choline, and betaine, with the presence and severity of NAFLD, the hepatic manifestation of the MetS [14], in a large sample of hospital- and community-based Chinese adults [13].

Nevertheless, controversy remains over the exact role of TMAO in the pathogenesis of MetS, a constellation of cardio-metabolic risk factors, including central obesity, hypertriglyceridemia, low high-density lipoprotein (HDL) cholesterol, hyperglycemia, and hypertension [15], which predispose T2DM and CVD [16], according to the definition of nascent MetS [17]. Very recently, a clinical study investigating several biogenic amines in urine, including TMAO in a sample of patients with MetS showed that these subjects presented higher levels of TMAO compared with their counterparts without MetS [18]. In addition, a further study investigating unselected white patients undergoing coronary angiography for the evaluation of suspected coronary artery disease showed a positive correlation between TMAO and MetS [19]. However, this association was lost after adjusting for impaired kidney function and poor metabolic control in this population sample.

On the other hand, this association was not found in a sample of patients with nascent MetS (without CVD or T2DM), but not with the commonly used surrogate index of insulin resistance, i.e., the HoMA-IR [9]. Again, in these recent studies, the population samples were not divided according to BMI classes.

The VAI, a gender-specific indicator of adipose distribution and dysfunction [20], and the FLI, an accurate predictor of the NAFLD [21], are two surrogate indices of cardio-metabolic risk and are linked to the inflammatory pathways [22,23]. Both indices are based on simple anthropometric and metabolic parameters, and are strictly correlated with MetS, representing early predictors of MetS [20,24]. VAI has been counted as an effective marker to assess insulin resistance and metabolic disturbances that contribute to CVD in primary-care non-obese subjects, with specific cut-off values depending on the population of interest [20]. Also, FLI has been proposed as a marker of insulin resistance [21] and recently the clinical utility of FLI as a predictor of incident T2DM has been reported [25]. As three of the variables making up VAI (waist circumference (WC), plasma triglycerides (TG), and HDL cholesterol) and FLI (BMI, WC, and TG) are used as continuous variables, and while they are dichotomically expressed in the criteria for MetS, VAI and FLI might represent useful indicators of early cardio-metabolic risk in all borderline conditions in which overt MetS is not present [22].

Considering the lack of evidence in humans of a progressive increase of TMAO levels across BMI classes and to gain further insight into the levels of TMAO in the setting of obesity, in this study we aimed to investigate the circulating levels of TMAO in a sample of the adult population stratified according to BMI. In addition, considering the still controversial role of TMAO in the pathogenesis of MetS and the predictive value of VAI and FLI as easy and early indicators of MetS, we investigated the association of circulating levels of TMAO with VAI and FLI and hypothesized that this association could serve as a biological marker of early metabolic derangement in subjects with overweight and obesity.

2. Materials and Methods

2.1. Design and Setting

This is a cross-sectional observational study carried out at the Department of Clinical Medicine and Surgery, Unit of Endocrinology, University Federico II, Naples (Italy), from January 2017 to August 2018. The work has been carried out in accordance with the Code of Ethics of the World Medical Association (Declaration of Helsinki) for experiments involving humans, and it has been approved by the Ethical Committee of the University of Naples "Federico II" Medical School (n. 173/16). The purpose of the protocol was explained to all the study participants, and written informed consent was obtained. This trial was registered at http://register.clinicaltrials.gov/. Unique identifier: NCT03060811.

2.2. Population Study

Recruitment strategies included a sample of 330 adult Caucasians subjects (20–63 years) of both genders consecutively enrolled among patients of our outpatient clinic, hospital volunteers, and employees from the same geographical area around Naples, Italy). All female subjects were non-pregnant and non-lactating. A full medical history, including drug use, was collected.

To increase the homogeneity of the subject sample, we included only adults of both genders with the following criteria of exclusion:

- Impaired renal function (normal values: estimated glomerular filtration rate $\geq$ 90 mL/min/1.73 m^2 calculated by chronic kidney disease epidemiology collaboration equation; CKD EPI) (15 patients)
- Presence of T2DM (defined by criteria of the American Diabetes Association as follows: basal plasma glucose level $\geq$ 126 mg/dL on two occasions, or glycated hemoglobin (HbA1c) $\geq$ 6.5% ($\geq$48 mmol/mol) on two occasions, or both at the same time (35 patients). Participants on antidiabetic medication were considered to have T2DM [26].
- Clinical atherosclerosis (coronary artery disease, peripheral vascular disease, CVD) (41 patients)
- Current therapy with anti-inflammatory drugs, statins and other hypolipidemic agents (34 patients);
- User of antibiotics or probiotics within 2 months of recruitment (19 subjects);
- Specific nutritional regimens, including vegan or vegetarian diets (eight subjects);
- Vitamin/mineral or antioxidant supplementation (34 subjects);
- Alcohol abuse according to the Diagnostic and Statistical Manual of Mental Disorders (DSM)-V diagnostic criteria (eleven subjects);

The flow chart of the study subjects is shown in Figure 1.

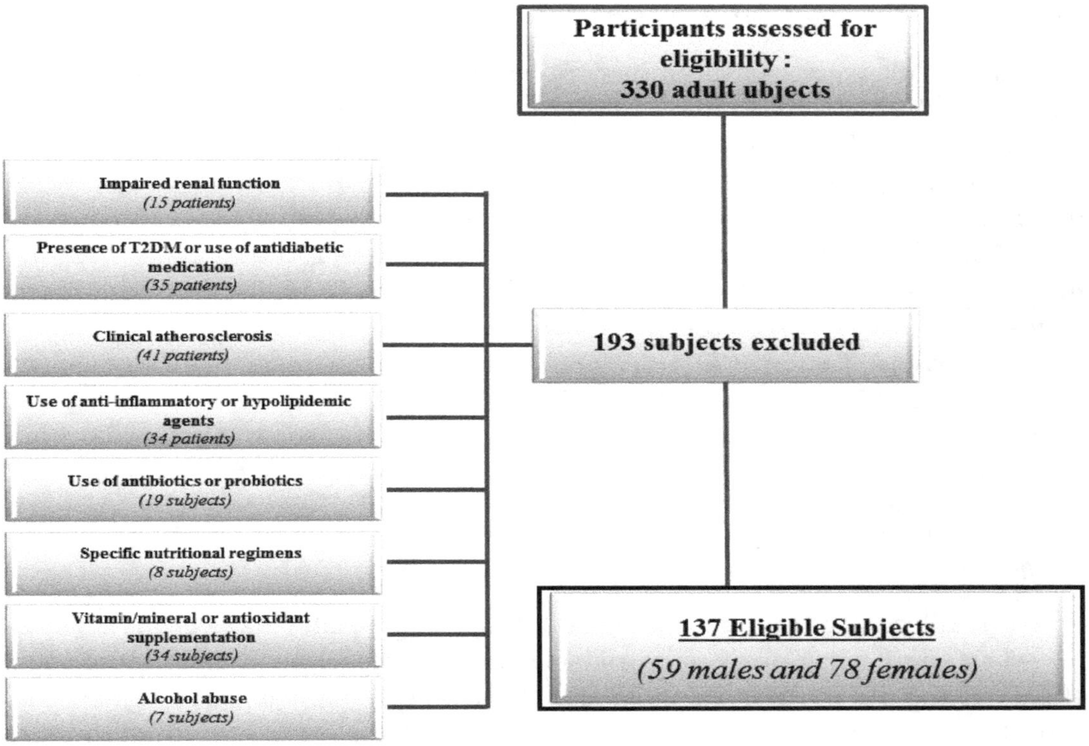

Figure 1. Flow chart of the studied subjects.

2.3. *Lifestyle Habits*

Lifestyle habits, including smoking and physical activity level, have been investigated as follows: subjects smoking at least one cigarette per day were considered current smokers, while former smokers were the subjects who stopped smoking at least one year before the interview. Remaining participants were defined as non-smokers. Physical activity levels were expressed according to whether the participant habitually engaged at least 30 min/day of aerobic exercise (YES/NO).

2.4. *Anthropometric Measurements and Blood Pressure*

Measurements were performed between 8 and 12 a.m. All subjects were measured after an overnight fast. The measurements were made in a standard way by the same operator (a nutritionist experienced in providing nutritional assessment and body composition). At the beginning of the study, all anthropometric measurements were taken with subjects wearing only light clothes and without shoes. In each subject, weight and height were measured to calculate the BMI [weight (kg) divided by height squared (m^2), kg/m^2]. Height was measured to the nearest 0.5 cm using a wall-mounted stadiometer (Seca 711; Seca, Hamburg, Germany). Body weight was determined to the nearest 0.1 kg using a calibrated balance beam scale (Seca 711; Seca, Hamburg, Germany). BMI was classified according to the World Health Organization (WHO)'s criteria with normal weight: 18.5–24.9 kg/m^2; overweight, 25.0–29.9 kg/m^2; grade I obesity, 30.0–34.9 kg/m^2; grade II obesity, 35.0–39.9 kg/m^2; grade III obesity $\geq$ 40.0 kg/m^2 [27]. WC was measured to the closest 0.1 cm using a non-stretchable measuring tape at the natural indentation or at a midway level between the lower edge of the rib cage and the iliac crest if no natural indentation was visible, as per the National Center for Health Statistics (NCHS) [28]. In all subjects Systolic Blood Pressure (SBP) and Diastolic Blood Pressure (DBP) were measured three times, two min apart, with a random zero sphygmomanometer (Gelman Hawksley Ltd., Sussex, UK) after the subject had been sitting for at least 10 min. The average of the second and third reading was recorded.

2.5. Determination of Circulating Levels of TMAO

TMAO serum levels were measured in samples stored at −80 °C. A previous study indicated that, under these conditions, TMAO is stable for several years [29]. The quantification of circulating TMAO levels has been performed using the method described by Beale and Airs [30], and reported in our previous study [4], with slight modifications. Briefly, serum proteins were precipitated with methanol (serum:methanol, 1:2, v/v); samples were vortex-mixed for 2 min, centrifuged at 14,000 g for 10 min (4 °C) [31] and supernatants were collected and analyzed by High-Performance Liquid Chromatography-Mass Spectrometry (HPLC-MS) method. Both HPLC-MS conditions and method optimization were performed in accordance with Beale and Airs [30]. The HPLC system Jasco Extrema LC-4000 system (Jasco Inc., Easton, MD, USA) was coupled to a single quadrupole mass spectrometer (Advion ExpressIonL CMS, Advion Inc., Ithaca, NY, USA) equipped with an Electrospray ionization (ESI) source, operating in positive ion mode. The chromatographic separation was performed with a Luna HILIC column (150 × 3 mm, 5 μm particles) in combination with a guard column (HILIC), both supplied by Phenomenex (Torrance, CA, USA).

2.6. Assay Methods

Samples were collected in the morning between 8 and 10 a.m., after an overnight fast of at least 8 h and stored at −80 °C until being processed. All biochemical analyses including fasting plasma glucose, total cholesterol, fasting plasma TG, Alanine Transaminase (ALT), Aspartate Aminotransferase (AST), and γ-Glutamyltransferase (γGT) were performed with a Roche Modular Analytics System in the Central Biochemistry Laboratory of our Institution. Low-Density Lipoprotein (LDL) cholesterol and HDL cholesterol were determined by a direct method (homogeneous enzymatic assay for the direct quantitative determination of LDL and HDL cholesterol). Fasting insulin levels were measured by a solid-phase chemiluminescent enzyme immunoassay using commercially available kits (Immunolite Diagnostic Products Co., Los Angeles, CA, USA). The intra-assay coefficients of variations (CV) was <5.5%, as already widely reported in our previous studies [32–36].

2.7. Cardio-Metabolic Indices

HoMA-IR was calculated according to Matthews et al. [37]. A value of HoMA-IR >2.5 was used as cut-off of insulin resistance. VAI score has been calculated by the following sex-specific formula, with TG levels expressed in mmol/L and HDL levels expressed in mmol/L:

$$\text{Males: VAI} = [\text{WC}/39.68 + (1.88 \times \text{BMI})] \times (\text{TG}/1.03) \times (1.31/\text{HDL}), \quad (1)$$

$$\text{Females: VAI} = [\text{WC}/36.58 + (1.89 \times \text{BMI})] \times (\text{TG}/0.81) \times (1.52/\text{HDL}), \quad (2)$$

Age-specific VAI cut-off values were used according to Amato et al. [22,38]. In detail, cut-offs in subjects aged ≤30, 31–42, 43–52, and 53–66 years old were 2.52, 2.23, 1.92, 1.93, respectively [22,38].

FLI was calculated with the formula:

$$[\text{FLI} = \text{eL}/(1 + \text{eL}) \times 100, \text{L} = 0.953 \times \text{loge triglycerides} + 0.139 \times \text{BMI} + 0.718 \times \text{loge}\gamma\text{GT} + 0.053 \times \text{WC} - 15.745]. \quad (3)$$

FLI of 30 was considered as the cut-off value based on Bedogni's criterion [21].

2.8. Criteria to Define MetS

According to the National Cholesterol Education Program Adult Treatment Panel (NCEP ATP) III definition, MetS is present if three or more of the following five criteria are met: WC ≥ 102 cm (men) or 88 cm (women), blood pressure ≥ 130/85 mmHg, fasting TG level ≥ 150 mg/dL, fasting HDL cholesterol level ≤ 40 mg/dL (men) or ≤50 mg/dL (women), and fasting glucose ≥ 100 mg/dL [39].

2.9. Dietary Assessment

As has been already widely reported in the literature [34–36,40], data were obtained during a face-to-face interview between the patient and a qualified nutritionist. Specifically, the dietary interview allowed the quantification of foods and drinks by using a photographic food atlas (≈1000 photographs) of known portion sizes to ensure accurate completion of the records [41]. On day 1, the diary nutritionists were trained to standardized protocols and provided participants with instructions on how to complete the diary at the health check, and asked participants to recall the previous day's intake. Participants prospectively completed the remaining 6 days and returned the records to the nutritionist [42]. Data were processed using a commercial software (Terapia Alimentare Dietosystem® DS-Medica, http://www.dsmedica.info). Considering quantities of foods consumed, the software can calculate the total energy intake, expressed in kilocalories (kcal).

2.10. Statistical Analysis

The data distribution was evaluated by Kolmogorov-Smirnov test and the abnormal data were normalized by logarithm. Skewed variables were back-transformed for presentation in tables and figures. Results are expressed as mean ± standard deviation (SD). The chi square (χ^2) test was used to determine the significance of differences in frequency distribution of smoking habit, physical activity, and presence/absence of MetS. Differences according to gender, lifestyle habits, cardio-metabolic indices, and MetS were analyzed by Student's unpaired *t*-test, while the differences among the classes of BMI were analyzed by ANOVA followed by the Bonferroni post-hoc test. The correlations between study variables were performed using Pearson *r* correlation coefficients and were estimated after adjusting for gender, BMI, smoking, physical activity, and total energy intake. Proportional Odds Ratio (OR) models, 95% Interval Confidence (IC), and R^2 were performed to assess the association between gender, lifestyle habits, classes of BMI, cardio-metabolic indices, and MetS. In addition, two multiple linear regression analysis models (stepwise method), expressed as R^2, Beta (β), and *t*, with circulating levels of TMAO as dependent variables were used to estimate the predictive value of: (a) cardio-metabolic indices; and (b) FLI and MetS. Receiver operator characteristic (ROC) curve analysis was performed to determine sensitivity and specificity, area under the curve (AUC), and IC, as well as cut-off values of circulating levels of TMAO in detecting FLI and MetS. Test AUC for ROC analysis was also performed. We wanted to show that AUC being 0.943 for a particular test is significant from the null hypothesis value 0.5 (meaning no discriminating power), so we entered 0.943 for AUC ROC and 0.5 for null hypothesis values. For α level we selected 0.05 type I error and for β level we selected 0.20 type II error. In these analyses, we entered only those variables that had a *p*-value < 0.05 in the univariate analysis (partial correlation). To avoid multicollinearity, variables with a variance inflation factor (VIF) >10 were excluded. Values ≤0.05% were considered statistically significant. Data were stored and analyzed using the MedCalc® package (Version 12.3.0 1993–2012 MedCalc Software bvba—MedCalc Software, Mariakerke, Belgium).

3. Results

The study population consisted of 137 participants, 59 males and 78 females, aged 21–56 years. Current smokers were 49.6% (68 subjects). A moderate-intensity aerobic activity at least 5 days per week was reported in 42.3% (58 subjects). BMIs ranged from 19.6 to 58.8 kg/m^2. Median values of HoMA-IR, VAI and FLI were 1.95 (0.1–15.16), 1.89 (0.60–13.85) and 75.30 (3.40–100.0), respectively. In particular, 64 subjects (46.7%) had HoMA-IR values higher than the cut-off. VAI was higher than sex- and age-specific cut-offs in 43.8% (60 subjects) and 59.9% (82 subjects) presented FLI values above the cut-off. MetS was present in 53 participants (38.7%).

In Table 1 we report the lifestyle habits, anthropometric measurements, blood pressure, metabolic profile, and cardio-metabolic indices in the total population grouped based on BMI categories. As shown in Table 1, no differences were observed in age (p = 0.292), while subjects with overweight and obesity exhibited statistical differences in all parameters compared with normal-weight subjects ($p < 0.001$). In particular, circulating levels of TMAO increased with the BMI classes, with the highest TMAO values in the class III obesity.

Table 1. Lifestyle habits, anthropometric characteristics, blood pressure, metabolic profile, cardio-metabolic indices, and total energy intake of participants grouped based on BMI categories.

Parameters	Normal Weight *n* = 34; 24.8%	Over Weight *n* = 29; 21.2%	Grade I Obesity *n* = 21; 15.3%	Grade II Obesity *n* = 15; 10.9%	Grade III Obesity *n* = 38; 27.7%	*p*-value
Lifestyle Habits						
Age (years)	35.71 ± 8.48	38.14 ± 7.58	38.24 ± 5.89	35.80 ± 8.20	35.00 ± 6.82	0.292
Smoking (yes)	16, 47.1%	19, 65.5%	4, 19.0%	2, 13.3%	22, 10.5%	χ^2 = 19.21, **p < 0.001**
Physical activity (yes)	22, 64.7%	11, 37.9%	3, 14.3%	5, 33.3%	4, 10.5%	χ^2 = 27.85, **p < 0.001**
Anthropometric measurement						
BMI (kg/m^2)	23.01 ± 1.49	27.32 ± 1.43	32.41 ± 1.37	37.48 ± 1.56	46.99 ± 5.16	**<0.001**
WC (cm)	85.12 ± 10.13	94.30 ± 12.38	109.65 ± 8.14	118.81 ± 13.40	139.47 ± 15.15	**<0.001**
Blood pressure						
SBP (mmHg)	115.44 ± 8.01	121.21 ± 10.90	129.52 ± 10.83	131.00 ± 16.38	133.68 ± 11.79	**<0.001**
DBP (mmHg)	71.33 ± 6.07	75.68 ± 7.41	81.67 ± 6.77	86.33 ± 11.25	89.61 ± 9.25	**<0.001**
Metabolic profile						
Circulating levels of TMAO (μM)	3.62 ± 2.37	8.23 ± 0.67	9.03 ± 0.97	9.89 ± 0.85	11.53 ± 0.96	**<0.001**
Fasting Glucose (mg/dL)	83.65 ± 10.25	93.17 ± 13.10	96.47 ± 12.11	97.73 ± 11.00	121.87 ± 10.91	**<0.001**
Insulin (μU/mL)	2.66 ± 1.23	7.01 ± 5.35	10.69 ± 5.83	14.85 ± 9.65	31.29 ± 8.87	**<0.001**
Total cholesterol (mg/dL)	146.8 ± 20.28	176.69 ± 29.17	170.76 ± 20.85	206.87 ± 39.57	221.37 ± 33.58	**<0.001**
HDL cholesterol (mg/dL)	57.59 ± 7.53	50.21 ± 8.19	41.95 ± 13.28	39.60 ± 10.60	37.05 ± 9.42	**<0.001**
LDL cholesterol (mg/dL)	69.92 ± 23.15	101.43 ± 30.05	103.37 ± 16.67	134.49 ± 41.49	150.17 ± 38.54	**<0.001**
Triglycerides (mg/dL)	96.71 ± 26.96	125.24 ± 28.30	155.52 ± 65.23	163.87 ± 33.78	170.74 ± 70.88	**<0.001**
ALT (U/L)	23.26 ± 6.87	24.89 ± 9.06	38.14 ± 12.16	40.73 ± 17.87	41.39 ± 22.49	**<0.001**
AST (U/L)	20.44 ± 5.57	26.58 ± 6.67	36.83 ± 18.25	39.07 ± 14.10	41.00 ± 20.12	**<0.001**
γGT (U/L)	25.64 ± 6.62	26.52 ± 12.48	42.42 ± 19.71	44.47 ± 19.65	49.53 ± 27.20	**<0.001**
Cardio-metabolic indices						
HoMA-IR	0.55 ± 0.28	1.49 ± 0.96	2.51 ± 1.32	3.55 ± 2.31	9.52 ± 3.13	**<0.001**
VAI	1.28 ± 0.54	2.09 ± 1.27	3.42 ± 2.91	3.55 ± 1.97	3.77 ± 2.18	**<0.001**
FLI	19.89 ± 12.37	43.70 ± 21.36	79.39 ± 10.26	90.98 ± 6.97	98.36 ± 2.30	**<0.001**
Metabolic Syndrome						
MetS (number parameter)	0.18 ± 0.52	1.24 ± 1.02	2.33 ± 1.06	2.67 ± 1.40	3.68 ± 1.07	**<0.001**
MetS (presence)	0, 0	4, 13.8%	9, 42.9%	9, 60%	31, 81.6%	χ^2 = 61.53, **p < 0.001**
Nutritional parameters						
Total energy intake (kcal)	2084.79 ± 304.05	2249.14 ± 433.86	2423.33 ± 211.27	2658.67 ± 244.80	2966.45 ± 365.69	**<0.001**

A *p*-value in bold type denotes a significant difference ($p < 0.05$).

Circulating levels of TMAO according to gender, lifestyle habits, and cut-off of the cardio-metabolic indices are reported in Table 2. As reported in Table 2, circulating levels of TMAO were significantly higher in males ($p = 0.015$), among current smokers or physically inactive individuals ($p < 0.001$), and in subjects with cardio-metabolic indices higher than cut-offs ($p < 0.001$). In addition, circulating levels of TMAO were significantly higher in presence of MetS ($p < 0.001$).

Table 2. Circulating levels of TMAO in the study population according to gender, lifestyle habits, cardio-metabolic indices, and MetS.

Parameters		**Circulating Levels of TMAO (μM)**	***p*-value**
Gender	Males (n 59)	9.11 ± 3.09	**0.015**
	Females (n 78)	7.70 ± 3.28	
Smoking	Yes (n 68)	9.38 ± 2.63	**<0.001**
	No (n 69)	7.24 ± 3.49	
Physical activity	Yes (n 58)	6.41 ± 3.52	**<0.001**
	No (n 79)	9.69 ± 2.21	
HoMA-IR	> cut-off (n 64)	10.53 ± 1.62	**<0.001**
	< cut-off (n 73)	6.36 ± 3.01	
VAI	> cut-off (n 60)	10.08 ± 2.13	**<0.001**
	< cut-off (n 77)	6.92 ± 3.33	
FLI	> cut-off (n 82)	10.24 ± 1.56	**<0.001**
	< cut-off (n 55)	5.42 ± 3.00	
MetS (parameters)			
WC	Yes (n 87)	9.88 ± 2.06	**<0.001**
	No (n 50)	5.56 ± 3.18	
SBP/DBP	Yes (n 37)	10.49 ± 1.72	**<0.001**
	No (n 100)	7.50 ± 3.33	
Fasting Glucose	Yes (n 43)	11.29 ± 1.22	**<0.001**
	No (n 94)	6.94 ± 2.98	
HDL cholesterol	Yes (n 59)	10.13 ± 2.09	**<0.001**
	No (n 78)	6.93 ± 3.33	
Triglycerides	Yes (n 45)	10.28 ± 2.20	**<0.001**
	No (n 92)	7.34 ± 3.27	
MetS (presence/absence)	Yes (n 53)	10.65 ± 1.62	**<0.001**
	No (n 84)	6.82 ± 3.17	

A *p*-value in bold type denotes a significant difference ($p < 0.05$).

Correlation Analysis

The correlations between circulating levels of TMAO, age, components of the MetS, metabolic profile, cardio-metabolic indices, are summarized in Table 3. Apart from the age, circulating levels of TMAO show significant correlations with all metabolic parameters. After adjusting for gender, BMI, smoking, physical activity, and total energy intake, correlations with almost all the components of MetS and cardio-metabolic indices were still evident, as shown in Table 3.

Table 3. Correlations among circulating levels of TMAO with age, anthropometric characteristics, blood pressure, metabolic profile, cardio-metabolic indices, and nutritional parameter.

Parameters	Circulating Levels of TMAO (μM)		Circulating Levels of TMAO (μM)	
	Simple Correlation		After Adjusting	
	r	*p*-value	r	*p*-value
Age (years)	0.103	0.232	0.169	0.054
Anthropometric measurements				
BMI (kg/m^2)	0.737	**<0.001**	-	-
WC (cm)	0.670	**<0.001**	−0.055	0.538
Blood pressure				
SBP (mmHg)	0.600	**<0.001**	0.273	**0.002**
DBP (mmHg)	0.532	**<0.001**	0.149	0.091
Metabolic profile				
Fasting Glucose (mg/dL)	0.656	**<0.001**	0.034	0.700
Insulin (μU/mL)	0.668	**<0.001**	0.202	**0.021**
Total cholesterol (mg/dL)	0.628	**<0.001**	0.236	**0.007**
HDL cholesterol (mg/dL)	−0.568	**<0.001**	−0.180	**0.041**
LDL cholesterol (mg/dL)	0.663	**<0.001**	0.356	**<0.001**
Triglycerides (mg/dL)	0.535	**<0.001**	0.224	**0.010**
ALT (U/L)	0.376	**0.001**	0.065	0.461
AST (U/L)	0.506	**<0.001**	0.176	**0.046**
γGT (U/L)	0.396	**0.001**	0.086	0.333
Cardio-metabolic indices				
HoMA-IR	0.699	**<0.001**	0.211	**0.016**
VAI	0.549	**<0.001**	0.255	**0.003**
FLI	0.820	**<0.001**	0.604	**<0.001**
Nutritional parameter				
Total energy intake (kcal)	0.592	**<0.001**	-	-

A *p*-value in bold type denotes a significant difference ($p < 0.05$).

The results of bivariate proportional OR model performed to assess the association of circulating levels of TMAO with quantitative variables are reported in Table 4. The highest circulating levels of TMAO are significantly associated with the severity of obesity (OR 9.59; $p < 0.001$), and insulin resistance (OR 2.82; $p < 0.001$). Moreover, the highest levels of TMAO are associated with the highest levels of VAI (OR 1.58; $p < 0.001$) and FLI (OR 4.31; $p < 0.001$), presence of MetS (OR 2.36; $p < 0.001$) and of all components of the MetS.

Table 4. Bivariate proportional odds ratio model to assess the association between circulating levels of TMAO and gender, lifestyle habits, cardio-metabolic indices, and MetS.

Parameters	Circulating Levels of TMAO (μM)			
	OR	***p*-value**	**95% IC**	R^2
Gender	1.15	**0.015**	1.029–1.295	0.047
Smoking	1.26	**0.001**	1.110–1.423	0.108
Physical activity	0.67	**<0.001**	0.576–0.788	0.240
BMI categories				
Normal weight	0.05	**0.001**	0.009–0.297	0.604
Overweight	0.27	**<0.001**	0.011–1.121	0.209
Grade I obesity	0.18	**<0.001**	0.010–0.099	0.237
Grade II obesity	1.25	**<0.001**	0.995–1.565	0.033
Grade III obesity	9.59	**<0.001**	3.946–23.344	0.561
HoMA-IR	2.82	**<0.001**	1.937–4.116	0.458
VAI	1.58	**<0.001**	1.308–1.912	0.248
FLI	4.31	**<0.001**	2.353–7.874	0.536
MetS (single parameters)				
WC	1.88	**<0.001**	1.490–2.375	0.378
SBP/DBP	1.64	**<0.001**	1.304–2.065	0.201
Fasting Glucose	5.84	**<0.001**	3.161–10.804	0.538
HDL cholesterol	1.61	**<0.001**	1.320–1.953	0.254
Triglycerides	1.57	**0.001**	1.278–1.919	0.205
MetS (presence/absence)	2.36	**<0.001**	1.727–3.227	0.389

A *p*-value in bold type denotes a significant difference ($p < 0.05$).

To compare the relative predictive power of the cardio-metabolic indices associated with the circulating levels of TMAO, we performed a multiple linear regression analysis using a model that included as HoMA-IR, VAI, and FLI. Using this model, FLI entered at the first step ($p < 0.001$), while HoMA-IR, VAI were excluded. To compare the relative predictive power of FLI and number of components of MetS associated with the circulating levels of TMAO, we performed a second multiple linear regression analysis model. Using this second model, FLI entered at the first step ($p < 0.001$), while the number of components of MetS were excluded. Results were reported in Table 5.

Table 5. Multiple regression analysis models (stepwise method) with the circulating levels of TMAO as dependent variable to estimate the predictive value of: (a) cardio-metabolic indices; (b) FLI and MetS.

Parameters	Multiple Regression Analysis			
Model 1	R^2	β	t	*p*-value
FLI	0.672	0.820	16.63	**<0.001**
Variables excluded: HoMA-IR and VAI				
Model 2				
FLI	0.469	0.685	9.2	**<0.001**
Variables excluded: MetS				

A *p*-value in bold type denotes a significant difference ($p < 0.05$).

A ROC analysis was then performed to determine the cut-off values of circulating levels of TMAO predictive of MetS and FLI. In particular, circulating levels of TMAO ≥8.74 μM ($p < 0.001$, AUC 0.876, standard error 0.029, 95% CI 0.808 to 0.926; Figure 2a), and circulating levels of TMAO ≥8.02 μM ($p < 0.001$, AUC 0.943, standard error 0.018, 95% CI 0.890 to 0.975; Figure 2b), could serve as thresholds for significantly increased risk of the presence of MetS and NAFLD, respectively.

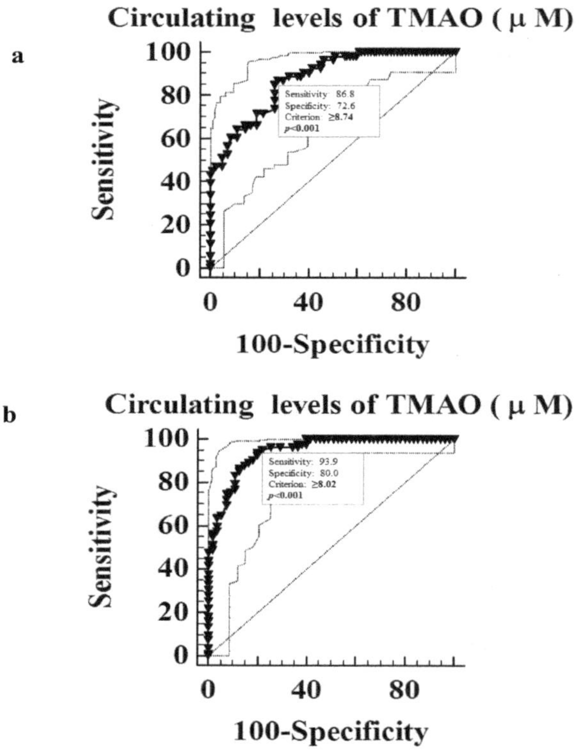

Figure 2. ROC for predictive values of circulating levels of TMAO in detecting FLI (**a**) and MetS (**b**). A p-value in bold type denotes a significant difference ($p < 0.05$).

4. Discussion

In this cross-sectional observational study, we evaluated the circulating levels of TMAO in a sample of adult population stratified according to categories of BMI. In addition, we investigated the association among circulating levels of TMAO and cardio-metabolic indices. The classification of the study population according to the BMI demonstrated that circulating levels of TMAO increased along with BMI. To the best of our knowledge, this is the first study that reported statistical differences in the circulating levels of TMAO across classes of BMI. Moreover, we confirmed the presence of a positive association of circulating levels of TMAO with MetS, the increasing number of its components, and HoMA-IR. Finally, a novel association was also reported among the circulating levels of TMAO and VAI and FLI, two surrogate indices of cardio-metabolic risk and early indicators of MetS, independently on common potential covariates.

There is a paucity of literature that has studied the relationship between TMAO and adiposity. A recent experimental study reported that both antisense oligonucleotide-mediated knockdown and genetic deletion of the TMAO-producing enzyme FMO3 protected mice against high-fat diet-induced obesity, thus highlighting a role of the gut microbe-driven TMA/FMO3/TMAO pathway in affecting specific transcriptional reprogramming in white adipocytes [11]. Of interest, in this study circulating levels of TMAO were positively associated with body weight, fat mass, mesenteric adiposity, and subcutaneous adiposity across the different mice-inbred strains; in addition, in cohorts of overweight or obese subjects with metabolic traits and different ethnicity the expression of FMO3 in liver biopsies was positively correlated with BMI and waist-to-hip ratio, and negatively correlated with the Matsuda Index, a measure of insulin sensitivity [11]. Consistent with these data, the findings of the present study show that there is a clear positive association of circulating TMAO levels and classes of BMI. Thus, besides its role as a risk factor for CVD and adverse event in risks subjects, emerging evidence suggests that gut microbiota-derived TMAO might represent per se a key environmental factor contributing to obesity and obesity-associated disorders.

VAI is a surrogate of adipocyte dysfunction independently correlated with insulin sensitivity, and cardio-metabolic risk in primary-care non-obese subjects [20]. In particular, VAI was proposed as a useful tool for the early detection of a condition of insulin resistance and cardio-metabolic risk before it develops into an overt MetS [38]. FLI is a surrogate marker of a fatty liver considered a screening tool to identify NAFLD, recognized as the liver manifestation of MetS, in subjects with insulin resistance and cardio-metabolic risk factors where ultrasound is unavailable [43]. In our population sample there was a positive association between circulating levels of TMAO and both indices. Of interest, the association of the circulating levels of TMAO with VAI and FLI was also shown independently on potential covariates, such as gender, BMI, smoking status, physical activity, and energy intake. In addition, among the cardio-metabolic indices included in this study, FLI, which incorporates BMI, WC, TG, and liver function, was a better predictor of TMAO variability than MetS per se. This finding was in line with the putative role of FLI as early predictor of MetS and likely reflects that the main site of expression of FMO3, the enzyme that metabolizes gut microbe-derived TMA to produce TMAO, is the liver. Based on ROC curve analysis, the most sensitive and specific cut-offs for circulating levels of TMAO to predict the presence of NAFLD-FLI and MetS were $\geq$8.02 μM and $\geq$8.74 μM, respectively. Experimental studies in mice fed with a high-fat diet showed that a high urinary excretion of TMAO was associated with insulin resistance and NAFLD in mice (129S6) prone to these diseases [44]. Miao et al. [45] found that liver insulin receptor knockout mice, characterized by a selective hepatic insulin resistance, have increased circulating TMAO levels associated with a strong up-regulation of the TMAO-producing enzyme FMO3 in the liver [45]. According to the proposed mechanism, TMAO may block the hepatic insulin signaling pathway, thereby exacerbating the impaired glucose tolerance, and promoting the development of fatty liver [46]. Turning to human studies, the above-mentioned study by Randrianarisoa et al. [12] reported a positive correlation between TMAO and liver fat content [12]. In addition, in a large sample of hospital and community-based Chinese adults, Chen et al. [13] showed positive associations of the circulating TMAO levels and two of its nutrient precursors, choline and betaine, with the presence and severity of NAFLD [13]. Choline can be oxidized to betaine, and betaine is generally regarded as safe for dietary ingestion due to its sparing effects on choline, a basic component for the synthesis of phosphatidylcholine, which in turn is necessary for promoting lipid exportation from the liver [47]. In this study, the authors suggested that TMAO may represent a possible risk factor for NAFLD due to its effect in altering the synthesis and transport of bile acids, with subsequent effects on lipid metabolism, intrahepatic triglycerides levels and glucose homeostasis [6]. More recently, Ntzouvani et al. [18] reported a strong positive association between liver function and a pattern of amino acids, which included TMAO, in a sample of Greek adult males with MetS [18].

The results of this study lend support to the evidence that circulating levels of TMAO were positively associated with body weight, thus concurring with an increased risk of developing MetS, through insulin resistance, adipocyte dysfunction, and fatty liver. In this context, it is tempting to hypothesize that circulating levels of TMAO could have a role of a biological marker of early metabolic derangement in subjects with overweight and obesity. Thus, it allows speculation on the possible beneficial and cost-effective effects to early address specific nutrition interventions aimed to reduce the excessive intake of TMAO precursors in subjects at risk of MetS and NAFLD.

Despite these very interesting results, the main limitation of this study is that the cross-sectional design does not allow identification of any causal association between the variables included. Thus, it is not possible to clearly determine the prognostic value of circulating levels of TMAO for predicting the early metabolic derangement in subjects with overweight and obesity. Second, although it is well known that the gut-derived origin of TMAO and dietary intake are important determinants of

TMAO levels, we did not include in this study the gut microbiota and single-nutrient analysis. In particular, Kühn et al. [48] reported also that both dietary habits and the composition of the intestinal microbiota may be prone to changes, despite a certain stability of both factors during adulthood. On the other hand, Krüger et al. [49] reported that the large inter-individual variations TMAO levels have been mainly attributed to intestinal microbiota differences, while the influence of diet on fasting TMAO concentrations, albeit statistically significant, could be considered rather moderate. However, there is a large consensus that the study of gut microbiota is burdened by a high intra-individual variability that might hinder the interpretation of the results [48,50–52]. Third, we did not include the evaluation of markers of inflammation, such as C-reactive protein, or metabolic precursor of TMAO such as choline, betaine or carnitine, and liver expression of FMO3. However, several studies have shown that the associations between plasma TMAO and disease outcomes were independent of TMAO precursors [53–55]. In addition, the adverse effects of FMO3 on metabolic disease may be driven by factors other than TMAO, and the expression of the FMO3 or markers of inflammation encompassed the design of the present study. Fourth, we are aware that the liver biopsy is the gold-standard technique for identifying NAFLD. Liver biopsy is an invasive and costly procedure burdened with rare but potentially life-threatening complications. On the contrary, FLI has proved to represent an easy screening tool to identify NAFLD in patients with cardio-metabolic risk factors where ultrasound is unavailable [21,56,57], which is associated with reduced insulin sensitivity, and increased risk of T2DM, atherosclerosis, and cardiovascular disease [43]. Nevertheless, a major strength of this study is the good characterization of our sample population across BMI classes, with the exclusion of impaired renal function and T2DM known factors that can affect TMA metabolism, and likely with similar nutrient availability and food consumption pattern, as they were living in the same geographical area. Furthermore, we included of a variety of potential covariates, such as the total energy intake, to minimize the effect of confounding factors on the association of TMAO with adiposity. However, since complete understanding of TMAO biology is still lacking, the potential translation application of the results of this study to the clinical practice requires large-scale data investigating the beneficial and cost-effective effects of specific nutrition intervention aimed to avoid the excessive intake of TMAO precursors in subjects at risk of MetS and NAFLD. The main results of our study, compared to the results of the general literature, is reported in Table 6.

Table 6. A summary table with the main results of our study compared to the results of the general literature.

Parameters	Methodology	Participants	Effects	Hypothesis	Studies	Concordance
Nascent Metabolic Syndrome (MetS)	Case-control clinical study	30 patients 20 controls	TMAO with a trend of positive correlation	TMAO levels rise only after MetS has advanced to the later stages including T2DM and/or CVD	[9]	Yes
HoMA-IR	Case-control clinical study	30 patients 20 controls	TMAO not significantly correlated	No major role for TMAO in glucose metabolism or insulin sensitivity	[9]	No
	Intervention Program	220 subjects	A negative correlation between circulating TMAO levels insulin sensitivity	In obese, hyperglycemic humans FMO3 expression and TMAO levels are increased in hepatic insulin resistance.	[12]	Yes
NAFLD	Experimental study	Mouse strain 129S6, documented for its susceptibility to IR or NAFLD	Mice 129S6 fed with a high-fat diet showed a high urinary excretion of TMAO associated with insulin resistance and NAFLD	A high-fat diet reduces the conversion and the bioavailability of choline by microbiota, causing NAFLD	[44]	Yes
	Experimental study	Male ob/ob mice and their lean, wild-type C57BL/6J controls	Liver insulin receptor knockout mice with selective hepatic insulin resistance have increased circulating TMAO levels associated with a strong up-regulation of the TMAO-producing enzyme FMO3 in the liver	TMAO may block the hepatic insulin signaling pathway promoting the development of fatty liver	[11]	Yes
	Case-control study (CCS) and cross-sectional study (CSS)	60 adult patients and 35 controls for CCS 1.628participants for CSS	TMAO is an independent risk marker for NAFLD in humans. in both the CCS and CSS studies	TMAO decreases the total bile acid pool size and influences the hepatic triglycerides levels, as a potential risk factor for fatty liver disease	[13]	Yes
	Intervention Program	220 subjects	A positive correlation between circulating TMAO levels and liver fat content	Fasting levels of TMAO are regulated by hepatic FMO3	[12]	Yes
	Cross-sectional study	One hundred middle-aged men	A strong positive association between liver function and a pattern of amino acids, which included TMAO	A pattern of amino acids, included TMAO, are regulated by liver enzymes	[18]	Yes

Abbreviations: MetS, Metabolic Syndrome; TMAO, Trimethylamine N-oxide; T2DM, Type 2 Diabetes Mellitus; CVD, Cardiovascular Diseases; HoMA-IR, Homeostatic Model Assessment Insulin Resistance; FMO3, Flavin-containing Monooxygenases; NAFLD, non-alcoholic fatty liver disease; IR, insulin Resistance; CCS, Case-control Study; CSS, Cross-sectional Study.

5. Conclusions

In conclusion, this study in a sample of adult subjects stratified according to their BMI: (i) reported a positive association between adiposity and circulating levels of TMAO; (ii) confirmed the positive association between circulating levels of TMAO and MetS; and (iii) further expanded the knowledge of the relationship of TMAO and MetS, as we reported novel associations between circulating levels of TMAO and two early indicators of MetS. In particular, in this study we demonstrated that FLI is more tightly associated with TMAO levels than the presence of MetS per se. These associations let us to hypothesize a role of TMAO as an early biomarker of NAFLD-FLI in all borderline conditions in which overt MetS is not present. Moreover, given the current performance of therapies for MetS, we suggest that a specific cut-off of TMAO might help in identifying subjects at high risk of NAFLD, who will require specific nutrition intervention strategies. Appropriate cross-validation studies in larger patient population samples are mandatory to validate the cut-off of TMAO for the identification of subjects at high risk of NAFLD-FLI.

Author Contributions: Conceptualization, L.B. and S.S.; Data curation, G.M.; Formal analysis, L.B., G.M., C.D.S. and S.S.; Funding acquisition, L.B. and G.C.T.; Investigation, L.B., G.A., C.D.S., D.L., G.d.A. and S.S.; Methodology, L.B., G.A. and C.D.S.; Project administration, L.B. and G.M.; Resources, L.B.; Software, L.B.; Supervision, L.B.; Validation, L.B.; Visualization, L.B. and M.M.; Writing—Original Draft, L.B. and S.S.; Writing—Review and Editing, L.B., G.M., A.C. and S.S.

Acknowledgments: We would like to thank Angela Arnone for data retrieval.

Abbreviations

TMAO	Trimethylamine-N-oxide
TMA	Trimethylamine
FMO3	Flavin-monooxygenase-3
T2DM	Type 2 Diabetes Mellitus
CVD	Cardiovascular diseases
MetS	Metabolic Syndrome
HDL	High-density Lipoprotein
HoMA-IR	Homeostatic Model Assessment of Insulin Resistance
BMI	body mass index
VAI	Visceral Adiposity Index
FLI	Fatty Liver Index
NAFLD	Non-alcoholic Fatty Liver Disease
WC	Waist Circumference
TG	Triglycerides
SBP	Systolic Blood Pressure
DBP	Diastolic Blood Pressure
ALT	Alanine Transaminase
AST	Aspartate Aminotransferase
γGT	γ-Glutamyltransferase
LDL	Low-Density Lipoprotein
SD	Standard Deviation
OR	Odds Ratio
IC	Interval Confidence
ROC	Receiver Operator Characteristic
AUC	Area Under Curve.

References

1. Wang, Z.; Klipfel, E.; Bennett, B.J.; Koeth, R.; Levison, B.S.; Dugar, B.; Feldstein, A.E.; Britt, E.B.; Fu, X.; Chung, Y.M.; et al. Gut flora metabolism of phosphatidylcholine promotes cardiovascular disease. *Nature* **2011**, *472*, 57–63. [CrossRef] [PubMed]
2. Schiattarella, G.G.; Sannino, A.; Toscano, E.; Giugliano, G.; Gargiulo, G.; Franzone, A.; Trimarco, B.; Esposito, G.; Perrino, C. Gut microbe-generated metabolite trimethylamine-N-oxide as cardiovascular risk biomarker: A systematic review and dose-response meta-analysis. *Eur. Heart J.* **2017**, *38*, 2948–2956. [CrossRef] [PubMed]
3. Kanitsoraphan, C.; Rattanawong, P.; Charoensri, S.; Senthong, V. Trimethylamine N-Oxide and Risk of Cardiovascular Disease and Mortality. *Curr. Nutr. Rep.* **2018**. [CrossRef] [PubMed]
4. Barrea, L.; Annunziata, G.; Muscogiuri, G.; Ludisio, D.; Di Somma, C.; Maisto, M.; Tenore, G.C.; Colao, A.; Savastano, S. Trimethylamine N-oxide (TMAO), Mediterranean Diet and Nutrition in Healthy, Normal-weight Subjects: Is It Also A Matter Of Gender? *Nutrition* **2018**, in press. [CrossRef]
5. Zeisel, S.H.; Wishnok, J.S.; Blusztajn, J.K. Formation of methylamines from ingested choline and lecithin. *J. Pharmacol. Exp. Ther.* **1983**, *225*, 320–324.
6. Koeth, R.A.; Wang, Z.; Levison, B.S.; Buffa, J.A.; Org, E.; Sheehy, B.T.; Britt, E.B.; Fu, X.; Wu, Y.; Li, L.; et al. Intestinal microbiota metabolism of L-carnitine, a nutrient in red meat, promotes atherosclerosis. *Nat. Med.* **2013**, *19*, 576–585. [CrossRef] [PubMed]
7. Tang, W.H.; Hazen, S.L. The contributory role of gut microbiota in cardiovascular disease. *J. Clin. Investig.* **2014**, *124*, 4204–4211. [CrossRef] [PubMed]
8. Ufnal, M.; Zadlo, A.; Ostaszewski, R. TMAO: A small molecule of great expectations. *Nutrition* **2015**, *31*, 1317–1323. [CrossRef] [PubMed]
9. Lent-Schochet, D.; Silva, R.; McLaughlin, M.; Huet, B.; Jialal, I. Changes to trimethylamine-N-oxide and its precursors in nascent metabolic syndrome. *Horm. Mol. Biol. Clin. Investig.* **2018**, *35*. [CrossRef]
10. Zhu, W.; Gregory, J.C.; Org, E.; Buffa, J.A.; Gupta, N.; Wang, Z.; Li, L.; Fu, X.; Wu, Y.; Mehrabian, M.; et al. Gut Microbial Metabolite TMAO Enhances Platelet Hyperreactivity and Thrombosis Risk. *Cell* **2016**, *165*, 111–124. [CrossRef]
11. Schugar, R.C.; Shih, D.M.; Warrier, M.; Helsley, R.N.; Burrows, A.; Ferguson, D.; Brown, A.L.; Gromovsky, A.D.; Heine, M.; Chatterjee, A.; et al. The TMAO-Producing Enzyme Flavin-Containing Monooxygenase 3 Regulates Obesity and the Beiging of White Adipose Tissue. *Cell Rep.* **2017**, *19*, 2451–2461. [CrossRef] [PubMed]
12. Randrianarisoa, E.; Lehn-Stefan, A.; Wang, X.; Hoene, M.; Peter, A.; Heinzmann, S.S.; Zhao, X.; Königsrainer, I.; Königsrainer, A.; Balletshofer, B.; et al. Relationship of Serum Trimethylamine N-Oxide (TMAO) Levels with early Atherosclerosis in Humans. *Sci. Rep.* **2016**, *6*, 26745. [CrossRef] [PubMed]
13. Chen, Y.M.; Liu, Y.; Zhou, R.F.; Chen, X.L.; Wang, C.; Tan, X.Y.; Wang, L.J.; Zheng, R.D.; Zhang, H.W.; Ling, W.H.; et al. Associations of gut-flora-dependent metabolite trimethylamine-N-oxide, betaine and choline with non-alcoholic fatty liver disease in adults. *Sci. Rep.* **2016**, *6*, 19076. [CrossRef] [PubMed]
14. Marchesini, G.; Brizi, M.; Bianchi, G.; Tomassetti, S.; Bugianesi, E.; Lenzi, M.; McCullough, A.J.; Natale, S.; Forlani, G.; Melchionda, N. Nonalcoholic fatty liver disease: A feature of the metabolic syndrome. *Diabetes* **2001**, *50*, 1844–1850. [CrossRef]
15. Grundy, S.M.; Cleeman, J.I.; Daniels, S.R.; Donato, K.A.; Eckel, R.H.; Franklin, B.A.; Gordon, D.J.; Krauss, R.M.; Savage, P.J.; Smith, S.C., Jr.; et al. National Heart, Lung, and Blood Institute. Diagnosis and management of the metabolic syndrome: An American Heart Association/National Heart, Lung, and Blood Institute Scientific Statement. *Circulation* **2005**, *112*, 2735–2752. [CrossRef] [PubMed]
16. Lorenzo, C.; Williams, K.; Hunt, K.J.; Haffner, S.M. The National Cholesterol Education Program–Adult Treatment Panel III, International Diabetes Federation, and World Health Organization definitions of the metabolic syndrome as predictors of incident cardiovascular disease and diabetes. *Diabetes Care* **2007**, *30*, 8–13. [CrossRef] [PubMed]
17. Jialal, I.; Devaraj, S.; Adams-Huet, B.; Chen, X.; Kaur, H. Increased cellular and circulating biomarkers of oxidative stress in nascent metabolic syndrome. *J. Clin. Endocrinol. Metab.* **2012**, *97*, E1844–E1850. [CrossRef]

18. Ntzouvani, A.; Nomikos, T.; Panagiotakos, D.; Fragopoulou, E.; Pitsavos, C.; McCann, A.; Ueland, P.M.; Antonopoulou, S. Amino acid profile and metabolic syndrome in a male Mediterranean population: A cross-sectional study. *Nutr. Metab. Cardiovasc. Dis.* **2017**, *27*, 1021–1030. [CrossRef]
19. Mueller, D.M.; Allenspach, M.; Othman, A.; Saely, C.H.; Muendlein, A.; Vonbank, A.; Drexel, H.; von Eckardstein, A. Plasma levels of trimethylamine-N-oxide are confounded by impaired kidney function and poor metabolic control. *Atherosclerosis* **2015**, *243*, 638–644. [CrossRef]
20. Amato, M.C.; Giordano, C.; Galia, M.; Criscimanna, A.; Vitabile, S.; Midiri, M.; Galluzzo, A.; AlkaMeSy Study Group. Visceral Adiposity Index: A reliable indicator of visceral fat function associated with cardiometabolic risk. *Diabetes Care* **2010**, *33*, 920–922. [CrossRef]
21. Bedogni, G.; Bellentani, S.; Miglioli, L.; Masutti, F.; Passalacqua, M.; Castiglione, A.; Tiribelli, C. The Fatty Liver Index: A simple and accurate predictor of hepatic steatosis in the general population. *BMC Gastroenterol.* **2006**, *6*, 33. [CrossRef] [PubMed]
22. Amato, M.C.; Giordano, C. Visceral adiposity index: An indicator of adipose tissue dysfunction. *Int. J. Endocrinol.* **2014**, *2014*, 730827. [CrossRef] [PubMed]
23. Klisic, A.; Isakovic, A.; Kocic, G.; Kavaric, N.; Jovanovic, M.; Zvrko, E.; Skerovic, V.; Ninic, A. Relationship between Oxidative Stress, Inflammation and Dyslipidemia with Fatty Liver Index in Patients with Type 2 Diabetes Mellitus. *Exp. Clin. Endocrinol. Diabetes* **2018**, *126*, 371–378. [CrossRef] [PubMed]
24. Rogulj, D.; Konjevoda, P.; Milić, M.; Mladinić, M.; Domijan, A.M. Fatty liver index as an indicator of metabolic syndrome. *Clin. Biochem.* **2012**, *45*, 68–71. [CrossRef] [PubMed]
25. Yadav, D.; Choi, E.; Ahn, S.V.; Koh, S.B.; Sung, K.C.; Kim, J.Y.; Huh, J.H. Fatty liver index as a simple predictor of incident diabetes from the KoGES-ARIRANG study. *Medicine* **2016**, *95*, E4447. [CrossRef] [PubMed]
26. American Diabetes Association. Standards of Medical Care in Diabetes-2017: Summary of Revisions. *Diabetes Care* **2017**, *40*, S4–S5. [CrossRef] [PubMed]
27. World Health Organization (WHO). Waist Circumference and Waist-Hip Ratio. Report of WHO Expert Consultation, Geneva. 8–11 December 2008. Available online: http://apps.who.int/iris/bitstream/10665/44583/1/9789241501491_eng.pdf (accessed on 10 November 2018).
28. National Center for Health Statistics. Anthropometry Procedures Manual—National Health and Nutrition Examination Survey (NHANES). Available online: http://www.cdc.gov/nchs/data/nhanes/nhanes_11_12/Anthropometry_Procedures_Manual.pdf (accessed on 10 November 2018).
29. Wang, Z.; Levison, B.S.; Hazen, J.E.; Donahue, L.; Li, X.M.; Hazen, S.L. Measurement of trimethylamine-N-oxide by stable isotope dilution liquid chromatography tandem mass spectrometry. *Anal. Biochem.* **2014**, *455*, 35–40. [CrossRef] [PubMed]
30. Beale, R.; Airs, R. Quantification of glycine betaine, choline and trimethylamine N-oxide in seawater particulates: Minimisation of seawater associated ion suppression. *Anal. Chim. Acta.* **2016**, *938*, 114–122. [CrossRef]
31. Yu, W.; Xu, C.; Li, G.; Hong, W.; Zhou, Z.; Xiao, C.; Zhao, Y.; Cai, Y.; Huang, M.; Jin, J. Simultaneous determination of trimethylamine N-oxide, choline, betaine by UPLC-MS/MS in human plasma: An application in acute stroke patients. *J. Pharm. Biomed. Anal.* **2018**, *152*, 179–187. [CrossRef]
32. Savastano, S.; Barbato, A.; Di Somma, C.; Guida, B.; Pizza, G.; Barrea, L.; Avallone, S.; Schiano di Cola, M.; Strazzullo, P.; Colao, A. Beyond waist circumference in an adult male population of Southern Italy: Is there any role for subscapular skinfold thickness in the relationship between insulin-like growth factor-I system and metabolic parameters? *J. Endocrinol. Investig.* **2012**, *35*, 925–929. [CrossRef]
33. Savastano, S.; Di Somma, C.; Colao, A.; Barrea, L.; Orio, F.; Finelli, C.; Pasanisi, F.; Contaldo, F.; Tarantino, G. Preliminary data on the relationship between circulating levels of Sirtuin 4, anthropometric and metabolic parameters in obese subjects according to growth hormone/insulin-like growth factor-1 status. *Growth Horm. IGF Res.* **2015**, *25*, 28–33. [CrossRef]
34. Barrea, L.; Tarantino, G.; Di Somma, C.; Muscogiuri, G.; Macchia, P.E.; Falco, A.; Colao, A.; Savastano, S. Adherence to the Mediterranean Diet and Circulating Levels of Sirtuin 4 in Obese Patients: A Novel Association. *Oxid. Med. Cell Longev.* **2017**, *2017*, 6101254. [CrossRef] [PubMed]
35. Barrea, L.; Di Somma, C.; Macchia, P.E.; Falco, A.; Savanelli, M.C.; Orio, F.; Colao, A.; Savastano, S. Influence of nutrition on somatotropic axis: Milk consumption in adult individuals with moderate-severe obesity. *Clin. Nutr.* **2017**, *36*, 293–301. [CrossRef] [PubMed]

36. Barrea, L.; Macchia, P.E.; Tarantino, G.; Di Somma, C.; Pane, E.; Balato, N.; Napolitano, M.; Colao, A.; Savastano, S. Nutrition: A key environmental dietary factor in clinical severity and cardio-metabolic risk in psoriatic male patients evaluated by 7-day food-frequency questionnaire. *J. Transl. Med.* **2015**, *13*, 303. [CrossRef] [PubMed]
37. Matthews, D.R.; Hosker, J.P.; Rudenski, A.S.; Naylor, B.A.; Treacher, D.F.; Turner, R.C. Homeostasis model assessment: Insulin resistance and beta-cell function from fasting plasma glucose and insulin concentrations in man. *Diabetologia* **1985**, *28*, 412–419. [CrossRef]
38. Amato, M.C.; Giordano, C.; Pitrone, M.; Galluzzo, A. Cut-off points of the visceral adiposity index (VAI) identifying a visceral adipose dysfunction associated with cardiometabolic risk in a Caucasian Sicilian population. *Lipids Health Dis.* **2011**, *10*, 183. [CrossRef] [PubMed]
39. Expert Panel on Detection, Evaluation, and Treatment of High Blood Cholesterol in Adults. Executive Summary of The Third Report of The National Cholesterol Education Program (NCEP) Expert Panel on Detection, Evaluation, And Treatment of High Blood Cholesterol in Adults (Adult Treatment Panel III). *JAMA* **2001**, *285*, 2486–2497. [CrossRef]
40. Barrea, L.; Muscogiuri, G.; Di Somma, C.; Annunziata, G.; Megna, M.; Falco, A.; Balato, A.; Colao, A.; Savastano, S. Coffee consumption, metabolic syndrome and clinical severity of psoriasis: Good or bad stuff? *Arch. Toxicol.* **2018**, *92*, 1831–1845. [CrossRef]
41. Turconi, G.; Guarcello, M.; Berzolari, F.G.; Carolei, A.; Bazzano, R.; Roggi, C. An evaluation of a colour food photography atlas as a tool for quantifying food portion size in epidemiological dietary surveys. *Eur. J. Clin. Nutr.* **2005**, *59*, 923–931. [CrossRef]
42. Lentjes, M.A.; McTaggart, A.; Mulligan, A.A.; Powell, N.A.; Parry-Smith, D.; Luben, R.N.; Bhaniani, A.; Welch, A.A.; Khaw, K.T. Dietary intake measurement using 7 d diet diaries in British men and women in the European Prospective Investigation into Cancer-Norfolk study: A focus on methodological issues. *Br. J. Nutr.* **2014**, *111*, 516–526. [CrossRef]
43. Yang, K.C.; Hung, H.F.; Lu, C.W.; Chang, H.H.; Lee, L.T.; Huang, K.C. Association of Non-alcoholic Fatty Liver Disease with Metabolic Syndrome Independently of Central Obesity and Insulin Resistance. *Sci. Rep.* **2016**, *6*, 27034. [CrossRef] [PubMed]
44. Dumas, M.E.; Barton, R.H.; Toye, A.; Cloarec, O.; Blancher, C.; Rothwell, A.; Fearnside, J.; Tatoud, R.; Blanc, V.; Lindon, J.C.; et al. Metabolic profiling reveals a contribution of gut microbiota to fatty liver phenotype in insulin-resistant mice. *Proc. Natl. Acad. Sci. USA* **2006**, *103*, 12511–12516. [CrossRef] [PubMed]
45. Miao, J.; Ling, A.V.; Manthena, P.V.; Gearing, M.E.; Graham, M.J.; Crooke, R.M.; Croce, K.J.; Esquejo, R.M.; Clish, C.B.; Torrecilla, E.; et al. Flavin-containing monooxygenase 3 as a potential player in diabetes-associated atherosclerosis. *Nat. Commun.* **2015**, *6*, 6498. [CrossRef]
46. Gao, X.; Liu, X.; Xu, J.; Xue, C.; Xue, Y.; Wang, Y. Dietary trimethylamine N-oxide exacerbates impaired glucose tolerance in mice fed a high fat diet. *J. Biosci. Bioeng.* **2014**, *118*, 476–481. [CrossRef] [PubMed]
47. Noga, A.A.; Vance, D.E. A gender-specific role for phosphatidylethanolamine N-methyltransferase-derived phosphatidylcholine in the regulation of plasma high density and very low density lipoproteins in mice. *J. Biol. Chem.* **2003**, *278*, 21851–21859. [CrossRef] [PubMed]
48. Kühn, T.; Rohrmann, S.; Sookthai, D.; Johnson, T.; Katzke, V.; Kaaks, R.; von Eckardstein, A.; Müller, D. Intra-individual variation of plasma trimethylamine-N-oxide (TMAO), betaine and choline over 1 year. *Clin. Chem. Lab. Med.* **2017**, *55*, 261–268. [CrossRef] [PubMed]
49. Krüger, R.; Merz, B.; Rist, M.J.; Ferrario, P.G.; Bub, A.; Kulling, S.E.; Watzl, B. Associations of current diet with plasma and urine TMAO in the KarMeN study: Direct and indirect contributions. *Mol. Nutr. Food Res.* **2017**, *61*. [CrossRef]
50. Rohrmann, S.; Linseisen, J.; Allenspach, M.; von Eckardstein, A.; Müller, D. Plasma Concentrations of Trimethylamine-N-oxide Are Directly Associated with Dairy Food Consumption and Low-Grade Inflammation in a German Adult Population. *J. Nutr.* **2016**, *146*, 283–289. [CrossRef]
51. Zhernakova, A.; Kurilshikov, A.; Bonder, M.J.; Tigchelaar, E.F.; Schirmer, M.; Vatanen, T.; Mujagic, Z.; Vila, A.V.; Falony, G.; Vieira-Silva, S.; et al. Population-based metagenomics analysis reveals markers for gut microbiome composition and diversity. *Science* **2016**, *352*, 565–569. [CrossRef]
52. Cho, C.E.; Caudill, M.A. Trimethylamine-N-Oxide: Friend, Foe, or Simply Caught in the Cross-Fire? *Trends Endocrinol. Metab.* **2017**, *28*, 121–130. [CrossRef] [PubMed]

53. Senthong, V.; Li, X.S.; Hudec, T.; Coughlin, J.; Wu, Y.; Levison, B.; Wang, Z.; Hazen, S.L.; Tang, W.H. Plasma Trimethylamine N-Oxide, a Gut Microbe-Generated Phosphatidylcholine Metabolite, Is Associated With Atherosclerotic Burden. *J. Am. Coll. Cardiol.* **2016**, *67*, 2620–2628. [CrossRef]
54. Tang, W.H.; Wang, Z.; Fan, Y.; Levison, B.; Hazen, J.E.; Donahue, L.M.; Wu, Y.; Hazen, S.L. Prognostic value of elevated levels of intestinal microbe-generated metabolite trimethylamine-N-oxide in patients with heart failure: Refining the gut hypothesis. *J. Am. Coll. Cardiol.* **2014**, *64*, 1908–1914. [CrossRef] [PubMed]
55. Wang, Z.; Tang, W.H.; Buffa, J.A.; Fu, X.; Britt, E.B.; Koeth, R.A.; Levison, B.S.; Fan, Y.; Wu, Y.; Hazen, S.L. Prognostic value of choline and betaine depends on intestinal microbiota-generated metabolite trimethylamine-N-oxide. *Eur. Heart J.* **2014**, *35*, 904–910. [CrossRef] [PubMed]
56. Silaghi, C.A.; Silaghi, H.; Colosi, H.A.; Craciun, A.E.; Farcas, A.; Cosma, D.T.; Hancu, N.; Pais, R.; Georgescu, C.E. Prevalence and predictors of non-alcoholic fatty liver disease as defined by the fatty liver index in a type 2 diabetes population. *Clujul. Med.* **2016**, *89*, 82–88. [CrossRef] [PubMed]
57. Fedchuk, L.; Nascimbeni, F.; Pais, R.; Charlotte, F.; Housset, C.; Ratziu, V.; LIDO Study Group. Performance and limitations of steatosis biomarkers in patients with nonalcoholic fatty liver disease. *Aliment Pharmacol. Ther.* **2014**, *40*, 1209–1222. [CrossRef] [PubMed]

14

Population Approaches Targeting Metabolic Syndrome Focusing on Japanese Trials

Hitoshi Nishizawa * and Iichiro Shimomura

Department of Metabolic Medicine, Graduate School of Medicine, Osaka University, 2-2-B5, Yamada-oka, Suita, Osaka 565-0871, Japan; ichi@endmet.med.osaka-u.ac.jp

* Correspondence: hitoshin1127@endmet.med.osaka-u.ac.jp

Abstract: The clinical importance of assessment of metabolic syndrome lies in the selection of individuals with multiple risk factors based on visceral fat accumulation, and helping them to reduce visceral fat. Behavioral modification by population approach is important, which adds support to the personal approach. The complexity of visceral fat accumulation requires multicomponent and multilevel intervention. Preparation of food and physical environments could be useful strategies for city planners. Furthermore, actions on various frameworks, including organizational, community, and policy levels, have been recently reported. There are universal public health screening programs and post-screening health educational systems in Japan, and diseases management programs in Germany. Understanding one's own health status is important for motivation for lifestyle modification. The U.S. Preventive Services Task Force recommends that primary care practitioners screen all adults for obesity and offer behavioral interventions and intensive counseling. Established evidence-based guidelines for behavioral counseling are needed within the primary care setting.

Keywords: atherosclerotic cardiovascular disease; visceral fat accumulation; universal public health screening program; health check-up; health guidance; city planning

---

1. Introduction

Visceral fat accumulation is associated with glucose intolerance, dyslipidemia, hypertension, and atherosclerotic cardiovascular diseases (ACVD), conceptualized as metabolic syndrome (Figure 1). Several definitions of metabolic syndrome have been used worldwide. Abdominal obesity is one of the risk factors in the harmonized criteria by AHA (American Heart Association), IDF (International Diabetes Federation), NHLBI (National Heart, Lung, and Blood Institute), and other organizations (2009) [1], while in the original criteria of IDF (2005) [2] and the Japanese criteria [3,4], abdominal obesity or visceral fat accumulation is an essential component of metabolic syndrome. The latter criteria consider visceral fat accumulation as the basal pathogenic component of metabolic syndrome. An important aspect of the diagnosis of visceral fat-based metabolic syndrome is to select subjects with multiple risk factors based on visceral fat accumulation, and enroll them in health educational programs conducted at health check-up and medical facilities. The cornerstone of effective improvement of multiple risk factors for ACVD is the reduction of visceral fat (Figure 2).

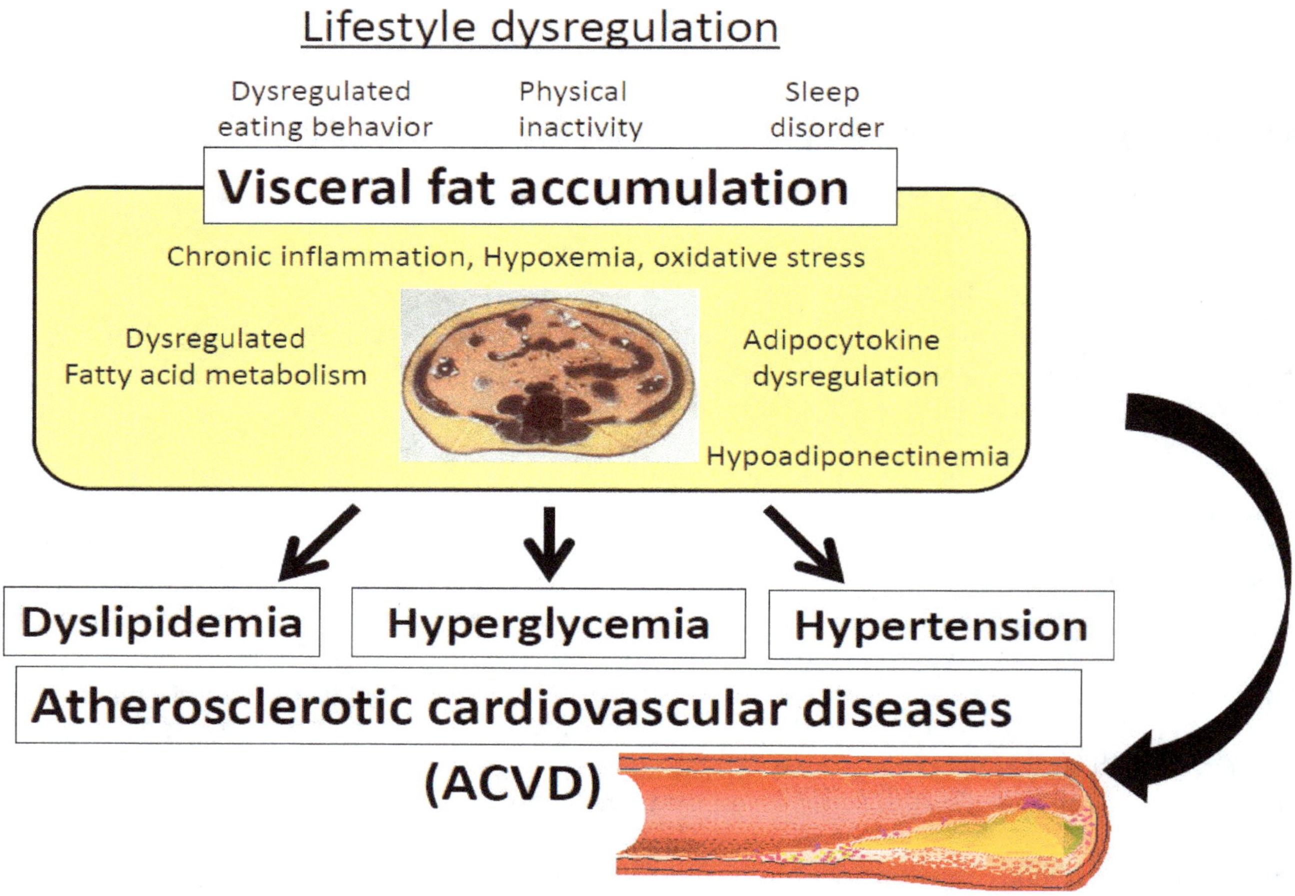

Figure 1. Concept of metabolic syndrome.

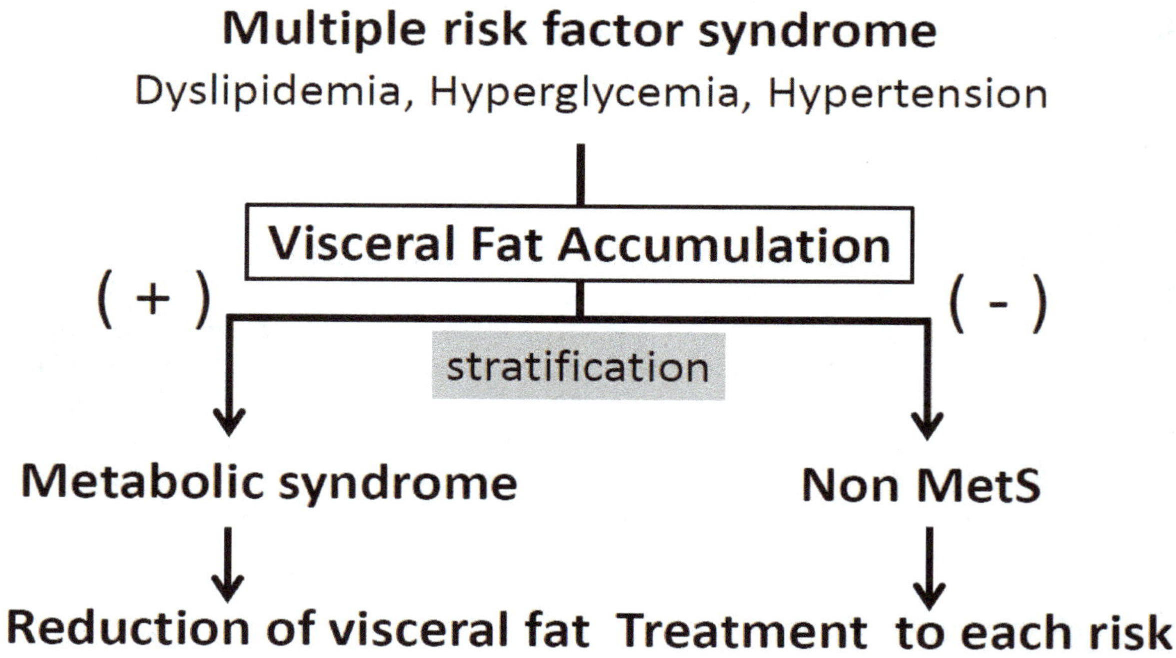

Figure 2. Management of multiple risk factor syndrome for prevention of atherosclerotic cardiovascular diseases (ACVD); "Metabolic syndrome (Mets)-oriented approach".

The cause of worldwide obesity and visceral fat accumulation is multifactorial at multiple levels, including food environment, physical activity levels, and policies. One of the important approaches to reduce visceral fat involves behavioral modification of individuals (personal approach), such as modifications to dietary and physical habits. Another is the population approach, which provides support to the personal approach, and could be even more important.

2. Obesity and Obesity Disease

Obesity is a state of excess body fat accumulation in individuals, and body mass index (BMI) is used as an index of obesity. Obesity is defined as BMI $\geq$ 30 kg/m^2 in Europe and the United States, and $\geq$ 25 kg/m^2 in Japan, where there are fewer obese individuals [5–7]. Obesity, per se, is not always clinically necessary to be subjected to aggressive medical intervention. On the other hand, "obesity disease" is defined in Japan as visceral fat obesity (BMI $\geq$ 25 kg/m^2 plus visceral fat area $\geq$ 100 cm^2), or obesity (BMI $\geq$ 25 kg/m^2) with obesity-related complications, such as metabolic or orthopedic disorders that require weight reduction for their improvement [7]. Therefore, "Obesity disease" should be dealt with as a clinical condition requiring medical intervention.

3. Visceral Fat and Subcutaneous Fat

It is well known that obesity is accompanied by glucose intolerance, dyslipidemia, and hypertension. Following the spread of the Western diet and motor vehicles, the prevalence of obesity and type 2 diabetes has increased worldwide [5,6]. East Asians, including Japanese, are more easily affected by metabolic disorders even with a mild degree of obesity, compared with Europeans and Americans. On the other hand, such disorders are not always accompanied by massive obesity. These disorders cannot be explained by the absolute value of BMI, and therefore understanding of body fat distribution is considerably important [8]. Analysis of body fat distribution using abdominal computed tomography (CT) has demonstrated that visceral fat obesity poses a higher risk for metabolic disorders and ACVD than subcutaneous obesity [9]. A recent Japanese study involving subjects who underwent health checks concluded that visceral fat area (VFA), but not subcutaneous fat area (SFA), correlated positively with the number of cardiovascular risk factors [10]. The same study also demonstrated that the mean number of risk factors exceeded one at 100 cm^2 of VFA, both in males and females. Therefore, the cutoff value of visceral fat accumulation was set to 100 cm^2 in Japan [10].

4. BMI and Visceral Fat Area

The BMI and VFA vary considerably among individuals, especially in males. In a study of Japanese male employees (mean age 48.0 ± 10.5 years, ±SD), 26.8% (n = 401/1497) of normal weight subjects (BMI < 25 kg/m^2) had visceral fat accumulation (VFA $\geq$10 0cm^2) (Figure 3) [11]. Irrespective of BMI, the mean number of metabolic risk factors in the subjects with visceral fat accumulation was significantly higher than those without (solid bars in Figure 3). Also, a study from the United Kingdom reported a relatively high mortality rate for individuals with central obesity, despite having normal weight (BMI <25 kg/m^2) [12]. Interestingly, reduction of body weight and VFA is closely associated with improvement of metabolic risk factors, such as diabetes, dyslipidemia, and hypertension [11,13]. These data suggest that assessment of visceral fat accumulation is important for selection of individuals who should avoid over-nutrition.

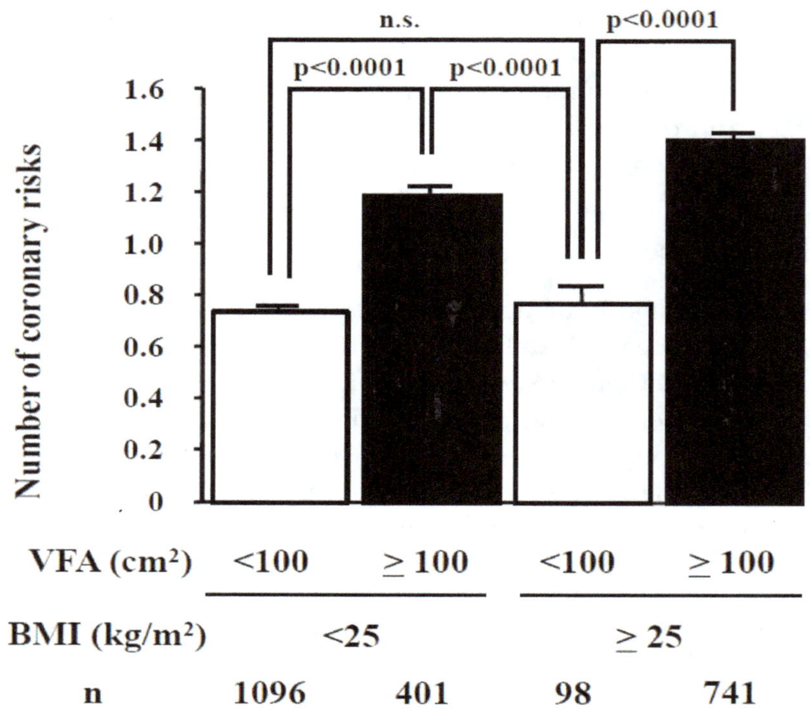

Figure 3. Relationship between number of metabolic risk factors and body fat distribution. Subjects were divided according to their BMI (cutoff value 25 kg/m^2) and VFA (cutoff value 100 cm^2). Data are mean ± SEM. BMI = body mass index; VFA = visceral fat area;. Data from Diabetes Care 2007; 30: 2392-94 [11], by permission of American Diabetes Association.

5. Clinical Significance of Metabolic Syndrome in Atherosclerotic Cardiovascular Diseases

It is important to take measures against individual risk factors, such as hypertension, smoking, and hypercholesterolemia, to prevent atherosclerotic cardiovascular diseases (ACVD). Since the 1990s, multiple risk factor syndrome and metabolic syndrome have been the focus of attention as residual risks, in which dysregulation of glucose and lipid metabolism, hypertension, and obesity coexisted in each individual [1,14,15]. Among them, the concept of metabolic syndrome was selected in the original criteria of IDF (2005) along with in Japan, stating that visceral fat accumulation is the basis of the pathogenesis of atherosclerosis complicated with dysregulation of glucose and lipid metabolism and elevated blood pressure (Figure 1). There are two types of arteriosclerosis—atherosclerosis that affects relatively large vessels, such as coronary arteries and middle cerebral arteries, and arteriosclerosis that affects relatively small vessels, such as cerebral perforating arteries. Atherosclerosis is the pathological process underlying myocardial infarction and cerebral thrombosis, whereas arteriosclerosis is that of cerebral hemorrhage and lacunar infarction. In Europe and the United States, atherosclerosis based on dyslipidemia and metabolic syndrome is more frequent due to over-intake of dietary fat. On the other hand, in East Asia, arteriosclerosis based on hypertension has been the predominant type due to over-intake of dietary salt [16]. Recently, even in East Asia and Japan, visceral fat based-metabolic syndrome has been increasing. However, hypertension and hypercholesterolemia should be important therapeutic targets in any clinical management program designed to prevent ACVD independent of the metabolic syndrome.

6. Pathogenesis of Visceral Fat Accumulation

Visceral fat is the adipose tissue that adheres and accumulates in the mesenterium and omentum, and acts as transient energy reservoir from gut to liver through the portal vein. In fasting and starvation, lipolysis efficiently occurs in visceral fat resulting in supply of free fatty acids and glycerol to hepatocytes. However, through excessive lipolysis in the accumulated visceral fat, large amounts of free fatty acids and glycerol overflow into the liver, resulting in the dysregulation of lipid metabolism and gluconeogenesis [17]. Although the weight of adipose tissue accounts for about 15–20% of total body weight, that of obese subjects reaches up to 30–50%. Therefore, the massive adipose tissue considerably affects the pathogenic condition of individuals.

Adipocyte precursor cells in visceral adipose tissue are relatively difficult to differentiate or proliferate compared to those in the subcutaneous adipose tissue [18]. Thus, visceral adipose cells, in parallel to over-nutrition, are considered hypertrophic adipocytes. Since the number of adipocytes can increase only during childhood and adolescence [19], over-nutrition in adulthood induces hypertrophy of visceral adipose cells, which are affected by hypoxia and inflammation, complicating the production of oxidative stress and dysregulation of adipocytokines and adipokines, such as hypoadiponectinemia. This is the pathogenic basis of visceral fat accumulation associated with metabolic syndrome (Figure 1) [20,21].

Fat distribution varies considerably between males and females and also among different ethnic groups. In Asian individuals, VFA is relatively larger than SFA [22,23]. This is probably related to genetic (ethnic) differences in the proliferative potential of subcutaneous adipose precursor cells, as well as differences in the duration of over-nutrition. Therefore, the susceptibility of Asian individuals to the metabolic syndrome could be higher, with visceral fat accumulation even in lower BMI relative to Europeans and Americans.

7. Population Approaches Targeting the Metabolic Syndrome

There is a need to reduce accumulated visceral fat in subjects with metabolic syndrome, rather than treat each metabolic risk factor with medications. To achieve this aim, it is important to provide health education about healthy diet and physical exercise to these individuals (personal approach). Next, improvement of various metabolic risk factors can be achieved through reduction of accumulated visceral fat [11,13]. Therefore, for assessment of the metabolic syndrome, it is clinically important to identify individuals with large amounts of visceral fat during medical or health check-ups, who are affected, or are supposed to be, by multiple metabolic disorders, even if each disorder is mild. Moreover, it is important to enroll the subjects with metabolic syndrome into the health education system. We will focus here on population approaches to combat metabolic syndrome (Figure 4), as individual programs on lifestyles, such as diet and physical exercise, are discussed in other chapters of this review and have also been described previously [24].

1. Strategies addressing lifestyle behavior and policies targeting the environment (diet, physical activity, sleep, and mental health)

a. Health education at school and for parents
b. Calorie labels on menus, taxation for "harmful" food
c. City planning (e.g. walking and cycling lane, sports facilities and training gym, green area, and TV program)

2. Screening and intervention program against the metabolic syndrome

a. Community or organization-based prevention
Multicomponent and multilevel intervention (e.g. city planning)

b. Healthcare program by public system
Health checkup and intervention program using public health insurance system (e.g. Japan)
Disease management program conducted on national level (e.g. German)

c. Behavioral approach including motivational interviewing

Figure 4. Population Approaches targeting the metabolic syndrome.

8. Strategies Addressing Lifestyle Behavior and Policies Targeting the Environment (Diet, Physical Activity, Sleep, and Mental Health)

For lifestyle modification, it is first important to have a clinical understanding of one's own health status. For this aim, health check-ups followed by health guidance is a good approach. Recent studies have provided evidence for the role of pictorial presentation of silent atherosclerosis in the prevention of cardiovascular diseases and its usefulness in reducing the low adherence to medications and lifestyle modification [25]. Therefore, scientific understanding of one's own health is the most important factor for motivation towards lifestyle modification. Once subjects are motivated to improve their lifestyle to reduce accumulated visceral fat, health promotion strategies, which address lifestyle behavior and policies targeting the environment, are potentially effective in the prevention of visceral fat accumulation.

Since dieting and disordered eating behaviors during childhood and adolescence are considered to continue to be present among young adults [26], some strategies were found to be useful, such as health education on nutrition for students and their parents in school and provision of healthy food at school (Figure 4) [27,28]. At the population level, public policies and economic strategies are important to improve food and physical environments. For example, calorie and nutritional information on food menus and packaging are useful for individuals who care about dietary modification and also to avoid harmful food components, such as saturated fatty acids and excess salt. In some countries, higher taxes have been enforced on harmful foods, such as fast foods, unhealthy fats, and sugar-sweetened drinks (Figure 4) [29].

High physical activity is reported to be associated with low risk of mortality and cardiovascular disease [30], and diet-plus-exercise was more effective in weight loss than diet-only interventions [31]. Strategies that encourage individuals to exercise are important. Walking and cycling can serve for both transportation and recreational purposes, and both can reduce motor vehicle dependency. Therefore, it should be important to support lifestyle choices through city planning, such as preparation for walking, running, and cycling lanes (Figure 4) [32]. In general, aerobic exercise several days per week (total: 150 min/week) has been recommended in physical activity guidelines [33]. However, it was recently reported that there was no significant difference in the likelihood of metabolic syndrome in the general population between frequently active participants (≥5 days per week) and infrequently active participants (1–4 days per week) after adjustment for total weekly moderate-to-vigorous physical activity [34], suggesting that only weekend exercise could be effective in preventing metabolic syndrome if sufficient weekly physical activity was performed. Preparation of sports gymnasiums, playing fields, and parks that are easily accessed by citizens are useful strategies that should be instituted in city planning.

Sleep is considerably associated with eating behaviors and physical activity. Insufficient sleep has been reported to be associated with dysregulation of leptin and ghrelin [35], resulting in hyperphagia and physical inactivity due to sleepiness. Moreover, a late bedtime with shorter sleep time were reported to be closely associated with weight gain and visceral fat accumulation [36,37]. To facilitate more sleeping hours, many communities have attempted to change TV programming [32]. Since control of psychological status is important to continue lifestyle modification, green areas in communities are useful for stress management (Figure 4) [28,32].

9. Screening and Intervention Program Against the Metabolic Syndrome

9.1. Community or Organization-Based Prevention

The complexity of visceral fat accumulation requires multicomponent and multilevel intervention [28]. Multicomponent intervention is effective in weight loss programs, which consist of changes that combine food choices, physical environments, sleep, and stress management, as described above (Figure 4). Furthermore, multilevel approaches focus on changing health behaviors by acting on multiple frameworks, including individual, interpersonal, organizational, community, and policy levels. Many intervention programs at the community level have been used to combat metabolic syndrome [28,38,39]. For instance, the healthy living program delivered by community coaching staff for overweight and obese me, who were football fans of the Scottish Premier League football clubs proved effective for weight loss of 4.94 kg (95% CI 3.95–5.94) after 12 months [39].

Step1 : Abdominal obesity and/or overweight
Waist circumference Male ≥ 85cm. Female ≥ 90 cm → Group (1)
Waist circumference Male < 85cm. Female < 90 cm, but Body Mass Index ≥ 25 → Group (2)

Step2 : Additional risk factors
1) Fasting Plasma glucose FPG ≥ 100 mg/dl and/or HbA1c ≥ 5.6%
2) TG and HDL-cholesterol TG ≥ 150 mg/dl and/or HDL-cholesterol < 40mg/dl
3) Blood pressure SBP ≥ 130 mmHg and/or DPB ≥85 mmHg
4) Smoking (counted only for those who have 1 risk or more from 1-3)

Step3 : Classification for Health guidance Program
Group (1) Additional risks at Step2
≥ 2 Intensive Health Guidance program
2 Motivational Health Guidance program
Group (2) Additional risks at Step2
≥ 3 Intensive Health Guidance program
1 or 2 Motivational Health Guidance program

Step4 :
People taking medication for diabetes, hypertension, or high cholesterol are excluded
People aged 65-74 who are eligible for health guidance are allocated to
Motivational Health Guidance program regardless of risk profile

Figure 5. Participant classification for the Health Guidance program by the Ministry of Health, Labor, and Welfare in Japan [40].

9.2. *Healthcare Program by the Public System*

Atherosclerotic cardiovascular diseases (ACVD) are life-threatening. Development of ACVD is often followed by serious complications. Therefore, it is important to detect asymptomatic cardiovascular risk factors and provide counter measures. For this purpose, a health check-up is a good opportunity to assess one's own health status and assess the risk for cardiovascular diseases. In many countries, individuals are left on their own to decide whether to receive health check-ups or not. However, in the case of Japan, there is a universal public health screening program and a post-screening health educational system in place at the nation level to deal with metabolic syndrome, as described below [4,40]. There is also a disease management program (DMP) nationally in Germany. The Japanese intervention program aims at primary disease prevention, while the German DMP aims at secondary disease prevention (Figure 4) [41].

The Japanese criteria for metabolic syndrome were established in 2005 [3,4], in which visceral fat accumulation was an essential component. In 2008, the Japanese government started a new screening and educational system for metabolic syndrome, focusing on visceral fat accumulation [40]. This new public health care system has the following features: (1) medical insurers are obliged to perform free health check-ups followed by health guidance to their subscribers aged 40 to 74 years; (2) methods of health check-ups and health guidance are standardized and health data are collected and assessed electronically; (3) subjects who need health guidance are stratified based on visceral fat accumulation and smoking habits (Figure 5). Participants who are thought to be "downstream" of metabolic syndrome are subjected to an intensive health guidance program with intermittent support over three months after the first interview followed by assessment six months later [40,42]. Recently, descriptive analysis in Japan has shown greater improvement in metabolic syndrome profiles in those individuals that participated in specific health guidance programs for three years than nonparticipants, although selection bias may be present [42]. Since it is difficult to set control conditions, there are only a few population-level or policy-level studies on health behaviors [42,43]. Further randomized control trials of health guidance programs are theoretically needed, which are now being undertaken in Japan [44].

9.3. Behavioral Approach Including Motivational Interviewing

In 2003, the U.S. Preventive Services Task Force recommended that primary care practitioners screen all adults for obesity and offer behavioral interventions and intensive counseling (Figure 4) [38]. Although a meta-analysis demonstrated that behavioral intervention resulted in a mean weight loss of 3.01 kg (95% CI: 4.02–2.01) [38], there are no established evidence-based guidelines for behavioral weight loss counseling in a primary care setting [28,38,45].

To encourage improvement of unhealthy lifestyles in health check-ups followed by health guidance, the following are important points: (1) individuals free of symptoms can assess their health status with regard to visceral fat accumulation to metabolic syndrome through what is called the "Where am I? chart" [46], for example using health data and pictorial presentation of carotid artery echograms; (2) individuals can go back to review their past and their own lifestyle using past health data, and understand the significance of reduction of accumulated visceral fat; (3) individuals can find out how to improve their lifestyle; and finally (4) individuals can appreciate improvement of health data, such as changes in blood glucose, lipid, and blood pressure, as well as weight loss and reduction of visceral fat in health check-ups to be conducted in subsequent years [42,46]. Behavioral modification in lifestyle by face-to-face individual counseling is important in reduction of visceral fat [40,42,46]. One recent innovation in improvement of face-to-face counseling is the implementation of online tools, including e-mail counseling and internet treatment programs (telemedicine) [47].

Health education (Figure 4) and preparation of food and physical environments (Figure 4) should be useful in facilitating behavioral modifications and practicing lifestyle improvements.

Since healthy living programs were reported to be effective for weight loss [39], recreational exercise might be useful as exercise therapy to combat metabolic syndrome. Recreational exercise and sports could be more feasible than the exercise therapy-based FITT (frequency, Intensity, time, type) principle, because recreation and sports are fun and encouraging for individuals. Therefore, recreational exercise and sports are suitable community-based strategies for physical activity and city planning [32].

It has been reported that on average, visceral fat accumulation is increasing in 20 to 30 year-old Japanese males, and exceeded 100 cm^2 in 40-year old individuals [10]. Therefore, for prevention of metabolic syndrome, it is important to approach younger individuals. One of the targets of management of metabolic syndrome should be prevention of ACVD in the community. In the community, health education on lifestyle modification is important, and health guidance for acceleration of referral to physicians is also important for high-risk individuals [44]. In the medical field, medical intervention by focusing on visceral fat accumulation should be more efficient, since the etiology of metabolic diseases is diverse (Figure 2). Diabetic patients with visceral fat accumulation have dysregulated eating or sleeping behavior and progression of atherosclerosis [37,48]. Therefore, it is important to improve multiple metabolic diseases comprehensively by persistent lifestyle modification targeting reduction of visceral fat (Figure 1) [11,13,42]. On the other hand, an individual approach to each metabolic disease is needed for individuals with multiple risks without visceral fat accumulation (Figure 1; Figure 2) [49]. Programs against smoking, hypertension, and hypercholesterolemia are also quite important for individuals with or without visceral fat accumulation.

10. Conclusions

Taken together, the clinical significance of assessment of the metabolic syndrome is to link individuals with visceral fat–related multiple risk factors to follow health guidance, and to prevent atherosclerotic cardiovascular diseases by reducing visceral fat. To achieve this aim, in addition to personal approaches, population approaches are important to combat metabolic syndrome. Established evidence-based guidelines and programs are needed within primary care setting.

Author Contributions: H.N. wrote the manuscript. I.S. reviewed the manuscript. The authors approved the final manuscript.

Acknowledgments: We thank Norikazu Maeda, Ken Kishida, Midori Noguchi, Tohru Funahashi (Osaka University), and Yuji Matsuzawa (Sumitomo Hospital) for the helpful discussion and direction.

Abbreviations

ACVD	atherosclerotic cardiovascular disease
BMI	body mass index
Mets	metabolic syndrome
SFA	subcutaneous fat area
VFA	visceral fat area

References

1. Alberti, K.G.; Eckel, R.H.; Grundy, S.M.; Zimmet, P.Z.; Cleeman, J.I.; Donato, K.A.; Fruchart, J.C.; James, W.P.; Loria, C.M.; Smith, S.C., Jr. Harmonizing the metabolic syndrome: A joint interim statement of the International Diabetes Federation Task Force on Epidemiology and Prevention; National Heart, Lung, and Blood Institute; American Heart Association; World Heart Federation; International Atherosclerosis Society; and International Association for the Study of Obesity. *Circulation* **2009**, *120*, 1640–1645. [PubMed]
2. Alberti, K.G.; Zimmet, P.; Shaw, J.; IDF Epidemiology Task Force Consensus Group. The metabolic syndrome—a new worldwide definition. *Lancet* **2005**, *366*, 1059–1062. [CrossRef]
3. Matsuzawa, Y. Metabolic syndrome–definition and diagnostic criteria in Japan. *J. Atheroscler. Thromb.* **2005**, *12*, 301. [CrossRef] [PubMed]
4. Yamagishi, K.; Iso, H. The criteria for metabolic syndrome and the national health screening and education system in Japan. *Epidemiol. Health* **2017**, *39*, e2017003. [CrossRef] [PubMed]
5. Malik, V.S.; Willett, W.C.; Hu, F.B. Global obesity: Trends, risk factors and policy implications. *Nat. Rev. Endocrinol.* **2013**, *9*, 13–27. [CrossRef] [PubMed]
6. González-Muniesa, P.; Mártinez-González, M.A.; Hu, F.B.; Després, J.P.; Matsuzawa, Y.; Loos, R.J.F.; Moreno, L.A.; Bray, G.A.; Martinez, J.A. Obesity. *Nat. Rev. Dis. Primers* **2017**, *3*, 17034. [CrossRef] [PubMed]
7. Examination Committee of Criteria for 'Obesity Disease' in Japan; Japan Society for the Study of Obesity. New criteria for 'obesity disease' in Japan. *Circ. J.* **2002**, *66*, 987–992. [CrossRef]
8. Neeland, I.J.; Poirier, P.; Després, J.P. Cardiovascular and metabolic heterogeneity of obesity: Clinical challenges and implications for management. *Circulation* **2018**, *137*, 1391–1406. [CrossRef]
9. Fujioka, S.; Matsuzawa, Y.; Tokunaga, K.; Tarui, S. Contribution of intra-abdominal fat accumulation to the impairment of glucose and lipid metabolism in human obesity. *Metabolism* **1987**, *36*, 54–59. [CrossRef]
10. Hiuge-Shimizu, A.; Kishida, K.; Funahashi, T.; Ishizaka, Y.; Oka, R.; Okada, M.; Suzuki, S.; Takaya, N.; Nakagawa, T.; Fukui, T.; et al. Absolute value of visceral fat area measured on computed tomography scans and obesity-related cardiovascular risk factors in large-scale Japanese general population (The VACATION-J study). *Ann. Med.* **2012**, *44*, 82–92. [CrossRef]
11. Okauchi, Y.; Nishizawa, H.; Funahashi, T.; Ogawa, T.; Noguchi, M.; Ryo, M.; Kihara, S.; Iwahashi, H.; Yamagata, K.; Nakamura, T.; et al. Reduction of visceral fat is associated with decrease in the number of metabolic risk factors in Japanese men. *Diabetes Care* **2007**, *30*, 2392–2394. [CrossRef] [PubMed]
12. Hamer, M.; O'Donovan, G.; Stensel, D.; Stamatakis, E. Normal-weight central obesity and risk for mortality. *Ann. Intern. Med.* **2017**, *166*, 917–918. [CrossRef] [PubMed]
13. Pi-Sunyer, X.; Blackburn, G.; Brancati, F.L.; Bray, G.A.; Bright, R.; Clark, J.M.; Curtis, J.M.; Espeland, M.A.; Foreyt, J.P.; Graves, K.; et al. Look AHEAD Research Group. Reduction in weight and cardiovascular disease risk factors in individuals with type 2 diabetes. *Diabetes Care* **2007**, *30*, 1374–1383. [PubMed]

14. Alberti, K.G.; Zimmet, P.Z. Definition, diagnosis and classification of diabetes mellitus and its complications. Part 1: Diagnosis and classification of diabetes mellitus provisional report of a WHO consultation. *Diabet. Med.* **1998**, *15*, 539–553. [CrossRef]
15. National Cholesterol Education Program (NCEP) Expert Panel on Detection, Evaluation, and Treatment of High Blood Cholesterol in Adults (Adult Treatment Panel III). Third Report of the National Cholesterol Education Program (NCEP)Expert Panel on Detection, Evaluation, and Treatment of High Blood Cholesterol in Adults (Adult Treatment Panel III) final report. *Circulation* **2002**, *106*, 3143–3421.
16. Iso, H. A Japanese health success story: Trends in cardiovascular diseases, their risk factors, and the contribution of public health and personalized approaches. *EPMA J.* **2011**, *2*, 49–57. [CrossRef] [PubMed]
17. Kuriyama, H.; Shimomura, I.; Kishida, K.; Kondo, H.; Furuyama, N.; Nishizawa, H.; Maeda, N.; Matsuda, M.; Nagaretani, H.; Kihara, S.; et al. Coordinated regulation of fat-specific and liver-specific glycerol channels, aquaporin adipose and aquaporin 9. *Diabetes* **2002**, *51*, 2915–2921. [CrossRef]
18. Tchkonia, T.; Thomou, T.; Zhu, Y.; Karagiannides, I.; Pothoulakis, C.; Jensen, M.D.; Kirkland, J.L. Mechanisms and metabolic implications of regional differences among fat depots. *Cell Metab.* **2013**, *17*, 644–656. [CrossRef]
19. Spalding, K.L.; Arner, E.; Westermark, P.O.; Bernard, S.; Buchholz, B.A.; Bergmann, O.; Blomqvist, L.; Hoffstedt, J.; Näslund, E.; Britton, T.; et al. Dynamics of fat cell turnover in humans. *Nature* **2008**, *453*, 783–787. [CrossRef]
20. Kusminski, C.M.; Bickel, P.E.; Scherer, P.E. Targeting adipose tissue in the treatment of obesity-associated diabetes. *Nat. Rev. Drug Discov.* **2016**, *15*, 639–660. [CrossRef]
21. Maeda, K.; Okubo, K.; Shimomura, I.; Mizuno, K.; Matsuzawa, Y.; Matsubara, K. Analysis of an expression profile of genes in the human adipose tissue. *Gene* **1997**, *190*, 227–235. [CrossRef]
22. Nyamdorj, R.; Pitkäniemi, J.; Tuomilehto, J.; Hammar, N.; Stehouwer, C.D.; Lam, T.H.; Ramachandran, A.; Janus, E.D.; Mohan, V.; Söderberg, S.; et al. Ethnic comparison of the association of undiagnosed diabetes with obesity. *Int. J. Obes.* **2010**, *34*, 332–339. [CrossRef]
23. Kadowaki, T.; Sekikawa, A.; Murata, K.; Maegawa, H.; Takamiya, T.; Okamura, T.; El-Saed, A.; Miyamatsu, N.; Edmundowicz, D.; Kita, Y.; et al. Japanese men have larger areas of visceral adipose tissue than Caucasian men in the same levels of waist circumference in a population-based study. *Int. J. Obes. (Lond)* **2006**, *30*, 1163–1165. [CrossRef] [PubMed]
24. De Toro-Martín, J.; Arsenault, B.J.; Després, J.P.; Vohl, M.C. Precision nutrition: A review of personalized nutritional approaches for the prevention and management of metabolic syndrome. *Nutrients* **2017**, *9*, E913. [CrossRef] [PubMed]
25. Näslund, U.; Ng, N.; Lundgren, A.; Fhärm, E.; Grönlund, C.; Johansson, H.; Lindahl, B.; Lindahl, B.; Lindvall, K.; Nilsson, S.K.; et al. VIPVIZA trial group. Visualization of asymptomatic atherosclerotic disease for optimum cardiovascular prevention (VIPVIZA): A pragmatic, open-label, randomised controlled trial. *Lancet* **2019**, *393*, 133–142.
26. Neumark-Sztainer, D.; Wall, M.; Larson, N.I.; Eisenberg, M.E.; Loth, K. Dieting and disordered eating behaviors from adolescence to young adulthood: Findings from a 10-year longitudinal study. *J. Am. Diet. Assoc.* **2011**, *111*, 1004–1011. [CrossRef]
27. Shah, R.; Kennedy, S.; Clark, M.D.; Bauer, S.C.; Schwartz, A. Primary care-based interventions to promote positive parenting behaviors: A meta-analysis. *Pediatrics* **2016**, *137*, e20153393. [CrossRef]
28. Ewart-Pierce, E.; Mejía Ruiz, M.J.; Gittelsohn, J. "Whole-of-Community" Obesity Prevention: A review of challenges and opportunities in multilevel, multicomponent interventions. *Curr. Obes. Rep.* **2016**, *5*, 361–374. [CrossRef]
29. Cornelsen, L.; Green, R.; Dangour, A.; Smith, R. Why fat taxes won't make us thin. *J. Public Health (Oxford)* **2015**, *37*, 18–23. [CrossRef]
30. Lear, S.A.; Hu, W.; Rangarajan, S.; Gasevic, D.; Leong, D.; Iqbal, R.; Casanova, A.; Swaminathan, S.; Anjana, R.M.; Kumar, R.; et al. The effect of physical activity on mortality and cardiovascular disease in 130,000 people from 17 high-income, middle-income, and low-income countries: The PURE study. *Lancet* **2017**, *390*, 2643–2654. [CrossRef]
31. Wu, T.; Gao, X.; Chen, M.; van Dam, R.M. Long-term effectiveness of diet-plus-exercise interventions vs. diet-only interventions for weight loss: A meta-analysis. *Obes. Rev.* **2009**, *10*, 313–323. [CrossRef] [PubMed]

32. Giles-Corti, B.; Vernez-Moudon, A.; Reis, R.; Turrell, G.; Dannenberg, A.L.; Badland, H.; Foster, S.; Lowe, M.; Sallis, J.F.; Stevenson, M.; et al. City planning and population health: A global challenge. *Lancet* **2016**, *388*, 2912–2924. [CrossRef]
33. World Health Organization. *Global Recommendations on Physical Activity for Health*; World Health Organization: Geneva, Switzerland, 2010.
34. Clarke, J.; Janssen, I. Is the frequency of weekly moderate-to-vigorous physical activity associated with the metabolic syndrome in Canadian adults? *Appl. Physiol. Nutr. Metab.* **2013**, *38*, 773–778. [CrossRef] [PubMed]
35. Taheri, S.; Lin, L.; Austin, D.; Young, T.; Mignot, E. Short sleep duration is associated with reduced leptin, elevated ghrelin, and increased body mass index. *PLoS Med.* **2004**, *1*, e62. [CrossRef] [PubMed]
36. Knutson, K.L. Sleep duration and cardiometabolic risk: A review of the epidemiologic evidence. *Best Pract. Res. Endcrinol. Metab.* **2010**, *24*, 731–743. [CrossRef] [PubMed]
37. Fukuda, S.; Hirata, A.; Nishizawa, H.; Nagao, H.; Kimura, T.; Fujishima, Y.; Yamaoka, M.; Kozawa, J.; Imagawa, A.; Funahashi, T.; et al. Characteristics of sleep-wake cycle and sleep duration in Japanese type 2 diabetes patients with visceral fat accumulation. *J. Diabetes Invest.* **2018**, *9*, 63–68. [CrossRef] [PubMed]
38. Leblanc, E.S.; O'Connor, E.; Whitlock, E.P.; Patnode, C.D.; Kapka, T. Effectiveness of primary care-relevant treatments for obesity in adults: A systematic evidence review for the U.S. Preventive Services Task Force. *Ann. Intern. Med.* **2011**, *155*, 434–447. [CrossRef] [PubMed]
39. Hunt, K.; Wyke, S.; Gray, C.M.; Anderson, A.S.; Brady, A.; Bunn, C.; Donnan, P.T.; Fenwick, E.; Grieve, E.; Leishman, J.; et al. A gender-sensitised weight loss and healthy living programme for overweight and obese men delivered by Scottish Premier League football clubs (FFIT): A pragmatic randomised controlled trial. *Lancet* **2014**, *383*, 1211–1221. [CrossRef]
40. Kohro, T.; Furui, Y.; Mitsutake, N.; Fujii, R.; Morita, H.; Oku, S.; Ohe, K.; Nagai, R. The Japanese national health screening and intervention program aimed at preventing worsening of the metabolic syndrome. *Int. Heart J.* **2008**, *49*, 193–203. [CrossRef] [PubMed]
41. Stock, S.A.; Redaelli, M.; Lauterbach, K.W. Disease management and health care reforms in Germany - does more competition lead to less solidarity? *Health Policy* **2007**, *80*, 86–96. [CrossRef] [PubMed]
42. Tsushita, K.; Hosler, A.S.; Miura, K.; Ito, Y.; Fukuda, T.; Kitamura, A.; Tatara, K. Rationale and descriptive analysis of specific health guidance: The nationwide lifestyle intervention program targeting metabolic syndrome in Japan. *J. Atheroscler. Thromb.* **2018**, *25*, 308–322. [CrossRef]
43. Gregg, E.W.; Ali, M.K.; Moore, B.A.; Pavkov, M.; Devlin, H.M.; Garfield, S.; Mangione, C.M. The importance of natural experiments in diabetes prevention and control and the need for better health policy research. *Prev. Chronic Dis.* **2013**, *10*, E14. [CrossRef] [PubMed]
44. Noguchi, M.; Kojima, S.; Sairenchi, T.; Kinuta, M.; Yamakawa, M.; Nishizawa, H.; Takahara, M.; Imano, H.; Kitamura, A.; Yoshida, T.; et al. Study Profile: Japan Trial in High-risk Individuals to Accelerate their Referral to Physicians (J-HARP)—A Nurse-led, Community-based Prevention Program of Lifestyle-related Disease. *J. Epidemiol.* in press.
45. Kelley, C.P.; Sbrocco, G.; Sbrocco, T. Behavioral modification for the management of obesity. *Prim. Care* **2016**, *43*, 159–175. [CrossRef]
46. Ryo, M.; Nakamura, T.; Funahashi, T.; Noguchi, M.; Kishida, K.; Okauchi, Y.; Nishizawa, H.; Ogawa, T.; Kojima, S.; Ohira, T.; et al. Health education "Hokenshido" program reduced metabolic syndrome in the Amagasaki visceral fat study. Three-year follow-up study of 3,174 Japanese employees. *Intern. Med.* **2011**, *50*, 1643–1648. [CrossRef] [PubMed]
47. Tate, D.F. A series of studies examining internet treatment of obesity to inform Internet interventions for substance use and misuse. *Subst. Use Misuse* **2011**, *46*, 57–65. [CrossRef] [PubMed]
48. Fukuda, S.; Hirata, A.; Nishizawa, H.; Nagao, H.; Kashine, S.; Kimura, T.; Inoue, K.; Fujishima, Y.; Yamaoka, M.; Kozawa, J.; et al. Systemic arteriosclerosis and eating behavior in Japanese type 2 diabetic patients with visceral fat accumulation. *Cardiovasc. Diabetol.* **2015**, *14*, 8. [CrossRef] [PubMed]
49. Kishida, K.; Funahashi, T.; Matsuzawa, Y.; Shimomura, I. Visceral adiposity as a target for the metabolic syndrome. *Ann. Med.* **2012**, *44*, 233–241. [CrossRef] [PubMed]

15

Dietary Fructose and the Metabolic Syndrome

Marja-Riitta Taskinen [1], Chris J Packard [2] and Jan Borén [3,*]

1. Research Program for Clinical and Molecular Medicine Unit, Diabetes and Obesity, University of Helsinki, 00029 Helsinki, Finland
2. Institute of Cardiovascular and Medical Sciences, University of Glasgow, Glasgow G12 8QQ, UK
3. Department of Molecular and Clinical Medicine, University of Gothenburg and Sahlgrenska University Hospital, 41345 Gothenburg, Sweden

* Correspondence: jan.boren@wlab.gu.se

Abstract: Consumption of fructose, the sweetest of all naturally occurring carbohydrates, has increased dramatically in the last 40 years and is today commonly used commercially in soft drinks, juice, and baked goods. These products comprise a large proportion of the modern diet, in particular in children, adolescents, and young adults. A large body of evidence associate consumption of fructose and other sugar-sweetened beverages with insulin resistance, intrahepatic lipid accumulation, and hypertriglyceridemia. In the long term, these risk factors may contribute to the development of type 2 diabetes and cardiovascular diseases. Fructose is absorbed in the small intestine and metabolized in the liver where it stimulates fructolysis, glycolysis, lipogenesis, and glucose production. This may result in hypertriglyceridemia and fatty liver. Therefore, understanding the mechanisms underlying intestinal and hepatic fructose metabolism is important. Here we review recent evidence linking excessive fructose consumption to health risk markers and development of components of the Metabolic Syndrome.

Keywords: fructose; metabolic syndrome; hypertriglyceridemia; metabolism

---

1. Introduction

Food patterns and diet have greatly changed during the last decades in both industrialized and developing countries together with sedentary lifestyle resulting in dramatic increases of obesity, Metabolic Syndrome (MetS), non-alcoholic fatty liver disease (NAFLD), and type 2 diabetes [1–4]. Importantly, the rapid increase in pediatric NAFLD has become the major concern globally [5,6]. As obesity is a driving force for NAFLD and type 2 diabetes, it is not surprising that the prevalence of the MetS is high in both disorders.

The main component of dietary changes is not only lack of physical activity in face of extra calories, but in particular increases of added sugar mainly in sugar sweetened beverages (SSBs). The common sweeteners are sucrose (containing 50% saccharose and 50% fructose) and high fructose corn syrup (containing up to 55% fructose). The consumption of SSBs, comprising fruit-flavored drinks and sport and energy drinks, is the main source of added sugar. It accounts for about 15–17% of the total daily energy intake in Western diets. Thus, it exceeds the recommended limit of 5% of added sugar (World Health Organization's guidelines 2018) [7]. Consequently, excess sugar consumption has become a major public health problem particularly in children and teen-age populations globally. This menace has initiated the call for the restriction of sugar consumptions [8].

There is substantial and consistent data evidence that exposure to excess fructose intake has detrimental effects on multiple cardiometabolic risk factors [9–13]. In fact, fructose consumption is considered to be a culprit in the MetS as a lipogenic compound that associates with excess ectopic fat accumulation, particularly in the liver. This review will focus on the links between fructose consumption and the MetS, highlighting specifically effects of fructose on hepatic lipid homeostasis and metabolism.

2. Metabolic Effects of Fructose Consumption

2.1. Fructose Metabolism in Enterocytes

Although fructose and glucose are both monosaccharides with closely similar formulas, their metabolism pathways are divergent in both enterocytes and in hepatocytes [14–17]. Fructose absorption is mainly mediated by glucose transporter 5 (GLUT-5), a fructose transporter expressed on the apical border of enterocytes in the small intestine across the lumen in enterocytes (Figure 1) [17,18]. Fructose trafficking from the enterocytes into the portal vein is partly also mediated by GLUT-2. Notably, a part of fructose is metabolized in the cytosol by fructokinase, an enzyme that catalyzes the transfer of a high-energy phosphate group to d-fructose. Notably, high flux of fructose into enterocytes induces GLUT-5 expression. This mechanism may respond to excess chronic fructose intake by increasing the capacity of the intestine for fructose absorption and transport to the liver. Thus, GLUT-5 activity is the key regulator of fructose concentration in the portal vein.

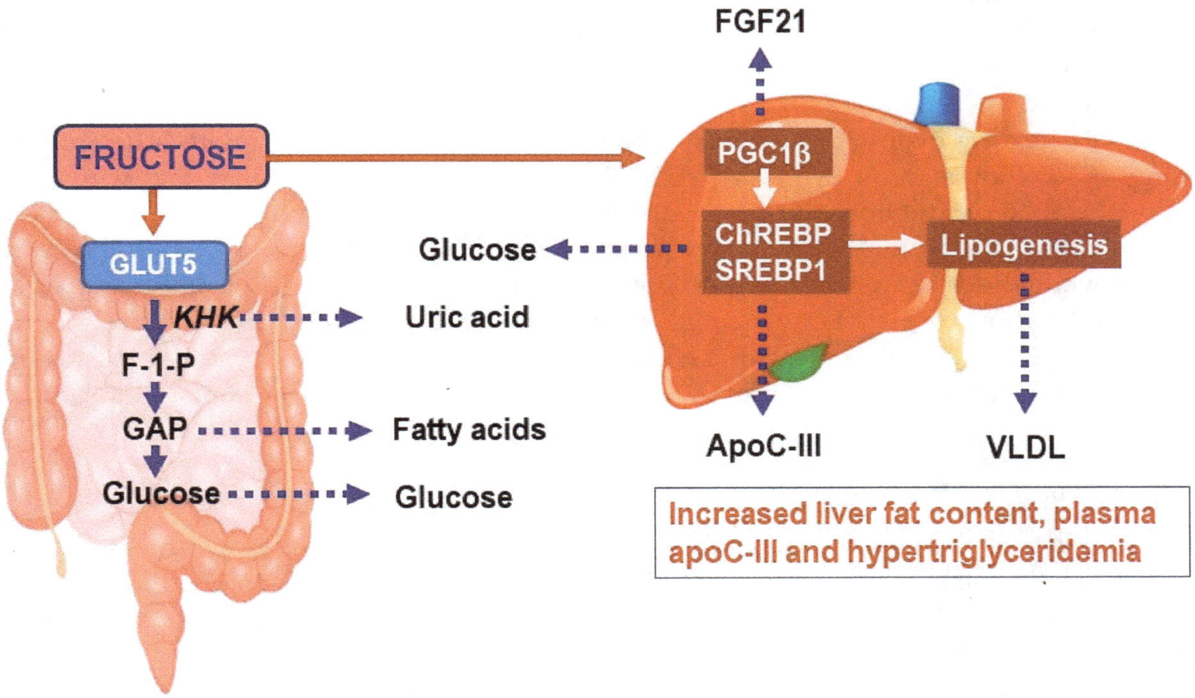

Figure 1. Metabolism of fructose in the intestine and liver. Fructose is in the small intestine metabolized by ketohexokinase (KHK) into fructose-1-phosphate (F-1-P) [19]. F-1-P is then cleaved by aldolase B into dihydroxyacetone phosphate and glyceraldehyde. Glyceraldehyde is phosphorylated by triokinase generating glyceraldehyde 3-phosphate (GAP). GAP and other triose phosphates are resynthesized into glucose via gluconeogenesis or metabolized into lactate or acetyl-CoA, which are oxidized or used for lipogenesis. In the liver, fructose activates the transcription factors carbohydrate-responsive element-binding protein (ChREBP) and sterol regulatory element-binding transcription factor 1c (SREBP1c) and their coactivator peroxisome proliferator-activated receptor-β (PGC1β) [16]. This results in upregulation of pathways that stimulate fructolysis, glycolysis, lipogenesis, and glucose production. Collectively, this results in increased hepatic glucose production, generation of lipid intermediates that may affect hepatic insulin sensitivity, increased expression of APOC3 and increased secretion of triglyceride-rich very-low density lipoproteins (VLDL). The increased APOC3 expression induces increased plasma apoC-III, an inhibitor of lipoprotein lipase and hepatic clearance of lipoprotein remnants [20]. This results in hypertriglyceridemia and accumulation of atherogenic triglyceride-rich lipoprotein (TRL) remnants.

Carbohydrate response element binding protein (ChREBP), a transcription factor responding to sugar intake, is recognized to be a key regulator of hepatic carbohydrate and lipid metabolism [21,22]. Recent data highlight the role of ChREBP in enterocytes as a regulator of intestinal GLUT-5 expression [19,23]. Interestingly, chronic fructose feeding in hamsters enhances lipid synthesis in enterocytes, resulting in increased synthesis of apoB48 and release of intestinal-derived chylomicrons, likely by activation of ChREBP and GLUT-5 [24]. In contrast, ChREBP-deficient mice fed a high fructose diet are reported to be fructose intolerant due to impaired fructose absorption and decreased expression of GLUT-5 [19]. These data highlight the role of intestinal ChREBP for fructose-induced impaired metabolism.

The liver is considered to be the major organ for fructose metabolism [16,25–27]. Plasma concentration of fructose are increased only trivially after fructose intake in humans as first pass metabolism by liver covers about 80–90% of the fructose load. Recently, this concept has been challenged by studies in mice utilizing isotope tracers and mass spectrometry [28]. The key finding suggests that the small intestine may be the major site for dietary fructose metabolism instead of the liver. Notably, the intestinal fructose metabolism seems to be a saturable process that allows high doses of dietary fructose to pass to the liver. The handling of dietary fructose in humans may be different due to the relatively smaller gut in humans than in mice [29]. This is supported by studies in healthy volunteers with stable isotope-labelled fructose to study the initial metabolism of ingested fructose [30]. The amount of dietary fructose escaping the splanchnic extraction averaged only about 14.5% and the first-pass extraction was 85.5%.

A study in healthy males ($n = 7$) demonstrated that fructose combined with Intralipid infusion (consisting of 10% soybean oil, 1.2% egg yolk phospholipids, 2.25% glycerin, and water) resulted in increased apoB48 production rate without any altered catabolism of chylomicrons [31]. Recently, we reported that in abdominally obese men, fructose consumption (75 g/per day served as fructose sweetened beverage) for 12 weeks increased postprandial responses of both plasma triglycerides and apoB48 to a fat rich meal [32]. How changes in fructose absorption and metabolism in enterocyte influence intestinal lipogenesis, reflected in handling of dietary fats and postprandial lipemia, remains to be established in future kinetic studies in humans as direct extrapolation from animal studies may be misleading.

2.2. *Fructose Metabolism in the Liver*

Hepatic fructose and glucose metabolism occurs via divergent pathways with consequences on hepatic lipid handling and insulin sensitivity reflected in metabolic diseases [15,27,33]. Fructose uptake from portal circulation into liver is mediated by GLUT2 via first pass metabolism by phosphorylation of fructose to fructose-1-phosphate, that is further metabolized to dihydroxyacetone phosphate and glyceraldehyde 3-phosphate. Notably only a small part of ingested fructose ends up in the circulation in contrast to glucose. These initial steps in fructose metabolism seem to be unregulated and bypass the hormonal control in contrast to the strictly regulated glucose uptake and glycolysis in the liver where insulin plays a central role. Glyceraldehyde 3-phosphate and other triose phosphate compounds derived from fructolysis are directed to the formation of pyruvate and acetyl-CoA and to lipogenesis. Consequently, fructose has effects on both glucose homeostasis and lipogenesis the partitioning depending on cellular energy needs [34].

2.3. *Evidence Linking Fructose Intake to Non-Alcoholic Fatty Liver Disease (NAFLD) and to Increased Cardiometabolic Risk*

The heterogeneity of obesity and its consequences on cardiometabolic risk has been addressed in several outstanding recent reviews that have recognized the importance of body fat distribution, in particular the ectopic fat in the liver as the critical link to cardiometabolic health [25,35–40]. The central role of non-alcoholic fatty liver disease (NAFLD) as the source for multiple cardiometabolic risk factors has raised the questions how the liver can handle extra influx of lipids and the consequences on lipoprotein metabolism and ultimately vascular health [9,10,13,41].

2.4. Effects of Fructose on Hepatic De Novo Lipogenesis

The hallmark of NAFLD is hepatic triglyceride accumulation. The disease develops when the influx of lipid into the liver (from circulating non-esterified fatty acids, diet-derived chylomicrons, and hepatic *de novo* lipogenesis(DNL)) exceeds hepatic lipid disposal (via β-oxidation in mitochondria and triglyceride secretion as lipoprotein particles) [42]. In the past decade, we have seen a remarkable increase in NAFLD [43–45]. It is already the most common cause of chronic liver disease in Western countries and may soon achieve this status in the rest of the world.

Accumulating evidence indicates that increased hepatic DNL is a significant pathway contributing to the development of NAFLD [6,46]. Dietary carbohydrates, in particular, fructose, have been shown to stimulate DNL and increase liver fat, although it is still debated whether this is due to excess energy or fructose per se [46]. Studies in humans are lacking but a comparison between fructose and glucose supplementation in rats for two months showed that, although total caloric consumption was higher in glucose-supplemented rats, fructose caused worse metabolic responses [47].

DNL is a highly regulated pathway, dependent upon several steps, in which key enzymes involved are upregulated in NAFLD [48–50]. Importantly, dietary fructose further increases levels of enzymes involved in DNL as fructose is absorbed via portal vein and delivered to the liver in much higher concentrations as compared to other tissues. Interestingly, in contrast to metabolism of glucose, the breakdown of fructose leads to the generation of metabolites that stimulate hepatic DNL [51–53].

Fructose drives lipogenesis in the setting of insulin resistance as fructose does not require insulin for its metabolism, and it directly stimulates sterol regulatory element-binding protein 1 (SREBP-1c), a major transcriptional regulator of DNL (Figure 1) [54]. Fructose also promotes hepatic DNL and lipid accumulation by suppressing hepatic β-oxidation and by inducing promotes ER stress and uric acid formation (see below). High-fructose feeding has also been shown to increase hepatic expression of ChREBP, a lipogenic transcription factor of carbohydrate metabolism and DNL. ChREBP regulates fructose-induced glucose production independently of insulin signaling [22], and the fructose-induced increases in circulating fibroblast growth factor 21 (FGF21) [55]. The fructose-induced FGF21 feeds back on the liver to enhance further ChREBP activity and hepatic DNL and VLDL secretion [55]. Consequently, circulating FGF21 levels correlate with rates of de novo lipogenesis in human subjects [55]. FGF21 has also been implemented in a signaling axis regulating carbohydrate consumption [11,16,27,33,46,56].

Despite convincing evidence in animals, whether fructose consumption increases DNL in humans to the extent that it induces metabolic disturbances has been more controversial [57]. However, Stanhope et al. reported that 10 weeks overfeeding of fructose (but not glucose), increased DNL (from 11% to 17%) [58]. Other studies have reported that a high fructose diet increased fasting DNL from 2% to 9% [59], and that fructose (75 g/day), served with their habitual diet over 12 weeks to abdominally obese men resulted in significant increases in DNL in both the fasting state (12.3% to 16.5%) and 4 to 8 h postprandially [32,60]. In line, 9 days of isocaloric fructose restriction in the context of an otherwise normal diet led to significant decreased DNL in 37 out of 40 children with obesity [61].

2.5. Clinical Evidence That Fructose Consumption Is Leading to Non-Alcoholic Fatty Liver Disease (NAFLD)

As fructose is recognized to be a lipogenic sugar, its contribution to the pathogenesis of NAFLD has been the focus of intensive research for more than a decade [16,27,33,54,58,62]. The ongoing interest is stimulated by the huge global burden of NAFLD as the potential driver of CVD and its clinical manifestations [11,15,16,63–65].

Although accumulated evidence has demonstrated a strong link between fructose consumption and NAFLD it is still unclear if the association is caused by fructose consumption per se, or by the increased energy intake [66]. An important reason for this is the technological problems associated with measuring liver fat content. Accurate non-invasively measurements of liver fat content require advanced equipment like magnetic resonance imaging and spectroscopy [66–69]. Notably, these technologies allow both quantitation and characterization of hepatic lipids [69,70]. NAFLD is commonly define as >5.5% hepatic fat fraction as determined by MRI [71].

Mot studies focusing on the association between fructose or saccharose overfeeding and liver fat steatosis (quantitated by MRI), have been performed in healthy or obese men [58,72–79]. Many of these studies have been positive [58,72–79]. For example, daily intake of one liter regular cola for 6 months in overweight subjects (n = 10) was shown to associate with significant increases of liver fat measured by MRI, but without significant changes of BMI or total fat mass [80]. However, many studies have also been negative [81–83].

Reasons for the different outcome from these earlier studies are the relatively smaller study cohorts, variable and short-duration less than 7 days) study designs, and differing doses of fructose. Despite these weaknesses, many studies seem to indicate that hypercaloric fructose feeding increases liver fat content and that this response is aggravated in obese subjects. For example, Ma et al. reported that the regular consumption of SSBs in overweight and obese subjects from the Framingham cohort (n = 2634) was associated with increases of liver fat content quantitated by computed tomography [84].

In line, we recently reported that fructose consumption (75 g/day as fructose sweetened beverage) for 12 weeks in abdominally obese men with cardiometabolic risk factors, significantly increased liver fat content measured by MRI despite relative low increases in weight and waist circumferences [32]. The study subjects were served their habitual diet with add on fructose feeding resulting in hypercaloric set up that also occurs in the real world with SSB intake [32].

Despite this study design, the average increase of liver fat content was modest (10%) in face of no significant change in visceral or subcutaneous fat depots and there was high variation in the response liver fat content. To better understand this variation, we genotyped all individuals for carrier status of the major risk alleles for hepatic steatosis; PNPLA3, TN6SF2, and MBOAT7. Results showed that the number of risk alleles associated with increased liver fat at the baseline. However, individuals without and with risk allele did not have differences in the response of liver fat during fructose feeding. In line with this, two other studies have confirmed increases of liver fat content during carbohydrate (simple sugars) overfeeding on hypercaloric diet for 3 weeks in overweight and obese subjects [85,86].

The key metabolic and mechanistic issues of fructose consumption has been studied during a nine days isocaloric feeding study (fructose restriction to less than 4% of calories) in obese children (n = 40) with MetS and a high habitual sugar consumption (>50 g/day) [61,87,88]. The metabolic assessment was extensive utilizing magnetic resonance imaging and stable isotope technology for DNL in addition to extensive biomarker platform. The first important message is that the dietary fructose restriction was associated with significant reductions of liver (from 7.2% to 3.8%, $p < 0.001$) and visceral fat content (from 123 cm^3 to 110 cm^3, $p < 0.001$). Notably, the reduction of liver fat content was not related to the baseline liver fat content. The diet intervention was also associated with a significant decrease of DNL and an improved lipoprotein profile. In addition, significant improvements were observed in biomarkers of insulin resistance and glucose metabolism. The authors also elucidated the impact of the diet intervention on the methylglyoxal (MG) pathway [15,63,89–91], and surprisingly found that fructose restriction associated with marked reduction of D-lactate, a biomarker of MG metabolism. This change of D-lactate correlated with reduction of liver fat content and DNL [88]. These observations open a new perspective of the adverse metabolic effects of excess fructose intake.

Thus, accumulating evidence supports the fact that fructose is an important mediator for the development of NAFLD and a main driver for DNL [64]. Indeed, this concept is supported by a recent meta-analysis including 6326 participants and 1361 cases with NAFLD [92]. However, it is still debated whether fructose, when consumed in isocaloric amounts, causes more liver fat accumulation than other energy-dense nutrients [93].

Kirk et al. investigated the effects of acute and chronic calorie restriction with either a low-fat, high-carbohydrate (>180 g/day) diet or a low-carbohydrate (<50 g/day) diet on hepatic and skeletal muscle insulin sensitivity in 22 obese subjects [94]. Interestingly, the low-carbohydrate diet lowered the hepatic lipids within 48 h by 30% (compared to ~10% in the low-fat, high-carbohydrate group). The mechanism for the rapid clearance of liver fat was not elucidated. After approximately 11 weeks (7% weight loss) a similar marked reduction of liver fat content was seen in both groups (38% vs. 44%). These results show that liver fat content is highly dynamic in response to energy balance and sugar intake. However, it is still debated whether a low-carbohydrate hypocaloric diet is more efficient than a low-fat hypocaloric diet in reducing intrahepatic lipid accumulation.

Haufe et al. compared the 6 months responses of a low-carbohydrate hypocaloric or a low-fat hypocaloric diet on intrahepatic lipid accumulation in overweight/obese subjects (n = 84 to 86 in each group) [95]. Results showed that both diets had the same beneficial effects on intrahepatic lipid accumulation, weight loss and insulin resistance. The decrease in intrahepatic fat was independent of visceral fat loss and not associated with changes in whole body insulin sensitivity. Interestingly, subjects with high baseline intrahepatic lipids (>5.6%) lost $\approx$ 7-fold more liver fat compared with those with low baseline values irrespective of the prolonged hypocaloric diet.

2.6. *Effects of Fructose on Uric Acid Metabolism and MG (Methyl Glyoxal) Pathways*

The role of fructose as a potential source of uric acid was recognized decades ago [96]. The rapid phosphorylation of fructose to fructose-1-phospate not only increases the fluxes of trioses for lipogenesis, but also depletes ATP stores leading to the degradation of AMP, resulting in increased generation of uric acid via purine pathway. Importantly, fructose seems to be the only carbohydrate that can generate uric acid. Cellular depletion of ATP has several adverse consequences on energy metabolism including increased ER stress and mitochondrial dysfunction [64]. ER stress has been linked to many metabolic diseases including NAFLD [97] and can be induced by a range of condition such as high protein demand, viral infection, mutant protein expression, hypoxia, energy deprivation, or exposure to excessive oxidative stress including ATP depletion [97–99]. The ER stress triggers an adaptive signaling pathway known as the Unfolded Protein Response (UPR) to restore normal ER function. If the UPR fail to restore normal ER function, the UPR aims towards apoptosis [97–99]. A sustained chronic UPR response may worsen the pathophysiological condition by inducing lipotoxicity, insulin resistance, inflammation, and apoptotic cell death [97–99].

ER stress activates the transcription factor X-box binding protein 1 (XBP1s), a key regulator of the unfolded protein response. Interestingly, XBP1 also regulates hepatic fatty acid synthesis [100]. Mitochondrial oxidative stress results in enhanced generation of citrate and acetyl coenzyme A AcCoA [101–103], two metabolites that stimulate lipogenesis. This may explain why fructose is lipogenic [16,104]. An additional nexus is that increased triose flux enhance the generation of methyl glyoxal (MG) and dicarbonyl stress. A key crossroad step is the inactivation of AMPK by MG and consequences on energy metabolism. This is a novel pathway linked to excess fructose intake and its metabolic relevance remains to be clarified [15]. In summary, fructose seems to influence multiple metabolic pathways in the liver that results in enhanced lipogenesis, generation of uric acid, ER stress, and inflammation. The association between uric acid and insulin resistance [105], raised the interest of uric acid as a potential biomarker in the Metabolic Syndrome [105]. Indeed, several studies have established that serum uric acid is a risk factor for the Metabolic Syndrome [106–113].

Substantial evidence suggest that uric acid also associates with NAFLD [114–117]. Several studies have reported that serum uric acid levels are higher in subjects with NAFLD than in those without NAFLD [64,118,119]. Importantly, hyperuricemia seems to associate with NAFLD independently of other features of the MetS and these associations are independent on body weight [120]. Thus, uric acid belongs to the cluster of biomarkers in Metabolic Syndrome and NAFLD.

Can excess intake of fructose and SSBs result in the elevation of plasma uric acid concentrations? Indeed, numerous studies have found an association between fructose/SSBs intake and uric acid levels [27,54,64,118,121,122]. For example, two large prospective cohort studies including American men (n = 46,393) or American women (n = 78,906) showed strong associations between consumption of SBBs and hyperuricemia [123,124]. Similar positive associations between SSBs intake and serum uric acid concentrations have been observed in Korean, Mexican, and Brazilian populations [125–127]. Likewise, in an adolescents cohort (n = 4867 aged 12 to 18 years) consumption of SSBs associated with higher serum uric acid and also higher systolic blood pressure [128].

So far, data from RCTs on fructose feeding trials have remained limited. Fructose feeding associated with increased uric acid in three smaller intervention studies [72,129,130]. Weaknesses of the study protocol are that the design and duration of feeding trials, as well as study cohorts, are highly variable. Unfortunately, data from available meta-analyses are not consistent. One meta-analysis reported that fructose intake as an apart of isocaloric diet did not raise uric acid levels but signaled that the hypercaloric intake of fructose may raise uric acid [131]. Although hyperuricemia is highly prevalent in patients with NAFLD and Met Syndrome, its clinical relevance remains debated. Recent French recommendations for sugar intake concluded that long-term consequences of potential small increases of uric acid by fructose/sugar intake remain insufficient [132], likewise critical analysis of the available data left open the casual link between fructose intake and hyperuricemia [133,134].

2.7. Consequences of Increased Lipid Synthesis to Very Low-Density Lipoproteins (VLDL) Metabolism and Release—Effects on Plasma Lipids, Lipoproteins, and Apolipoproteins

The association of blood lipid levels and consumption of added sugars was studied in the adult population in the National Health and Nutrition Examination Survey (NHANES) (n = 6113) [135]. In this American cross-sectional study higher fructose consumers had more unfavorable lipid levels, namely significantly lower HDL cholesterol, higher triglycerides, and a high ratio of triglycerides to high density lipoproteins (HDL), whereas women also had higher low-density lipoprotein (LDL) cholesterol levels. Likewise, in the Framingham study, daily soft drink consumers had higher incidence of elevated triglycerides and low HDL cholesterol than non-consumers (relative risk: 1.22 and 1.22, respectively) [136].

Several studies have consistently reported increased responses of fasting and postprandial triglyceride levels and 24 h. profiles to short term feeding of fructose as compared to glucose in both lean and obese subjects [8,53]. These perturbations directly lead to other lipid abnormalities including elevation of apoB levels, accumulation of small dense LDL, and increased remnant lipoproteins, combined with reduced HDL cholesterol which all are components of the atherogenic lipid triad, a strong risk factor for CVD. Interestingly, the deleterious effect of fructose on lipid metabolism is directly linked to the daily intake; a fructose intake >50 g/day is associated with postprandial hyperlipemia whereas intake above 100 g/day also results in elevation of fasting serum triglycerides [137]. Collectively, these results clearly show that fructose intake is directly linked to an atherogenic dyslipidemia.

The recent increased focus on plasma triglycerides and postprandial hyperlipidemia not only as markers but also as causal drivers of CVD has partly been driven by improved understanding of the biology and genetics of triglyceride heritability. Of particular interest is *APOC3*, which has emerged as a novel therapeutic target to reduce dyslipidemia and CVD risk [20,138–140]. Interestingly, fructose feeding is linked to a significant rise of plasma apoC-III levels (Figure 1) [32,141].

2.8. Interactions between Fructose Consumption and Changes in Gut Microbiota

High consumption of fructose, artificial sweeteners, and sugar alcohols have been shown to affect host-gastrointestinal microbe interactions and possibly contribute to the development of metabolic disorders and obesity. Multiple studies have also reported fructose as a critical factor contributing to NAFLD progression by modulating intestinal microbiota (see review [142]). Gut microbiota interacts with its host, and influences both the energy homeostasis and the immunity of the host [142]. Shifts in this composition can result in alterations of the symbiotic relationship, which can promote metabolic diseases [143]. Indeed, the microbial composition have been shown to differ between healthy individuals and NAFLD patients [144], and a diet enriched in fructose not only induced NAFLD but also negatively affected the gut barrier and the microbiota composition, leading to impaired microbiota [145]. The underlying mechanisms are complex and still unclear, but Oh et al. recently showed that dietary fructose activates the Ack-pathway, involved in generating acetic acid, which in turn triggers the bacterial stress response that promotes phage production [146]. Thus, prophages in a gut symbiont can be induced by diet and metabolites affected by diet, which provides a potential mechanistic explanation for the effects of diet on the intestinal phage community [147].

The complex interaction between dietary carbohydrates and gut microbiota was recently demonstrated in a two-week intervention with an isocaloric low-carbohydrate diet in obese subjects with NAFLD [148]. The authors observed rapid and marked reductions of liver fat paralleled by marked decreases in hepatic DNL and increases in hepatic β-oxidation. Interestingly, the marked reduction in cardiometabolic risk factors paralleled with rapid increases in the folate-producing gut microbiota Streptococcus, serum folate concentrations, and hepatic one-carbon metabolism.

3. Conclusions

Consistent data evidence that excess fructose intake as a central component of unhealthy lifestyle has detrimental effects on multiple cardiovascular risk factors. Consequently, it is not surprising that links between fructose consumption with MetS and NAFLD are strong. Fructose is a lipogenic sugar as it increases hepatic *de novo* lipogenesis in the liver through several metabolic pathways resulting in a vicious circle that further aggravates DNL. Increased DNL favors excess fat accumulation in the liver, being a driving force for increased secretion of VLDL particles leading to the atherogenic lipid profile and other metabolic derangements associated with CVD risk. The global health burden of MetS together with NAFLD is growing rapidly, sweeping across the world. It is clear that added sugars have become a threat to cardiometabolic health. These facts call for the restriction of dietary sugars, especially SSB consumption to limit fructose intake to achieve better cardiometabolic health.

References

1. GBD 2015 Obesity Collaborators; Afshin, A.; Forouzanfar, M.H.; Reitsma, M.B.; Sur, P.; Estep, K.; Lee, A.; Marczak, L.; Mokdad, A.H.; Moradi-Lakeh, M.; et al. Health Effects of Overweight and Obesity in 195 Countries over 25 Years. *N. Engl. J. Med.* **2017**, *377*, 13–27. [CrossRef] [PubMed]
2. Bluher, M. Obesity: Global epidemiology and pathogenesis. *Nat. Rev. Endocrinol.* **2019**, *15*, 288–298. [CrossRef] [PubMed]
3. Malik, V.S.; Li, Y.; Pan, A.; De Koning, L.; Schernhammer, E.; Willett, W.C.; Hu, F.B. Long-Term Consumption of Sugar-Sweetened and Artificially Sweetened Beverages and Risk of Mortality in US Adults. *Circulation* **2019**. [CrossRef] [PubMed]
4. Younossi, Z.M. Non-alcoholic fatty liver disease—A global public health perspective. *J. Hepatol.* **2019**, *70*, 531–544. [CrossRef] [PubMed]
5. Vos, M.B.; Abrams, S.H.; Barlow, S.E.; Caprio, S.; Daniels, S.R.; Kohli, R.; Mouzaki, M.; Sathya, P.; Schwimmer, J.B.; Sundaram, S.S.; et al. NASPGHAN Clinical Practice Guideline for the Diagnosis and Treatment of Nonalcoholic Fatty Liver Disease in Children: Recommendations from the Expert Committee on NAFLD (ECON) and the North American Society of Pediatric Gastroenterology, Hepatology and Nutrition (NASPGHAN). *J. Pediatr. Gastroenterol. Nutr.* **2017**, *64*, 319–334. [CrossRef] [PubMed]
6. Younossi, Z.; Tacke, F.; Arrese, M.; Chander Sharma, B.; Mostafa, I.; Bugianesi, E.; Wai-Sun Wong, V.; Yilmaz, Y.; George, J.; Fan, J.; et al. Global Perspectives on Nonalcoholic Fatty Liver Disease and Nonalcoholic Steatohepatitis. *Hepatology* **2019**, *69*, 2672–2682. [CrossRef] [PubMed]
7. Powell, E.S.; Smith-Taillie, L.P.; Popkin, B.M. Added Sugars Intake Across the Distribution of US Children and Adult Consumers: 1977–2012. *J. Acad. Nutr. Diet.* **2016**, *116*, 1543–1550. [CrossRef] [PubMed]
8. Johnson, R.K.; Lichtenstein, A.H.; Anderson, C.A.M.; Carson, J.A.; Despres, J.P.; Hu, F.B.; Kris-Etherton, P.M.; Otten, J.J.; Towfighi, A.; Wylie-Rosett, J.; et al. Low-Calorie Sweetened Beverages and Cardiometabolic Health: A Science Advisory From the American Heart Association. *Circulation* **2018**, *138*, e126–e140. [CrossRef] [PubMed]

9. Lim, S.; Taskinen, M.R.; Boren, J. Crosstalk between nonalcoholic fatty liver disease and cardiometabolic syndrome. *Obes. Rev.* **2019**, *20*, 599–611. [CrossRef]
10. Santos, R.D.; Valenti, L.; Romeo, S. Does nonalcoholic fatty liver disease cause cardiovascular disease? Current knowledge and gaps. *Atherosclerosis* **2019**, *282*, 110–120. [CrossRef]
11. Mirtschink, P.; Jang, C.; Arany, Z.; Krek, W. Fructose metabolism, cardiometabolic risk, and the epidemic of coronary artery disease. *Eur. Heart J.* **2018**, *39*, 2497–2505. [CrossRef] [PubMed]
12. Stanhope, K.L.; Goran, M.I.; Bosy-Westphal, A.; King, J.C.; Schmidt, L.A.; Schwarz, J.M.; Stice, E.; Sylvetsky, A.C.; Turnbaugh, P.J.; Bray, G.A.; et al. Pathways and mechanisms linking dietary components to cardiometabolic disease: Thinking beyond calories. *Obes. Rev.* **2018**, *19*, 1205–1235. [CrossRef] [PubMed]
13. Stahl, E.P.; Dhindsa, D.S.; Lee, S.K.; Sandesara, P.B.; Chalasani, N.P.; Sperling, L.S. Nonalcoholic Fatty Liver Disease and the Heart: JACC State-of-the-Art Review. *J. Am. Coll. Cardiol.* **2019**, *73*, 948–963. [CrossRef] [PubMed]
14. Ferraris, R.P.; Choe, J.Y.; Patel, C.R. Intestinal Absorption of Fructose. *Annu. Rev. Nutr.* **2018**, *38*, 41–67. [CrossRef] [PubMed]
15. Mortera, R.R.; Bains, Y.; Gugliucci, A. Fructose at the crossroads of the metabolic syndrome and obesity epidemics. *Front. Biosci. (Landmark Ed.)* **2019**, *24*, 186–211.
16. Hannou, S.A.; Haslam, D.E.; McKeown, N.M.; Herman, M.A. Fructose metabolism and metabolic disease. *J. Clin. Investig.* **2018**, *128*, 545–555. [CrossRef]
17. Hoffman, S.; Alvares, D.; Adeli, K. Intestinal lipogenesis: How carbs turn on triglyceride production in the gut. *Curr. Opin. Clin. Nutr. Metab. Care* **2019**, *22*, 284–288. [CrossRef]
18. Patel, C.; Douard, V.; Yu, S.; Gao, N.; Ferraris, R.P. Transport, metabolism, and endosomal trafficking-dependent regulation of intestinal fructose absorption. *FASEB J.* **2015**, *29*, 4046–4058. [CrossRef]
19. Lee, H.J.; Cha, J.Y. Recent insights into the role of ChREBP in intestinal fructose absorption and metabolism. *BMB Rep.* **2018**, *51*, 429–436. [CrossRef]
20. Taskinen, M.R.; Packard, C.J.; Boren, J. Emerging Evidence that ApoC-III Inhibitors Provide Novel Options to Reduce the Residual CVD. *Curr. Atheroscler. Rep.* **2019**, *21*, 27. [CrossRef]
21. Abdul-Wahed, A.; Guilmeau, S.; Postic, C. Sweet Sixteenth for ChREBP: Established Roles and Future Goals. *Cell Metab.* **2017**, *26*, 324–341. [CrossRef] [PubMed]
22. Kim, M.S.; Krawczyk, S.A.; Doridot, L.; Fowler, A.J.; Wang, J.X.; Trauger, S.A.; Noh, H.L.; Kang, H.J.; Meissen, J.K.; Blatnik, M.; et al. ChREBP regulates fructose-induced glucose production independently of insulin signaling. *J. Clin. Investig.* **2016**, *126*, 4372–4386. [CrossRef] [PubMed]
23. Kim, M.; Astapova, I.I.; Flier, S.N.; Hannou, S.A.; Doridot, L.; Sargsyan, A.; Kou, H.H.; Fowler, A.J.; Liang, G.; Herman, M.A. Intestinal, but not hepatic, ChREBP is required for fructose tolerance. *JCI Insight* **2017**, *2*. [CrossRef] [PubMed]
24. Haidari, M.; Leung, N.; Mahbub, F.; Uffelman, K.D.; Kohen-Avramoglu, R.; Lewis, G.F.; Adeli, K. Fasting and postprandial overproduction of intestinally derived lipoproteins in an animal model of insulin resistance. Evidence that chronic fructose feeding in the hamster is accompanied by enhanced intestinal de novo lipogenesis and ApoB48-containing lipoprotein overproduction. *J. Biol. Chem.* **2002**, *277*, 31646–31655. [CrossRef] [PubMed]
25. Stanhope, K.L. Sugar consumption, metabolic disease and obesity: The state of the controversy. *Crit. Rev. Clin. Lab. Sci.* **2016**, *53*, 52–67. [CrossRef] [PubMed]
26. Sun, S.Z.; Empie, M.W. Fructose metabolism in humans—What isotopic tracer studies tell us. *Nutr. Metab. (Lond.)* **2012**, *9*, 89. [CrossRef] [PubMed]
27. Softic, S.; Cohen, D.E.; Kahn, C.R. Role of Dietary Fructose and Hepatic De Novo Lipogenesis in Fatty Liver Disease. *Dig. Dis. Sci.* **2016**, *61*, 1282–1293. [CrossRef] [PubMed]
28. Jang, C.; Hui, S.; Lu, W.; Cowan, A.J.; Morscher, R.J.; Lee, G.; Liu, W.; Tesz, G.J.; Birnbaum, M.J.; Rabinowitz, J.D. The Small Intestine Converts Dietary Fructose into Glucose and Organic Acids. *Cell Metab.* **2018**, *27*, 351–361. [CrossRef] [PubMed]
29. Gonzalez, J.T.; Betts, J.A. Dietary Fructose Metabolism By Splanchnic Organs: Size Matters. *Cell Metab.* **2018**, *27*, 483–485. [CrossRef]
30. Francey, C.; Cros, J.; Rosset, R.; Creze, C.; Rey, V.; Stefanoni, N.; Schneiter, P.; Tappy, L.; Seyssel, K. The extra-splanchnic fructose escape after ingestion of a fructose-glucose drink: An exploratory study in healthy humans using a dual fructose isotope method. *Clin. Nutr. ESPEN* **2019**, *29*, 125–132. [CrossRef]

31. Xiao, C.; Dash, S.; Morgantini, C.; Lewis, G.F. Novel role of enteral monosaccharides in intestinal lipoprotein production in healthy humans. *Arterioscler. Thromb. Vasc. Biol.* **2013**, *33*, 1056–1062. [CrossRef] [PubMed]
32. Taskinen, M.R.; Soderlund, S.; Bogl, L.H.; Hakkarainen, A.; Matikainen, N.; Pietilainen, K.H.; Rasanen, S.; Lundbom, N.; Bjornson, E.; Eliasson, B.; et al. Adverse effects of fructose on cardiometabolic risk factors and hepatic lipid metabolism in subjects with abdominal obesity. *J. Intern. Med.* **2017**, *282*, 187–201. [CrossRef] [PubMed]
33. Herman, M.A.; Samuel, V.T. The Sweet Path to Metabolic Demise: Fructose and Lipid Synthesis. *Trends Endocrinol. Metab.* **2016**, *27*, 719–730. [CrossRef] [PubMed]
34. Tappy, L. Fructose-containing caloric sweeteners as a cause of obesity and metabolic disorders. *J. Exp. Biol.* **2018**, *221*. [CrossRef] [PubMed]
35. Spalding, K.L.; Bernard, S.; Naslund, E.; Salehpour, M.; Possnert, G.; Appelsved, L.; Fu, K.Y.; Alkass, K.; Druid, H.; Thorell, A.; et al. Impact of fat mass and distribution on lipid turnover in human adipose tissue. *Nat. Commun.* **2017**, *8*, 15253. [CrossRef] [PubMed]
36. Kim, S.H.; Despres, J.P.; Koh, K.K. Obesity and cardiovascular disease: Friend or foe? *Eur. Heart J.* **2016**, *37*, 3560–3568. [CrossRef] [PubMed]
37. Karpe, F.; Pinnick, K.E. Biology of upper-body and lower-body adipose tissue—Link to whole-body phenotypes. *Nat. Rev. Endocrinol.* **2015**, *11*, 90–100. [CrossRef] [PubMed]
38. Schulze, M.B. Metabolic health in normal-weight and obese individuals. *Diabetologia* **2019**, *62*, 558–566. [CrossRef] [PubMed]
39. Neeland, I.J.; Poirier, P.; Despres, J.P. Cardiovascular and Metabolic Heterogeneity of Obesity: Clinical Challenges and Implications for Management. *Circulation* **2018**, *137*, 1391–1406. [CrossRef]
40. Piche, M.E.; Vasan, S.K.; Hodson, L.; Karpe, F. Relevance of human fat distribution on lipid and lipoprotein metabolism and cardiovascular disease risk. *Curr. Opin. Lipidol.* **2018**, *29*, 285–292. [CrossRef]
41. Stefan, N.; Haring, H.U.; Cusi, K. Non-alcoholic fatty liver disease: Causes, diagnosis, cardiometabolic consequences, and treatment strategies. *Lancet Diabetes Endocrinol.* **2019**, *7*, 313–324. [CrossRef]
42. Stefan, N.; Kantartzis, K.; Haring, H.U. Causes and metabolic consequences of Fatty liver. *Endocr. Rev.* **2008**, *29*, 939–960. [CrossRef] [PubMed]
43. Vernon, G.; Baranova, A.; Younossi, Z.M. Systematic review: The epidemiology and natural history of non-alcoholic fatty liver disease and non-alcoholic steatohepatitis in adults. *Aliment. Pharmacol. Ther.* **2011**, *34*, 274–285. [CrossRef] [PubMed]
44. Bellentani, S.; Scaglioni, F.; Marino, M.; Bedogni, G. Epidemiology of non-alcoholic fatty liver disease. *Dig. Dis.* **2010**, *28*, 155–161. [CrossRef] [PubMed]
45. Estes, C.; Anstee, Q.M.; Arias-Loste, M.T.; Bantel, H.; Bellentani, S.; Caballeria, J.; Colombo, M.; Craxi, A.; Crespo, J.; Day, C.P.; et al. Modeling NAFLD disease burden in China, France, Germany, Italy, Japan, Spain, United Kingdom, and United States for the period 2016–2030. *J. Hepatol.* **2018**, *69*, 896–904. [CrossRef]
46. Chiu, S.; Mulligan, K.; Schwarz, J.M. Dietary carbohydrates and fatty liver disease: De novo lipogenesis. *Curr. Opin. Clin. Nutr. Metab. Care* **2018**, *21*, 277–282. [CrossRef]
47. Sanguesa, G.; Shaligram, S.; Akther, F.; Roglans, N.; Laguna, J.C.; Rahimian, R.; Alegret, M. Type of supplemented simple sugar, not merely calorie intake, determines adverse effects on metabolism and aortic function in female rats. *Am. J. Physiol. Heart Circ. Physiol.* **2017**, *312*, H289–H304. [CrossRef]
48. Dorn, C.; Riener, M.O.; Kirovski, G.; Saugspier, M.; Steib, K.; Weiss, T.S.; Gabele, E.; Kristiansen, G.; Hartmann, A.; Hellerbrand, C. Expression of fatty acid synthase in nonalcoholic fatty liver disease. *Int. J. Clin. Exp. Pathol.* **2010**, *3*, 505–514.
49. Mitsuyoshi, H.; Yasui, K.; Harano, Y.; Endo, M.; Tsuji, K.; Minami, M.; Itoh, Y.; Okanoue, T.; Yoshikawa, T. Analysis of hepatic genes involved in the metabolism of fatty acids and iron in nonalcoholic fatty liver disease. *Hepatol. Res.* **2009**, *39*, 366–373. [CrossRef]
50. Paglialunga, S.; Dehn, C.A. Clinical assessment of hepatic de novo lipogenesis in non-alcoholic fatty liver disease. *Lipids Health Dis.* **2016**, *15*, 159. [CrossRef]
51. Tappy, L.; Le, K.A. Metabolic effects of fructose and the worldwide increase in obesity. *Physiol. Rev.* **2010**, *90*, 23–46. [CrossRef]
52. Rutledge, A.C.; Adeli, K. Fructose and the metabolic syndrome: Pathophysiology and molecular mechanisms. *Nutr. Rev.* **2007**, *65*, S13–S23. [CrossRef]

53. Stanhope, K.L.; Havel, P.J. Fructose consumption: recent results and their potential implications. *Ann. N. Y. Acad. Sci.* **2010**, *1190*, 15–24. [CrossRef]
54. Malik, V.S.; Hu, F.B. Fructose and Cardiometabolic Health: What the Evidence From Sugar-Sweetened Beverages Tells Us. *J. Am. Coll. Cardiol.* **2015**, *66*, 1615–1624. [CrossRef]
55. Fisher, F.M.; Kim, M.; Doridot, L.; Cunniff, J.C.; Parker, T.S.; Levine, D.M.; Hellerstein, M.K.; Hudgins, L.C.; Maratos-Flier, E.; Herman, M.A. A critical role for ChREBP-mediated FGF21 secretion in hepatic fructose metabolism. *Mol. Metab.* **2017**, *6*, 14–21. [CrossRef]
56. Solinas, G.; Boren, J.; Dulloo, A.G. De novo lipogenesis in metabolic homeostasis: More friend than foe? *Mol. Metab.* **2015**, *4*, 367–377. [CrossRef]
57. Stanhope, K.L. Role of fructose-containing sugars in the epidemics of obesity and metabolic syndrome. *Annu. Rev. Med.* **2012**, *63*, 329–343. [CrossRef]
58. Stanhope, K.L.; Schwarz, J.M.; Keim, N.L.; Griffen, S.C.; Bremer, A.A.; Graham, J.L.; Hatcher, B.; Cox, C.L.; Dyachenko, A.; Zhang, W.; et al. Consuming fructose-sweetened, not glucose-sweetened, beverages increases visceral adiposity and lipids and decreases insulin sensitivity in overweight/obese humans. *J. Clin. Investig.* **2009**, *119*, 1322–1334. [CrossRef]
59. Faeh, D.; Minehira, K.; Schwarz, J.M.; Periasamy, R.; Park, S.; Tappy, L. Effect of fructose overfeeding and fish oil administration on hepatic de novo lipogenesis and insulin sensitivity in healthy men. *Diabetes* **2005**, *54*, 1907–1913. [CrossRef]
60. Stanhope, K.L. More pieces of the fructose puzzle. *J. Intern. Med.* **2017**, *282*, 202–204. [CrossRef]
61. Schwarz, J.M.; Noworolski, S.M.; Erkin-Cakmak, A.; Korn, N.J.; Wen, M.J.; Tai, V.W.; Jones, G.M.; Palii, S.P.; Velasco-Alin, M.; Pan, K.; et al. Effects of Dietary Fructose Restriction on Liver Fat, De Novo Lipogenesis, and Insulin Kinetics in Children With Obesity. *Gastroenterology* **2017**, *153*, 743–752. [CrossRef]
62. Vos, M.B.; Lavine, J.E. Dietary fructose in nonalcoholic fatty liver disease. *Hepatology* **2013**, *57*, 2525–2531. [CrossRef]
63. Jegatheesan, P.; De Bandt, J.P. Fructose and NAFLD: The Multifaceted Aspects of Fructose Metabolism. *Nutrients* **2017**, *9*, 230. [CrossRef]
64. Jensen, T.; Abdelmalek, M.F.; Sullivan, S.; Nadeau, K.J.; Green, M.; Roncal, C.; Nakagawa, T.; Kuwabara, M.; Sato, Y.; Kang, D.H.; et al. Fructose and sugar: A major mediator of non-alcoholic fatty liver disease. *J. Hepatol.* **2018**, *68*, 1063–1075. [CrossRef]
65. Moore, J.B. From sugar to liver fat and public health: Systems biology driven studies in understanding non-alcoholic fatty liver disease pathogenesis. *Proc. Nutr. Soc.* **2019**. [CrossRef]
66. Alexander, M.; Loomis, A.K.; Fairburn-Beech, J.; van der Lei, J.; Duarte-Salles, T.; Prieto-Alhambra, D.; Ansell, D.; Pasqua, A.; Lapi, F.; Rijnbeek, P.; et al. Real-world data reveal a diagnostic gap in non-alcoholic fatty liver disease. *BMC Med.* **2018**, *16*, 130. [CrossRef]
67. Lee, S.S.; Park, S.H.; Kim, H.J.; Kim, S.Y.; Kim, M.Y.; Kim, D.Y.; Suh, D.J.; Kim, K.M.; Bae, M.H.; Lee, J.Y.; et al. Non-invasive assessment of hepatic steatosis: Prospective comparison of the accuracy of imaging examinations. *J. Hepatol.* **2010**, *52*, 579–585. [CrossRef]
68. Reeder, S.B.; Cruite, I.; Hamilton, G.; Sirlin, C.B. Quantitative assessment of liver fat with magnetic resonance imaging and spectroscopy. *J. Magn. Reson. Imaging* **2011**, *34*, 729–749. [CrossRef]
69. Szczepaniak, L.S.; Nurenberg, P.; Leonard, D.; Browning, J.D.; Reingold, J.S.; Grundy, S.; Hobbs, H.H.; Dobbins, R.L. Magnetic resonance spectroscopy to measure hepatic triglyceride content: Prevalence of hepatic steatosis in the general population. *Am. J. Physiol. Endocrinol. Metab.* **2005**, *288*, E462–E468. [CrossRef]
70. van de Weijer, T.; Schrauwen-Hinderling, V.B. Application of Magnetic Resonance Spectroscopy in metabolic research. *Biochim. Biophys. Acta Mol. Basis Dis.* **2019**, *1865*, 741–748. [CrossRef]
71. European Association for the Study of the Liver; European Association for the Study of Diabetes; European Association for the Study of Obesity. EASL-EASD-EASO Clinical Practice Guidelines for the management of non-alcoholic fatty liver disease. *Diabetologia* **2016**, *59*, 1121–1140. [CrossRef]
72. Le, K.A.; Ith, M.; Kreis, R.; Faeh, D.; Bortolotti, M.; Tran, C.; Boesch, C.; Tappy, L. Fructose overconsumption causes dyslipidemia and ectopic lipid deposition in healthy subjects with and without a family history of type 2 diabetes. *Am. J. Clin. Nutr.* **2009**, *89*, 1760–1765. [CrossRef]
73. Sobrecases, H.; Le, K.A.; Bortolotti, M.; Schneiter, P.; Ith, M.; Kreis, R.; Boesch, C.; Tappy, L. Effects of short-term overfeeding with fructose, fat and fructose plus fat on plasma and hepatic lipids in healthy men. *Diabetes Metab.* **2010**, *36*, 244–246. [CrossRef]

74. Lecoultre, V.; Egli, L.; Carrel, G.; Theytaz, F.; Kreis, R.; Schneiter, P.; Boss, A.; Zwygart, K.; Le, K.A.; Bortolotti, M.; et al. Effects of fructose and glucose overfeeding on hepatic insulin sensitivity and intrahepatic lipids in healthy humans. *Obesity (Silver Spring)* **2013**, *21*, 782–785. [CrossRef]
75. Theytaz, F.; Noguchi, Y.; Egli, L.; Campos, V.; Buehler, T.; Hodson, L.; Patterson, B.W.; Nishikata, N.; Kreis, R.; Mittendorfer, B.; et al. Effects of supplementation with essential amino acids on intrahepatic lipid concentrations during fructose overfeeding in humans. *Am. J. Clin. Nutr.* **2012**, *96*, 1008–1016. [CrossRef]
76. Johnston, R.D.; Stephenson, M.C.; Crossland, H.; Cordon, S.M.; Palcidi, E.; Cox, E.F.; Taylor, M.A.; Aithal, G.P.; Macdonald, I.A. No difference between high-fructose and high-glucose diets on liver triacylglycerol or biochemistry in healthy overweight men. *Gastroenterology* **2013**, *145*, 1016–1025. [CrossRef]
77. Surowska, A.; Jegatheesan, P.; Campos, V.; Marques, A.S.; Egli, L.; Cros, J.; Rosset, R.; Lecoultre, V.; Kreis, R.; Boesch, C.; et al. Effects of Dietary Protein and Fat Content on Intrahepatocellular and Intramyocellular Lipids during a 6-Day Hypercaloric, High Sucrose Diet: A Randomized Controlled Trial in Normal Weight Healthy Subjects. *Nutrients* **2019**, *11*, 209. [CrossRef]
78. Schwarz, J.M.; Noworolski, S.M.; Wen, M.J.; Dyachenko, A.; Prior, J.L.; Weinberg, M.E.; Herraiz, L.A.; Tai, V.W.; Bergeron, N.; Bersot, T.P.; et al. Effect of a High-Fructose Weight-Maintaining Diet on Lipogenesis and Liver Fat. *J. Clin. Endocrinol. Metab.* **2015**, *100*, 2434–2442. [CrossRef]
79. Cox, C.L.; Stanhope, K.L.; Schwarz, J.M.; Graham, J.L.; Hatcher, B.; Griffen, S.C.; Bremer, A.A.; Berglund, L.; McGahan, J.P.; Havel, P.J.; et al. Consumption of fructose-sweetened beverages for 10 weeks reduces net fat oxidation and energy expenditure in overweight/obese men and women. *Eur. J. Clin. Nutr.* **2012**, *66*, 201–208. [CrossRef]
80. Maersk, M.; Belza, A.; Stodkilde-Jorgensen, H.; Ringgaard, S.; Chabanova, E.; Thomsen, H.; Pedersen, S.B.; Astrup, A.; Richelsen, B. Sucrose-sweetened beverages increase fat storage in the liver, muscle, and visceral fat depot: A 6-mo randomized intervention study. *Am. J. Clin. Nutr.* **2012**, *95*, 283–289. [CrossRef]
81. Silbernagel, G.; Machann, J.; Unmuth, S.; Schick, F.; Stefan, N.; Haring, H.U.; Fritsche, A. Effects of 4-week very-high-fructose/glucose diets on insulin sensitivity, visceral fat and intrahepatic lipids: An exploratory trial. *Br. J. Nutr.* **2011**, *106*, 79–86. [CrossRef]
82. Chung, M.; Ma, J.; Patel, K.; Berger, S.; Lau, J.; Lichtenstein, A.H. Fructose, high-fructose corn syrup, sucrose, and nonalcoholic fatty liver disease or indexes of liver health: A systematic review and meta-analysis. *Am. J. Clin. Nutr.* **2014**, *100*, 833–849. [CrossRef]
83. Chiu, S.; Sievenpiper, J.L.; de Souza, R.J.; Cozma, A.I.; Mirrahimi, A.; Carleton, A.J.; Ha, V.; Di Buono, M.; Jenkins, A.L.; Leiter, L.A.; et al. Effect of fructose on markers of non-alcoholic fatty liver disease (NAFLD): a systematic review and meta-analysis of controlled feeding trials. *Eur. J. Clin. Nutr.* **2014**, *68*, 416–423. [CrossRef]
84. Ma, J.; Fox, C.S.; Jacques, P.F.; Speliotes, E.K.; Hoffmann, U.; Smith, C.E.; Saltzman, E.; McKeown, N.M. Sugar-sweetened beverage, diet soda, and fatty liver disease in the Framingham Heart Study cohorts. *J. Hepatol.* **2015**, *63*, 462–469. [CrossRef]
85. Sevastianova, K.; Santos, A.; Kotronen, A.; Hakkarainen, A.; Makkonen, J.; Silander, K.; Peltonen, M.; Romeo, S.; Lundbom, J.; Lundbom, N.; et al. Effect of short-term carbohydrate overfeeding and long-term weight loss on liver fat in overweight humans. *Am. J. Clin. Nutr.* **2012**, *96*, 727–734. [CrossRef]
86. Luukkonen, P.K.; Sadevirta, S.; Zhou, Y.; Kayser, B.; Ali, A.; Ahonen, L.; Lallukka, S.; Pelloux, V.; Gaggini, M.; Jian, C.; et al. Saturated Fat Is More Metabolically Harmful for the Human Liver Than Unsaturated Fat or Simple Sugars. *Diabetes Care* **2018**, *41*, 1732–1739. [CrossRef]
87. Gugliucci, A.; Lustig, R.H.; Caccavello, R.; Erkin-Cakmak, A.; Noworolski, S.M.; Tai, V.W.; Wen, M.J.; Mulligan, K.; Schwarz, J.M. Short-term isocaloric fructose restriction lowers apoC-III levels and yields less atherogenic lipoprotein profiles in children with obesity and metabolic syndrome. *Atherosclerosis* **2016**, *253*, 171–177. [CrossRef]
88. Erkin-Cakmak, A.; Bains, Y.; Caccavello, R.; Noworolski, S.M.; Schwarz, J.M.; Mulligan, K.; Lustig, R.H.; Gugliucci, A. Isocaloric Fructose Restriction Reduces Serum d-Lactate Concentration in Children With Obesity and Metabolic Syndrome. *J. Clin. Endocrinol. Metab.* **2019**, *104*, 3003–3011. [CrossRef]
89. Lee, O.; Bruce, W.R.; Dong, Q.; Bruce, J.; Mehta, R.; O'Brien, P.J. Fructose and carbonyl metabolites as endogenous toxins. *Chem. Biol. Interact.* **2009**, *178*, 332–339. [CrossRef]

90. Pickens, M.K.; Yan, J.S.; Ng, R.K.; Ogata, H.; Grenert, J.P.; Beysen, C.; Turner, S.M.; Maher, J.J. Dietary sucrose is essential to the development of liver injury in the methionine-choline-deficient model of steatohepatitis. *J. Lipid Res.* **2009**, *50*, 2072–2082. [CrossRef]
91. Masania, J.; Malczewska-Malec, M.; Razny, U.; Goralska, J.; Zdzienicka, A.; Kiec-Wilk, B.; Gruca, A.; Stancel-Mozwillo, J.; Dembinska-Kiec, A.; Rabbani, N.; et al. Dicarbonyl stress in clinical obesity. *Glycoconj. J.* **2016**, *33*, 581–589. [CrossRef] [PubMed]
92. Asgari-Taee, F.; Zerafati-Shoae, N.; Dehghani, M.; Sadeghi, M.; Baradaran, H.R.; Jazayeri, S. Association of sugar sweetened beverages consumption with non-alcoholic fatty liver disease: A systematic review and meta-analysis. *Eur. J. Nutr.* **2018**. [CrossRef] [PubMed]
93. Ter Horst, K.W.; Serlie, M.J. Fructose Consumption, Lipogenesis, and Non-Alcoholic Fatty Liver Disease. *Nutrients* **2017**, *9*, 981. [CrossRef] [PubMed]
94. Kirk, E.; Reeds, D.N.; Finck, B.N.; Mayurranjan, S.M.; Patterson, B.W.; Klein, S. Dietary fat and carbohydrates differentially alter insulin sensitivity during caloric restriction. *Gastroenterology* **2009**, *136*, 1552–1560. [CrossRef] [PubMed]
95. Haufe, S.; Engeli, S.; Kast, P.; Bohnke, J.; Utz, W.; Haas, V.; Hermsdorf, M.; Mahler, A.; Wiesner, S.; Birkenfeld, A.L.; et al. Randomized comparison of reduced fat and reduced carbohydrate hypocaloric diets on intrahepatic fat in overweight and obese human subjects. *Hepatology* **2011**, *53*, 1504–1514. [CrossRef] [PubMed]
96. Perheentupa, J.; Raivio, K. Fructose-induced hyperuricaemia. *Lancet* **1967**, *2*, 528–531. [CrossRef]
97. Sozen, E.; Ozer, N.K. Impact of high cholesterol and endoplasmic reticulum stress on metabolic diseases: An updated mini-review. *Redox Biol.* **2017**, *12*, 456–461. [CrossRef] [PubMed]
98. Lebeaupin, C.; Vallee, D.; Hazari, Y.; Hetz, C.; Chevet, E.; Bailly-Maitre, B. Endoplasmic reticulum stress signalling and the pathogenesis of non-alcoholic fatty liver disease. *J. Hepatol.* **2018**, *69*, 927–947. [CrossRef]
99. Henkel, A.; Green, R.M. The unfolded protein response in fatty liver disease. *Semin. Liver Dis.* **2013**, *33*, 321–329. [CrossRef]
100. Lee, A.H.; Scapa, E.F.; Cohen, D.E.; Glimcher, L.H. Regulation of hepatic lipogenesis by the transcription factor XBP1. *Science* **2008**, *320*, 1492–1496. [CrossRef]
101. Lanaspa, M.A.; Sanchez-Lozada, L.G.; Choi, Y.J.; Cicerchi, C.; Kanbay, M.; Roncal-Jimenez, C.A.; Ishimoto, T.; Li, N.; Marek, G.; Duranay, M.; et al. Uric acid induces hepatic steatosis by generation of mitochondrial oxidative stress: Potential role in fructose-dependent and -independent fatty liver. *J. Biol. Chem.* **2012**, *287*, 40732–40744. [CrossRef] [PubMed]
102. Abdelmalek, M.F.; Lazo, M.; Horska, A.; Bonekamp, S.; Lipkin, E.W.; Balasubramanyam, A.; Bantle, J.P.; Johnson, R.J.; Diehl, A.M.; Clark, J.M.; et al. Higher dietary fructose is associated with impaired hepatic adenosine triphosphate homeostasis in obese individuals with type 2 diabetes. *Hepatology* **2012**, *56*, 952–960. [CrossRef] [PubMed]
103. Satapati, S.; Kucejova, B.; Duarte, J.A.; Fletcher, J.A.; Reynolds, L.; Sunny, N.E.; He, T.; Nair, L.A.; Livingston, K.A.; Fu, X.; et al. Mitochondrial metabolism mediates oxidative stress and inflammation in fatty liver. *J. Clin. Investig.* **2015**, *125*, 4447–4462. [CrossRef] [PubMed]
104. Softic, S.; Gupta, M.K.; Wang, G.X.; Fujisaka, S.; O'Neill, B.T.; Rao, T.N.; Willoughby, J.; Harbison, C.; Fitzgerald, K.; Ilkayeva, O.; et al. Divergent effects of glucose and fructose on hepatic lipogenesis and insulin signaling. *J. Clin. Investig.* **2017**, *127*, 4059–4074. [CrossRef] [PubMed]
105. Facchini, F.; Chen, Y.D.; Hollenbeck, C.B.; Reaven, G.M. Relationship between resistance to insulin-mediated glucose uptake, urinary uric acid clearance, and plasma uric acid concentration. *JAMA* **1991**, *266*, 3008–3011. [CrossRef] [PubMed]
106. Choi, H.K.; Ford, E.S. Prevalence of the metabolic syndrome in individuals with hyperuricemia. *Am. J. Med.* **2007**, *120*, 442–447. [CrossRef]
107. Yu, T.Y.; Jee, J.H.; Bae, J.C.; Jin, S.M.; Baek, J.H.; Lee, M.K.; Kim, J.H. Serum uric acid: A strong and independent predictor of metabolic syndrome after adjusting for body composition. *Metabolism* **2016**, *65*, 432–440. [CrossRef]
108. Lee, Y.J.; Cho, S.; Kim, S.R. A possible role of serum uric acid as a marker of metabolic syndrome. *Intern. Med. J.* **2014**, *44*, 1210–1216. [CrossRef]
109. Sun, H.L.; Pei, D.; Lue, K.H.; Chen, Y.L. Uric Acid Levels Can Predict Metabolic Syndrome and Hypertension in Adolescents: A 10-Year Longitudinal Study. *PLoS ONE* **2015**, *10*, e0143786. [CrossRef]

110. Johnson, R.J.; Nakagawa, T.; Sanchez-Lozada, L.G.; Shafiu, M.; Sundaram, S.; Le, M.; Ishimoto, T.; Sautin, Y.Y.; Lanaspa, M.A. Sugar, uric acid, and the etiology of diabetes and obesity. *Diabetes* **2013**, *62*, 3307–3315. [CrossRef]
111. Zurlo, A.; Veronese, N.; Giantin, V.; Maselli, M.; Zambon, S.; Maggi, S.; Musacchio, E.; Toffanello, E.D.; Sartori, L.; Perissinotto, E.; et al. High serum uric acid levels increase the risk of metabolic syndrome in elderly women: The PRO.V.A study. *Nutr. Metab. Cardiovasc. Dis.* **2016**, *26*, 27–35. [CrossRef] [PubMed]
112. Babio, N.; Martinez-Gonzalez, M.A.; Estruch, R.; Warnberg, J.; Recondo, J.; Ortega-Calvo, M.; Serra-Majem, L.; Corella, D.; Fito, M.; Ros, E.; et al. Associations between serum uric acid concentrations and metabolic syndrome and its components in the PREDIMED study. *Nutr. Metab. Cardiovasc. Dis.* **2015**, *25*, 173–180. [CrossRef] [PubMed]
113. Yuan, H.; Yu, C.; Li, X.; Sun, L.; Zhu, X.; Zhao, C.; Zhang, Z.; Yang, Z. Serum Uric Acid Levels and Risk of Metabolic Syndrome: A Dose-Response Meta-Analysis of Prospective Studies. *J. Clin. Endocrinol. Metab.* **2015**, *100*, 4198–4207. [CrossRef] [PubMed]
114. Ouyang, X.; Cirillo, P.; Sautin, Y.; McCall, S.; Bruchette, J.L.; Diehl, A.M.; Johnson, R.J.; Abdelmalek, M.F. Fructose consumption as a risk factor for non-alcoholic fatty liver disease. *J. Hepatol.* **2008**, *48*, 993–999. [CrossRef] [PubMed]
115. Zhang, S.; Du, T.; Li, M.; Lu, H.; Lin, X.; Yu, X. Combined effect of obesity and uric acid on nonalcoholic fatty liver disease and hypertriglyceridemia. *Medicine (Baltimore)* **2017**, *96*, e6381. [CrossRef] [PubMed]
116. Liu, Z.; Que, S.; Zhou, L.; Zheng, S. Dose-response Relationship of Serum Uric Acid with Metabolic Syndrome and Non-alcoholic Fatty Liver Disease Incidence: A Meta-analysis of Prospective Studies. *Sci. Rep.* **2015**, *5*, 14325. [CrossRef] [PubMed]
117. Yang, C.; Yang, S.; Xu, W.; Zhang, J.; Fu, W.; Feng, C. Association between the hyperuricemia and nonalcoholic fatty liver disease risk in a Chinese population: A retrospective cohort study. *PLoS ONE* **2017**, *12*, e0177249. [CrossRef]
118. Lee, J.W.; Cho, Y.K.; Ryan, M.; Kim, H.; Lee, S.W.; Chang, E.; Joo, K.J.; Kim, J.T.; Kim, B.S.; Sung, K.C. Serum uric Acid as a predictor for the development of nonalcoholic Fatty liver disease in apparently healthy subjects: A 5-year retrospective cohort study. *Gut Liver* **2010**, *4*, 378–383. [CrossRef]
119. Lonardo, A.; Loria, P.; Leonardi, F.; Borsatti, A.; Neri, P.; Pulvirenti, M.; Verrone, A.M.; Bagni, A.; Bertolotti, M.; Ganazzi, D.; et al. Fasting insulin and uric acid levels but not indices of iron metabolism are independent predictors of non-alcoholic fatty liver disease. A case-control study. *Dig. Liver Dis.* **2002**, *34*, 204–211. [CrossRef]
120. Sirota, J.C.; McFann, K.; Targher, G.; Johnson, R.J.; Chonchol, M.; Jalal, D.I. Elevated serum uric acid levels are associated with non-alcoholic fatty liver disease independently of metabolic syndrome features in the United States: Liver ultrasound data from the National Health and Nutrition Examination Survey. *Metabolism* **2013**, *62*, 392–399. [CrossRef]
121. Li, Y.; Xu, C.; Yu, C.; Xu, L.; Miao, M. Association of serum uric acid level with non-alcoholic fatty liver disease: A cross-sectional study. *J. Hepatol.* **2009**, *50*, 1029–1034. [CrossRef] [PubMed]
122. Xu, C.; Yu, C.; Xu, L.; Miao, M.; Li, Y. High serum uric acid increases the risk for nonalcoholic Fatty liver disease: A prospective observational study. *PLoS ONE* **2010**, *5*, e11578. [CrossRef] [PubMed]
123. Choi, H.K.; Curhan, G. Soft drinks, fructose consumption, and the risk of gout in men: Prospective cohort study. *BMJ* **2008**, *336*, 309–312. [CrossRef] [PubMed]
124. Choi, H.K.; Willett, W.; Curhan, G. Fructose-rich beverages and risk of gout in women. *JAMA* **2010**, *304*, 2270–2278. [CrossRef] [PubMed]
125. Bae, J.; Chun, B.Y.; Park, P.S.; Choi, B.Y.; Kim, M.K.; Shin, M.H.; Lee, Y.H.; Shin, D.H.; Kim, S.K. Higher consumption of sugar-sweetened soft drinks increases the risk of hyperuricemia in Korean population: The Korean Multi-Rural Communities Cohort Study. *Semin. Arthritis Rheum.* **2014**, *43*, 654–661. [CrossRef] [PubMed]
126. Meneses-Leon, J.; Denova-Gutierrez, E.; Castanon-Robles, S.; Granados-Garcia, V.; Talavera, J.O.; Rivera-Paredez, B.; Huitron-Bravo, G.G.; Cervantes-Rodriguez, M.; Quiterio-Trenado, M.; Rudolph, S.E.; et al. Sweetened beverage consumption and the risk of hyperuricemia in Mexican adults: A cross-sectional study. *BMC Public Health* **2014**, *14*, 445. [CrossRef] [PubMed]
127. Siqueira, J.H.; Mill, J.G.; Velasquez-Melendez, G.; Moreira, A.D.; Barreto, S.M.; Bensenor, I.M.; Molina, M. Sugar-Sweetened Soft Drinks and Fructose Consumption Are Associated with Hyperuricemia: Cross-Sectional Analysis from the Brazilian Longitudinal Study of Adult Health (ELSA-Brasil). *Nutrients* **2018**, *10*, 981. [CrossRef]

128. Nguyen, S.; Choi, H.K.; Lustig, R.H.; Hsu, C.Y. Sugar-sweetened beverages, serum uric acid, and blood pressure in adolescents. *J. Pediatr.* **2009**, *154*, 807–813. [CrossRef]
129. Ngo Sock, E.T.; Le, K.A.; Ith, M.; Kreis, R.; Boesch, C.; Tappy, L. Effects of a short-term overfeeding with fructose or glucose in healthy young males. *Br. J. Nutr.* **2010**, *103*, 939–943. [CrossRef]
130. Cox, C.L.; Stanhope, K.L.; Schwarz, J.M.; Graham, J.L.; Hatcher, B.; Griffen, S.C.; Bremer, A.A.; Berglund, L.; McGahan, J.P.; Keim, N.L.; et al. Consumption of fructose- but not glucose-sweetened beverages for 10 weeks increases circulating concentrations of uric acid, retinol binding protein-4, and gamma-glutamyl transferase activity in overweight/obese humans. *Nutr. Metab. (Lond.)* **2012**, *9*, 68. [CrossRef]
131. Wang, D.D.; Sievenpiper, J.L.; de Souza, R.J.; Chiavaroli, L.; Ha, V.; Cozma, A.I.; Mirrahimi, A.; Yu, M.E.; Carleton, A.J.; Di Buono, M.; et al. The effects of fructose intake on serum uric acid vary among controlled dietary trials. *J. Nutr.* **2012**, *142*, 916–923. [CrossRef]
132. Tappy, L.; Morio, B.; Azzout-Marniche, D.; Champ, M.; Gerber, M.; Houdart, S.; Mas, E.; Rizkalla, S.; Slama, G.; Mariotti, F.; et al. French Recommendations for Sugar Intake in Adults: A Novel Approach Chosen by ANSES. *Nutrients* **2018**, *10*, 989. [CrossRef] [PubMed]
133. Caliceti, C.; Calabria, D.; Roda, A.; Cicero, A.F.G. Fructose Intake, Serum Uric Acid, and Cardiometabolic Disorders: A Critical Review. *Nutrients* **2017**, *9*, 395. [CrossRef] [PubMed]
134. Kanbay, M.; Jensen, T.; Solak, Y.; Le, M.; Roncal-Jimenez, C.; Rivard, C.; Lanaspa, M.A.; Nakagawa, T.; Johnson, R.J. Uric acid in metabolic syndrome: From an innocent bystander to a central player. *Eur. J. Intern. Med.* **2016**, *29*, 3–8. [CrossRef] [PubMed]
135. Welsh, J.A.; Sharma, A.; Abramson, J.L.; Vaccarino, V.; Gillespie, C.; Vos, M.B. Caloric sweetener consumption and dyslipidemia among US adults. *JAMA* **2010**, *303*, 1490–1497. [CrossRef] [PubMed]
136. Dhingra, R.; Sullivan, L.; Jacques, P.F.; Wang, T.J.; Fox, C.S.; Meigs, J.B.; D'Agostino, R.B.; Gaziano, J.M.; Vasan, R.S. Soft drink consumption and risk of developing cardiometabolic risk factors and the metabolic syndrome in middle-aged adults in the community. *Circulation* **2007**, *116*, 480–488. [CrossRef] [PubMed]
137. Livesey, G.; Taylor, R. Fructose consumption and consequences for glycation, plasma triacylglycerol, and body weight: Meta-analyses and meta-regression models of intervention studies. *Am. J. Clin. Nutr.* **2008**, *88*, 1419–1437. [CrossRef] [PubMed]
138. Adiels, M.; Taskinen, M.R.; Bjornson, E.; Andersson, L.; Matikainen, N.; Soderlund, S.; Kahri, J.; Hakkarainen, A.; Lundbom, N.; Sihlbom, C.; et al. Role of apolipoprotein C-III overproduction in diabetic dyslipidaemia. *Diabetes Obes. Metab.* **2019**. [CrossRef]
139. Taskinen, M.R.; Boren, J. Why Is Apolipoprotein CIII Emerging as a Novel Therapeutic Target to Reduce the Burden of Cardiovascular Disease? *Curr. Atheroscler. Rep.* **2016**, *18*, 59. [CrossRef]
140. Borén, J.; Watts, G.F.; Adiels, M.; Söderlund, S.; Chan, D.C.; Hakkarainen, A.; Lundbom, N.; Matikainen, N.; Kahri, J.; Vergès, B.; et al. Kinetic and Related Determinants of Plasma Triglyceride Concentration in Abdominal Obesity. Multicenter Tracer Kinetic Study. *Arterioscler. Thromb. Vasc. Biol.* **2015**, *35*, 2218–2224. [CrossRef] [PubMed]
141. Stanhope, K.L.; Medici, V.; Bremer, A.A.; Lee, V.; Lam, H.D.; Nunez, M.V.; Chen, G.X.; Keim, N.L.; Havel, P.J. A dose-response study of consuming high-fructose corn syrup-sweetened beverages on lipid/lipoprotein risk factors for cardiovascular disease in young adults. *Am. J. Clin. Nutr.* **2015**, *101*, 1144–1154. [CrossRef]
142. Lambertz, J.; Weiskirchen, S.; Landert, S.; Weiskirchen, R. Fructose: A Dietary Sugar in Crosstalk with Microbiota Contributing to the Development and Progression of Non-Alcoholic Liver Disease. *Front. Immunol.* **2017**, *8*, 1159. [CrossRef] [PubMed]
143. den Besten, G.; Lange, K.; Havinga, R.; van Dijk, T.H.; Gerding, A.; van Eunen, K.; Muller, M.; Groen, A.K.; Hooiveld, G.J.; Bakker, B.M.; et al. Gut-derived short-chain fatty acids are vividly assimilated into host carbohydrates and lipids. *Am. J. Physiol Gastrointest. Liver Physiol.* **2013**, *305*, G900–G910. [CrossRef] [PubMed]
144. Mouzaki, M.; Comelli, E.M.; Arendt, B.M.; Bonengel, J.; Fung, S.K.; Fischer, S.E.; McGilvray, I.D.; Allard, J.P. Intestinal microbiota in patients with nonalcoholic fatty liver disease. *Hepatology* **2013**, *58*, 120–127. [CrossRef] [PubMed]
145. Jegatheesan, P.; Beutheu, S.; Ventura, G.; Sarfati, G.; Nubret, E.; Kapel, N.; Waligora-Dupriet, A.J.; Bergheim, I.; Cynober, L.; De-Bandt, J.P. Effect of specific amino acids on hepatic lipid metabolism in fructose-induced non-alcoholic fatty liver disease. *Clin. Nutr.* **2016**, *35*, 175–182. [CrossRef] [PubMed]

146. Oh, J.H.; Alexander, L.M.; Pan, M.; Schueler, K.L.; Keller, M.P.; Attie, A.D.; Walter, J.; van Pijkeren, J.P. Dietary Fructose and Microbiota-Derived Short-Chain Fatty Acids Promote Bacteriophage Production in the Gut Symbiont Lactobacillus reuteri. *Cell Host Microbe* **2019**, *25*, 273–284. [CrossRef] [PubMed]
147. Chatterjee, A.; Duerkop, B.A. Sugar and Fatty Acids Ack-celerate Prophage Induction. *Cell Host Microbe* **2019**, *25*, 175–176. [CrossRef]
148. Mardinoglu, A.; Wu, H.; Bjornson, E.; Zhang, C.; Hakkarainen, A.; Rasanen, S.M.; Lee, S.; Mancina, R.M.; Bergentall, M.; Pietilainen, K.H.; et al. An Integrated Understanding of the Rapid Metabolic Benefits of a Carbohydrate-Restricted Diet on Hepatic Steatosis in Humans. *Cell Metab.* **2018**, *27*, 559–571. [CrossRef]

16

Associations Between Dietary Protein Sources, Plasma BCAA and Short-Chain Acylcarnitine Levels in Adults

Michèle Rousseau [1,2], Frédéric Guénard [1,2], Véronique Garneau [1,2], Bénédicte Allam-Ndoul [1,2], Simone Lemieux [1,2], Louis Pérusse [1,3] and Marie-Claude Vohl [1,2,*]

1 Institute of Nutrition and Functional Foods (INAF), Laval University, Quebec City, QC G1V 0A6, Canada; michele.rousseau.1@ulaval.ca (M.R.); frederic.guenard@fsaa.ulaval.ca (F.G.); veronique.garneau@fsaa.ulaval.ca (V.G.); benedicte.allam-ndoul@criucpq.ulaval.ca (B.A.-N.); simone.lemieux@fsaa.ulaval.ca (S.L.); louis.perusse@kin.ulaval.ca (L.P.)
2 School of Nutrition, Laval University, Quebec City, QC G1V 0A6, Canada
3 Department of Kinesiology, Laval University, Quebec City, QC G1V 0A6, Canada
* Correspondence: marie-claude.vohl@fsaa.ulaval.ca

Abstract: Elevated plasma branched-chain amino acids (BCAA) and C3 and C5 acylcarnitines (AC) levels observed in individuals with insulin resistance (IR) might be influenced by dietary protein intakes. This study explores the associations between dietary protein sources, plasma BCAA levels and C3 and C5 ACs in normal weight (NW) or overweight (OW) individuals with or without metabolic syndrome (MS). Data from 199 men and women aged 18–55 years with complete metabolite profile were analyzed. Associations between metabolic parameters, protein sources, plasma BCAA and AC levels were tested. OW/MS+ consumed significantly more animal protein ($p = 0.0388$) and had higher plasma BCAA levels ($p < 0.0001$) than OW/MS− or NW/MS− individuals. Plasma BCAA levels were not associated with BCAA intakes in the whole cohort, while there was a trend for an association between plasma BCAA levels and red meat or with animal protein in OW/MS+. These associations were of weak magnitude. In NW/MS− individuals, the protein sources associated with BCAA levels varied greatly with adjustment for confounders. Plasma C3 and C5 ACs were associated with plasma BCAA levels in the whole cohort ($p < 0.0001$) and in subgroups based on OW and MS status. These results suggest a modest association of meat or animal protein intakes and an association of C3 and C5 ACs with plasma BCAA levels, obesity and MS.

Keywords: branched-chain amino acids; acylcarnitines; dietary protein sources; meat; metabolic syndrome; metabolite profiling; diet

---

1. Introduction

Branched-chain amino acids (BCAA) are comprised of leucine, isoleucine and valine [1]. Their plasma levels have been positively associated with features of the metabolic syndrome (MS), such as insulin resistance (IR) and pre-diabetes [2,3], and thus with an increased risk of type 2 diabetes (T2D) and cardiovascular diseases (CVD) [4–8]. Controversies still remain on whether an increase in plasma BCAA levels is a cause or a consequence of IR. The latter is the most strongly supported hypothesis [9,10], since plasma BCAAs elevation could be the result of an impaired metabolism caused by the decreased gene expression of BCAA aminotransferase (*BCAT*) and branched-chain a-keto acid dehydrogenase (*BCKD*), as seen in mice models [11].

Most dietary BCAAs are metabolized in the skeletal muscle after passing through systemic circulation, whereas other amino acids (AA) are metabolized in the liver [12–15]. This reinforces the potential impact of BCAAs on circulating metabolites, hormones or nutrients [15]. Some studies also relate the increase of plasma BCAAs to the amount or the type (animal or vegetal) of protein ingested [16,17]. Moreover, diets high in red meat [18], animal protein or BCAAs [8,19,20] are associated with an increased risk of T2D in contrast to diets high in vegetal protein, which appears to be associated with a lower risk of T2D [19,20]. In addition, acylcarnitines (AC), a by-product of incomplete mitochondrial fatty acid oxidation, are acyl esters of carnitine that can also result from the degradation of other compounds, such as BCAAs into C3 and C5 ACs [21]. More specifically, isoleucine and leucine catabolism generate 2-methylbutyryl-CoA and isovaleryl-CoA, which will transfer their acyl group to carnitine to form C5 ACs. Isoleucine and valine catabolism will generate propionyl-CoA to be incorporated into C3 ACs [22,23]. These short-chain ACs have previously been associated with IR [21,22] along with western-type dietary habits [24], and are considered as a potential marker of animal products and meat consumption [25].

Changes in plasma BCAA levels according to dietary profiles and dietary protein intakes have been investigated. While higher BCAA intakes have been related to plasma BCAA levels in some studies [16,26], others found no or an inverse association between these two factors [27–29]. One possible explanation for this discrepancy may be related to the source of protein, either animal or vegetal [4]. Protein source might also influence the relationship between plasma BCAA levels and IR. Accordingly, red meat, poultry, fish and whole milk were reported to be the main sources of dietary BCAAs in the US [8] and UK [28] populations, two countries for which a positive association between IR and plasma BCAAs has been reported. An association between IR and plasma BCAAs have also been observed in population from Brazil where red meat, poultry, bread, rice and beans were the principal dietary sources of BCAAs [30]. In contrast, cereal, potatoes and starches, followed by fish, shellfish and finally meats were the main sources of BCAAs in a Japanese cohort where an inverse relationship between BCAA intakes and T2D risk was observed, but only in women [29]. However, up to now, no study has explored the associations between the principal dietary sources of protein and plasma BCAAs, as well as its association with C3 and C5 AC levels in one single cohort.

As such, the main objective of this study was to investigate the relationship between dietary protein source—either animal or vegetal—intakes and fasting plasma BCAA levels in adults with diverse BMI and obesity-associated metabolic perturbations. The second objective was to describe the association between plasma BCAA levels and C3 and C5 AC levels in the same subgroups according to overweight (OW) MS status. We found plasma BCAA levels to be associated with animal protein consumption, with red meat being the main source of proteins that correlates in OW/MS+ individuals. C3 and C5 plasma concentrations were also associated with plasma BCAA levels in the whole cohort, and by subgroups defined on the basis of BMI and the metabolic status.

2. Materials and Methods

2.1. Study Population

INFOGENE is a cross-sectional study investigating the familial history of obesity [31–33]. The recruitment took place in the Quebec City metropolitan area between May 2004 and March 2007 via advertisements in local newspaper and radio stations. Electronic group messages were also sent to university and hospital employees. In the first period of recruitment, only normal weight (NW) individuals were accepted while in the second phase, only OW individuals were recruited. No other criteria of exclusion were applied. After a phone interview where a trained research assistant asked the participants to report their weight and height, eligible individuals were given an appointment at the clinical investigation unit. At this appointment, anthropometric measurements were taken, and participants had to complete a food frequency questionnaire (FFQ), as well as other questionnaires assessing socio-demographic level and lifestyle habits. Individuals who were homeless (1), pregnant (1), older than 55 years (1), had acquired immune deficiency syndrome (AIDS) (1), total energy intakes greater than 4 SD (4), fibre intakes greater than 4 SD (1) or who reported unreliable data (1), were excluded. The final sample consisted of 664 adults—of which 245 men and 372 women—aged 18 to 55 years who gave their written consent to participate. Of those individuals [34], 100 men and 100 women were randomly selected for metabolic profiling of their blood samples [35]. One individual missing biochemical information was excluded from the following analyses. This study has been approved by the Université Laval Ethics Committee.

2.2. Dietary Assessment and Food Grouping

Dietary intakes over the past month were assessed using a 91-item FFQ administered by a registered dietitian. This FFQ was previously validated in French Canadian men and women, and was structured to reflect nutritional habits of the Quebec population [36]. Nutritional intakes were evaluated using the Nutrition Data System for Research (NDS-R) software version 4.03 (Nutrition Coordination Center, Minneapolis, MN, USA). For each item in the FFQ, participants were asked to report their consumption either in days, weeks or months. Many portion size examples were provided for a better estimation of the consumption. Thirty-seven food groups were made, based on the nutrient profile of each item or on its culinary usage. Some groups consisted of only one food (e.g., eggs or beer) because of their particular composition. Twelve groups typically providing most of the dietary proteins in Canada were kept for the current analysis [37]. These are red meat, processed meat, organ meat, fish and other seafood, poultry, eggs, reduced or low-fat dairy products, regular or high-fat dairy products, legumes, nuts, refined grain products and whole grains products. Total animal protein and total vegetal protein (in grams) were also available from the database by calculating the sum of each food sources and mixed dishes. Nutritional information from foods missing in the database was derived from nutritional food labels and entered manually.

2.3. Anthropometric Measurements

Participants were asked to wear light indoor clothes on the day of their appointment. All measurements were made by a trained research assistant. Weight and height were measured using a beam scale with rod graduated in centimetres (Detecto, Webb City, MO USA). Weight was measured to the nearest 0.1 kg and height was measured to the nearest 0.5 cm. Body mass index (BMI) was computed as weight in kilograms divided by height in meters squared (kg/m^2). OW was defined as having BMI over 25 kg/m^2 while individuals with a BMI below 25 kg/m^2 were defined as having a NW. Waist (WC) and hip circumferences were measured according to the procedures recommended by the Airlie Conference [38]. For the measure of systolic (SBP) and diastolic blood pressure (DBP), participants were asked to sit straight with arms and legs uncrossed. The measures were taken after a 5-minute rest.

2.4. Biochemical Parameters

Blood samples were collected from an antecubital vein into vacutainer tubes containing EDTA after a 12-h overnight fast. Blood samples were immediately centrifuged. Total cholesterol (total-C) and triglyceride (TG) concentrations were determined from plasma and lipoprotein fractions using the Olympus AU400e system (Olympus America Inc., Melville, NY, USA). A precipitation of low-density lipoprotein cholesterol (LDL-C) fraction in the infranatant with heparin-manganese chloride was used to obtain the high-density lipoprotein cholesterol (HDL-C) fraction. LDL-C concentrations were estimated using the Friedewald's equation [39]. Radioimmunoassay with polyethylene glycol separation was used to measure fasting insulin. Fasting glucose concentrations were enzymatically measured. Homeostasis model assessment of IR (HOMA-IR) was obtained using (fasting glucose $\times$ fasting insulin)/22.5. MS was defined as having three or more of the following risk factors: WC >88 cm for women and 102 cm for men, fasting plasma TG $\geq$1.7 mmol/L, HDL-C levels $\leq$1.29 mmol/L for women and 1.03 mmol/L for men, glucose levels $\geq$5.6 mmol/L and resting SBP/DBP $\geq$130/85 mmHg. Participants taking medication for lipidemia, diabetes or hypertension control were considered as having abnormal values for their respective parameters.

2.5. Metabolite Profiling

As previously described [35], the Absolute ID p180 Kit (Biocrates Life Sciences AG, Innsbruck, Australia) for mass spectrometry was used for the metabolic profiling measurements for two-hundred participants. Ninety-five metabolites were quantified. They include: 67 Glycerophospholipids (GPs), 12 AC, 10 Sphingolipids (SGs) and 6 AAs. For GPs, ACs and SGs x:y notation was used, x denoting the number of carbons in the side chain and y the number of double bonds. All metabolite concentrations are presented in μM. A metabolite would have been excluded if more than half of the values obtained were below the limit of detection or with standard out of range.

2.6. Statistical Analyses

Variables not normally distributed were transformed using $\log_{10}$ (TG, HDL-C, insulin, animal protein, processed meat, eggs, low-fat dairy), square root (legumes) or inverse transformation (nuts). Organ meat intakes were still not normally distributed after transformation and were then used as a categorical variable (eater or non-eater of organ meat). BCAA dietary intakes or plasma levels were defined as the sum of valine, leucine and isoleucine respectively calculated in FFQ or following plasma metabolite profiling. The General Linear Model (GLM) procedure with the type-III sum of squares was used to assess the association between plasma BCAA levels and age, sex, BMI, WC, BCAA intakes, energy from proteins and total energy intakes. Different models were computed to further assess the associations between plasma BCAA levels, vegetal protein and animal protein and their constituents, as well as to take into account adjustments for total daily energy intakes, age and sex. Associations between different protein sources, as well as BCAA intakes and plasma BCAA levels, were tested with and without adjustments for confounding factors. The associations between ACs levels and plasma BCAA levels were finally assessed. The same models were tested when subdividing study participants based on OW status and the absence/presence of MS (MS−/MS+). Four groups were consequently created: NW/MS−, NW/MS+, OW/MS− and OW/MS+. The NW/MS+ group was excluded from dietary, BCAAs and ACs analyses since this group was composed of only one woman and one man. The GLM procedure was also used to compare mean intakes between groups. All data analyses were performed using SAS statistical software University edition (SAS Institute Inc, Cary, NC, USA). A p-value < 0.05 was considered as statistically significant.

3. Results

3.1. Study Population

Characteristics of study participants are presented in Table 1. Mean values for the four groups are presented. Mean age of participants was 34.2 years and 49.7% of them were women. There were significant differences between groups for all anthropometric and metabolic parameters except for men/women proportions and LDL-C levels. OW individuals were older and had higher BMI, WC, total-C, TG, insulin, SBP and DBP, as well as lower HDL-C than NW/MS− subjects.

3.2. Dietary Intakes

As shown in Table 2, mean daily protein intakes were 104.2 g, which represents 16.8% of total daily energy intakes. Proteins were mainly provided by animal-based foods, with a mean intake of 70.5g versus 32.0g from plant-based sources. There were some differences between groups for total energy (p = 0.0172), total carbohydrates (p = 0.0446), % of kcal from carbohydrates (p = 0.0340), total protein (p = 0.0303), animal protein (p = 0.0086), BCAA intakes (0.0310), total fat (p = 0.0102), total SFA (p = 0.0173), total monounsaturated fatty acids (MUFA) (p = 0.0131) and total polyunsaturated fatty acids (PUFA) (p = 0.0347) intakes. These differences were no longer significant after adjustments for age, sex and energy intake except for significantly greater animal protein intakes in both OW groups (p = 0.0388). Table 3 presents mean intakes, expressed in portions/day, of the food subgroups providing most dietary proteins. OW individuals either MS- or MS+ consumed less fish (p = 0.0106) and more eggs (p = 0.0166) than NW/MS− individuals, but the difference in eggs consumption did not remain significant after adjustments for age, sex and total energy intake. OW/MS+ also consumed more red meat ($p = 0.0027$) and this was still observed, but only as a trend, after adjustments for age, sex and total energy intake ($p = 0.0899$). A detailed list of foods included in each category is provided in Supplementary Table S1.

Table 1. Characteristics of participants.

Characteristics	Total Subjects (n = 199)	NW/MS− (n = 65)	NW/MS+ (n = 2)	OW/MS− (n = 84)	OW/MS+ (n = 48)	p-Value
Women (%)	49.7	58.5	50.0	51.1	35.4	0.1130
Age (years)	34.2 ± 10.2	28.9 ± 7.4 [a]	39.1 ± 17.8 [a]	35.7 ± 10.4 [b]	38.4 ± 10.1 [b,c]	**<0.0001**
BMI (kg/m^2)	29.0 ± 6.2	22.2 ± 1.8 [a]	24.5 ± 0.66 [a]	31.4 ± 4.2 [b]	34.3 ± 4.8 [c]	**<0.0001**
WC (cm)	92.7 ± 16.5	74.7 ± 5.7 [a]	83.1 ± 0.64 [a]	97.7 ± 10.7 [b]	109.0 ± 11.8 [c]	**<0.0001**
Total-C (mmol)	4.49 ± 1.00	4.13 ± 0.67 [a]	3.58 ± 0.76 [a,b]	4.57 ± 1.0 [b]	4.88 ± 1.19 [b]	**0.0003**
TG (mmol)	1.29 ± 0.91	0.77 ± 0.31 [a]	0.88 ± 0.03 [a,b]	1.15 ± 0.56 [b,c]	2.23 ± 1.22 [d]	**<0.0001** *
HDL-C (mmol)	1.33 ± 0.41	1.60 ± 0.45[c]	1.07 ± 0.21 [a,b]	1.32 ± 0.30 [b]	0.99 ± 0.24 [a]	**<0.0001** *
LDL-C (mmol)	2.76 ± 0.94	2.52 ± 0.70	2.51 ± 0.55	2.81 ± 0.91	3.00 ± 1.21	0.0545
Fasting glycemia (mmol/L)	5.65 ± 0.74	5.68 ± 0.74 [a]	6.90 ± 1.13 [b]	5.43 ± 0.52 [c]	5.94 ± 1.92 [a,b]	**0.0001**
Insulin (pM)	85.1 ± 60.6	48.7 ± 17.1 [a]	68.5 ± 21.9 [a,b,c]	86.1 ± 56.3 [b]	134.5 ± 72.2 [c]	**<0.0001** *
SBP (mmHg)	121.3 ± 11.1	115.9 ± 9.8 [a]	130.5 ± 4.9 [b,c,d]	119.9 ± 8.9 [c]	130.5 ± 10.6 [d]	**<0.0001**
DBP (mmHg)	77.9 ± 9.5	74.0 ± 9.9 [a]	74.0 ± 5.7 [a,b,c]	77.7 ± 7.7 [b]	83.6 ± 9.4 [c]	**<0.0001**
BCAAs (μM)	455.6 ± 92.3	413.8 ± 83.5 [a]	378.8 ± 83.3 [a,b]	460.0 ± 83.2 [a,b]	507.7 ± 92.3 [b]	**<0.0001**
C3 ACs (μM)	0.325 ± 0.115	0.281 ± 0.104 [a]	0.181 ± 0.011 [a,b]	0.327 ± 0.100 [b]	0.387 ± 0.125 [c]	**<0.0001**
C5 ACs (μM)	0.137 ±0.048	0.118±0.036 [a]	0.094± 0.005 [a,b]	0.137 ± 0.045 [b]	0.163 ± 0.056 [c]	**<0.0001**

Values are means ± SD. Model p-values of comparisons between NW/MS−, NW/MS+, OW/MS− and MW/MS+ are shown. Between-groups comparisons were made using the LS means procedure. Results who do not share the same letter ([a,b,c,d]) are significantly different ($p < 0.05$) from each other. * indicates that the p-value was obtained with the transformed variables. Significant values ($p < 0.05$) are presented in bold. Abbreviations, NW, normal weight; OW, overweight; MS, metabolic syndrome; BMI, body mass index; WC, waist circumference; Total-C, total cholesterol; TG, triglycerides; HDL-C, high-density lipoproteins; LDL-C, low-density lipoproteins; SBP, systolic blood pressure; DBP, diastolic blood pressure; BCAAs, branched-chain amino-acids; ACs, acylcarnitines; SD, standard deviation.

Table 2. Daily dietary energy and macronutrients intakes of participants.

Nutrients	Total Subjects (n = 197)	NW/MS− (n = 65)	OW/MS− (n = 84)	OW/MS+ (n = 48)	p-Value [1]	p-Value [2]
Total energy (kcal)	2474 ± 790	2412 ± 853 [a]	2364 ± 695 [a]	2754 ± 809 [b]	**0.0172**	
Total carbohydrates (g)	297.5 ± 92.5	298.8 ± 95.7 [a,c]	281.7 ± 87.0 [a,b]	323.3 ± 93.5 [c]	**0.0446**	0.5447
Carbohydrates (%kcal)	46.7 ± 6.0	48.23 ± 6.54 [a]	45.9 ± 5.3 [b]	45.8 ± 6.1 [b]	**0.0340**	0.2229
Total dietary fiber (g)	23.5 ± 7.9	23.6 ± 8.7	22.8 ± 7.3	24.6 ± 7.7	0.4495	0.7690
Soluble dietary fibers (g)	7.8 ± 2.5	7.6 ± 2.6	7.5 ± 2.3	8.5 ± 2.7	0.0745	0.7736
Insoluble dietary fibers (g)	15.5 ± 5.5	15.7 ± 6.2	15.2 ± 5.2	15.9 ± 5.1	0.7463	0.5677
Total protein (g)	104.2 ± 37.1	99.9 ± 43.2 [a]	100.4 ± 29.9 [a]	116.4 ± 37.7 [b]	**0.0303**	0.6209
Protein (%kcal)	16.8 ± 2.4	16.4 ± 2.6	17.1 ± 2.0	17.0 ± 2.5	0.2580	0.3762
Vegetal protein (g)	32.0 ± 11.8	31.9 ± 12.5	31.0 ± 11.6	34.1 ± 11.1	0.3459	0.6093
Animal protein (g)	70.5 ± 30.3	66.2 ± 35.9 [a]	68.0 ± 23.7 [a]	80.7 ± 30.9 [b]	**0.0086** *	0.0388 *
BCAA intakes (g)	18.5 ± 6.8	17.6 ± 7.8 [a]	17.9 ± 5.5 [a]	20.7 ± 7.0 [b]	**0.0310**	0.3789
Total fat (g)	93.4 ± 37.3	88.4 ± 39.9 [a]	89.2 ± 30.6 [a]	107.4 ± 41.3 [b]	**0.0102**	0.8410
Fat (%kcal)	33.6 ± 5.3	32.4 ± 5.7	33.8 ± 4.7	34.7 ± 5.6	0.0649	0.5095
Total SFA (g)	32.6 ± 14.7	30.6 ± 15.9 [a]	31.1 ± 12.3 [a]	37.8 ± 16.0 [b]	**0.0173**	0.8734
SFA (%kcal)	11.6 ± 2.6	11.1 ± 2.7	11.8 ± 2.6	12.1 ± 2.6	0.0902	0.4312
Total MUFA (g)	38.3 ± 15.7	36.3 ± 16.7 [a]	36.5 ± 12.5 [a]	44.0 ± 18.1 [b]	**0.0131**	0.9269
MUFA (%kcal)	13.8 ± 2.6	13.3 ± 2.9	13.9 ± 2.2	14.2 ± 2.8	0.2203	0.7753
Total PUFA (g)	15.2 ± 6.2	14.5 ± 6.3 [a]	14.7 ± 5.6 [a]	17.3 ± 6.9 [b]	**0.0347**	0.9148
PUFA (%kcal)	5.5 ± 1.4	5.4 ± 1.3	5.6 ± 1.3	5.6 ± 1.5	0.6765	0.9631
Total alcohol (g)	10.5 ± 12.1	9.8 ± 9.0	11.1 ± 13.0	10.5 ± 14.0	0.2968 *	0.1406 *
Alcohol (%kcal)	3.0 ± 2.9	2.9 ± 2.5	3.2 ± 3.2	2.5 ± 2.9	0.4770	0.3919

Values are means ± SD. %kcal from carbohydrates was calculated by difference. Model p-values of comparisons between NW/MS−, OW/MS− and MW/MS+ are shown [1]unadjusted and [2]adjusted for age, sex and total energy intakes. Between-groups comparisons were made using the LS means procedure. Results who do not share the same letter ([a,b,c]) are significantly different ($p < 0.05$) from each other. * indicates that the p-value was obtained with the transformed variables. Significant values ($p < 0.05$) are presented in bold. Abbreviations: NW, normal weight; OW, overweight; MS, metabolic syndrome; BCAA, branched-chain amino-acids; SFA, saturated fatty acids; MUFA, monounsaturated fatty acids; PUFA, polyunsaturated fatty acids.

Table 3. Mean intakes (standard portions/day) of the principal food groups contributing to protein intakes

Food Groups	Total Subjects (n = 197)	NW/MS− (n = 65)	OW/MS− (n = 84)	OW/MS+ (n = 48)	p-Value [1]	p-Value [2]
Red meat	2.25 ± 1.78	1.93 ± 1.95 [a]	2.07 ± 1.40 [a]	3.01 ± 1.94 [b]	**0.0027**	0.0899
Processed meat	0.85 ± 0.95	0.78 ± 0.83	0.72 ± 0.60	1.16 ± 1.44	0.0660 *	0.4325 *
Organ meat	0.02 ± 0.09	0.01 ± 0.04	0.03 ± 0.10	0.04 ± 0.11	0.1009 *	0.2641 *
Fish	1.21 ± 1.19	1.56 ± 1.56 [b]	1.11 ± 0.97 [a]	0.92 ± 0.81 [a]	0.0106	**0.0119**
Poultry	1.17 ± 0.91	1.13 ± 0.94	1.23 ± 0.89	1.12 ± 0.90	0.7332	0.1337
Eggs	0.36 ± 0.30	0.28 ± 0.23 [a]	0.38 ± 0.29 [b]	0.43 ± 0.37 [b]	**0.0166**	0.1431
Low fat dairy	1.60 ± 1.34	1.42 ± 1.08	1.59 ± 1.24	1.86 ± 1.77	0.5081 *	0.5713 *
High fat dairy	1.80 ± 1.29	1.73 ± 1.27	1.77 ± 1.17	1.95 ± 1.51	0.6389	0.7883
Legumes	0.28 ± 0.49	0.28 ± 0.41	0.31 ± 0.62	0.21 ± 0.32	0.4132 *	0.2473 *
Nuts	0.97 ± 2.99	0.75 ± 0.81	0.80 ± 1.00	1.58 ± 5.84	0.9254 *	0.9691 *
Refined grain products	2.78 ± 1.95	2.72 ± 1.65	2.54 ± 1.83	3.28 ± 2.41	0.1028	0.7890
Whole grain products	2.43 ± 1.85	2.64 ± 2.13	2.34 ± 1.63	2.29 ± 1.82	0.5212	0.1007

Values are means ± SD. [1] p-value unadjusted, [2] p-value adjusted for age, sex and total energy intakes. Results who do not share the same letter ([a,b]) are significantly different ($p < 0.05$) from each other. * indicates that the p-value was obtained with the transformed variables. Significant values ($p < 0.05$) are presented in bold. Abbreviations: NW, normal weight; OW, overweight; MS, metabolic syndrome.

3.3. Plasma BCAAs and Protein Intakes

The associations between total protein intake, total energy, BCAA intakes, age, sex and BMI with plasma BCAA levels have also been investigated. Sex and BMI or WC contributed significantly to the variance of plasma BCAA levels ($p < 0.0001$ for both), while total protein, total energy and BCAA intakes and age did not. We also investigated plasma BCAA levels according to obesity and MS status. As shown in Figure 1, there was an increase of plasma BCAA levels with obesity and the presence of MS ($p < 0.0001$) that remained significant after adjustments for age, sex and energy intake ($p < 0.0001$). A concomitant increase in BCAA intakes was also seen ($p = 0.0310$), with OW/MS+ consuming more BCAAs than the other groups (Figure 1). However, the difference in BCAA intakes was no longer significant after adjustments for confounding factors, including age, sex and energy intake ($p = 0.3789$).

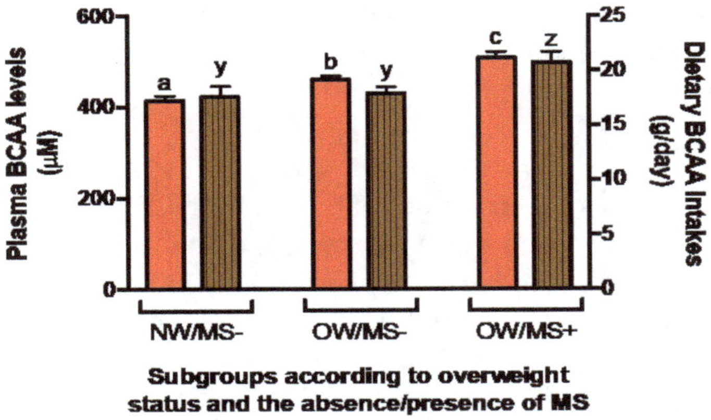

Figure 1. Mean plasma and dietary BCAA levels between subgroups of NW/OW individuals with or without MS. Plasma BCAA levels are shown in plain salmon; BCAA intakes calculated from food frequency questionnaire are shown in lined brown. Whiskers represent standard error. Results who do not share the same letter ([a,b,c] for plasma BCAA levels and [y,z] for dietary BCAA intakes) are significantly different ($p < 0.05$) from each other. Values presented are unadjusted.

The association of each of the 12 principal protein sources (red meat, processed meat, fish, poultry, eggs, legumes, nuts, high and low-fat dairy and whole and refined grain products) with plasma BCAA levels was also tested in a GLM model. Considering all 197 study participants, the only trend observed was with red meat ($p = 0.0575$). This trend was lost after adjustments for age, sex, BMI and total energy intake (data not shown).

When looking at food correlates of plasma BCAA levels in groups defined on the basis of OW and MS status (Table 4), refined and whole grain products were positively associated with plasma BCAA levels (β = 16.07, p = 0.0338 and β = 13.04, p = 0.0279, respectively) in NW/MS− subjects. Their respective contribution to the variance of plasma BCAA levels was of 5.55% and 5.97%, respectively. None of the food group was significantly associated with plasma BCAA levels in OW/MS+ subjects, but a positive trend was seen for red meat (β = 15.40, p = 0.0713). After adjustments for age, sex and energy intake, a negative association between red meat consumption and plasma BCAA levels (β = −26.15, p = 0.0013) was found in NW/MS, explaining 9.64% of its variance. When looking at men and women separately, this negative association was only found in NW/MS− men (β = −49.75.16, p = 0.0039) and not in NW/MS− women (β = −11.81, p = 0.4715). As for OW/MS+ individuals, red meat showed a trend toward a positive relationship (β = 16.16, p = 0.0548), and a negative association was observed with eggs (β = −310.14, p = 0.0272).

Finally, in a model testing the association between total animal and vegetal protein intakes and plasma BCAA levels, only animal protein intake was associated with plasma BCAA levels (p = 0.0002) with a weak contribution of 6.89% to the variance of the trait (not shown). After adjustments for age, sex and energy, the positive association between animal protein intakes and plasma BCAA levels remained significant (R^2 = 0.0193, p = 0.0297, not shown). When analysed by sex, this association was significant in women (β = 177.16, p = 0.0164), but not in men (β = 98.12, p = 0.2908). In subgroups, there was a positive association between total animal protein intakes and plasma BCAA levels for NW/MS− (R^2 = 0.0675, p = 0.0292), as well as a trend toward relationship for OW/MS+ (R^2 = 0.0664, p = 0.0786) individuals. After adjustments for age, sex and energy intake, the positive association between animal protein intakes and plasma BCAA levels was significant in OW/MS+ (R^2 = 0.0422, p = 0.0422), but was lost in NW/MS− individuals (not shown).

As animal protein is the main nutritional correlate of plasma BCAA levels, we further tested the association with its constituents, thus including red meat, processed and organ meats, fish, poultry, eggs and low and high fat dairy in the model. Again, red meat was the single constituent significantly and positively associated with plasma BCAA levels (p = 0.0388) while a positive trend was also observed with poultry (p = 0.0801). These associations (with respective R^2 of 0.0209 and 0.0150) were no longer significant after adjustments for age, sex and total energy intake (data not shown).

3.4. Acylcarnitines

As shown in Figure 2, plasma concentrations of both C3 and C5 ACs increased in parallel to plasma BCAA levels according to OW status and MS even after adjustments for age, sex and total energy intake ($p < 0.001$) (not shown). The associations between plasma BCAA and plasma C3 and C5 AC levels were also tested. With or without adjustments for age, sex and total energy intake, associations between plasma BCAAs and C3 and C5 ACs were significant in the whole cohort ($p < 0.0001$ for all), and in subgroups based on obesity and MS presence ($p < 0.002$ for all) (Table 5). After further adjustments for dietary BCAAs, red meat and total protein intakes, only the association between plasma BCAAs and C5 ACs in OW/MS+ was lost. The contribution of C3 and C5 ACs to the variance was weak to moderate, with R^2 values ranging from 0.0466 to 0.3817.

Table 4. Associations between all 12 principal protein sources and plasma BCAA levels in subgroups based on OW and MS status without and with adjustments for confounders.

Group	NW/MS− (*n* = 65)				OW/MS− (*n* = 84)				OW/MS+ (*n* = 48)			
Model	Unadjusted		Adjusted [2]		Unadjusted		Adjusted [2]		Unadjusted		Adjusted [2]	
Parameters	R^2	*p*-value	R^2	*p*-value	R^2	*p*-value	R^2	*p*-value	R^2	*p*-value	R^2	*p*-value
Red meat	0.0087	0.3910	0.0964	**0.0013**	0.0113	0.3408	0.0072	0.4330	0.0771	0.0713	0.0602	0.0548
Processed meat *	0.0088	0.3892	0.0047	0.4571	0.0004	0.8625	0.0005	0.8336	0.0025	0.7380	0.0002	0.9061
Organ meat *	0.0007	0.8112	0.0006	0.7977	0.0028	0.6313	0.0002	0.8871	0.0293	0.2591	0.0449	0.0948
Fish	0.0258	0.1429	0.0306	0.0607	0.0105	0.3589	0.0037	0.5756	0.0151	0.4160	0.0149	0.3288
Poultry	0.0197	0.1999	0.0219	0.1108	0.0046	0.5410	0.0004	0.8479	0.0397	0.1902	0.0429	0.1022
Eggs *	0.0203	0.1936	0.0214	0.1153	0.0076	0.4324	0.0074	0.4275	0.0578	0.1161	0.0812	**0.0272**
Legumes *	0.0140	0.2787	0.0003	0.8594	0.0072	0.4453	0.0066	0.4543	0.0047	0.6496	0.0424	0.1039
Nuts *	0.0164	0.2418	0.0065	0.3820	0.0045	0.5485	0.0032	0.6039	0.0049	0.6432	0.0001	0.9438
Hf dairy	0.0071	0.4395	0.0058	0.4077	0.0296	0.1248	0.0344	0.0904	0.0105	0.4973	0.0099	0.4244
Lf dairy *	0.0010	0.7721	0.0006	0.7817	0.0013	0.7469	0.0088	0.3890	0.0001	0.9434	0.0054	0.5539
Refined gp	0.0555	**0.0338**	0.0016	0.6596	0.0146	0.2785	0.0000	0.9857	0.0207	0.3415	0.0108	0.4047
Whole gp	0.0597	**0.0279**	0.0002	0.8773	0.0161	0.2552	0.0020	0.6791	0.0250	0.2963	0.0053	0.5576

Protein sources were analysed in portions/day. [2] The model is adjusted for age, sex and total energy intakes. * indicates that the values was obtained with the transformed variables. Significant values ($p < 0.05$) are presented in bold. Abbreviations: NW, normal weight; OW, overweight; MS, metabolic syndrome; Hf dairy, high fat dairy; Lf dairy, Low fat dairy; Refined gp, refined grain products; Whole gp, whole grain products.

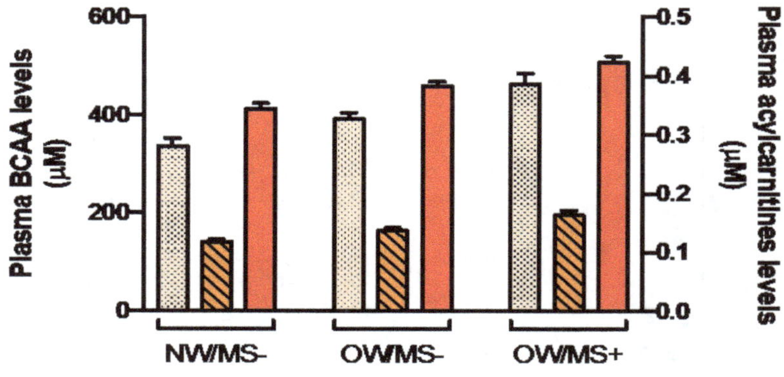

Figure 2. Mean plasma concentrations of C3 and C5 ACs in relation with mean plasma BCAA levels between subgroups of NW/OW individual with or without MS. Plasma BCAA levels are shown in salmon; C3 ACs are shown in dotted light orange; C5 ACs are shown in striped medium orange. Whiskers represent standard error. Values presented are unadjusted. All mean values are significantly different ($p < 0.05$) between groups.

Table 5. Associations between plasma BCAA and C3 and C5 ACs plasma levels in the whole cohort and by subgroups based on OW and MS status without and with adjustments for confounders. All lines were computed individually.

		Total cohort (n = 197)		**NW/MS− (n = 65)**		**OW/MS− (n = 84)**		**OW/MS+ (n = 48)**	
Parameters	Model	R^2	p-value	R^2	p-value	R^2	p-value	R^2	p-value
C3 ACs	Unadjusted	0.3804	**<0.0001**	0.3529	**<0.0001**	0.3069	**<0.0001**	0.2812	**0.0001**
	Adjusted [2]	0.2080	**<0.0001**	0.0909	**0.0020**	0.2356	**<0.0001**	0.2181	**0.0002**
	Adjusted [3]	0.1932	**<0.0001**	0.0775	**0.0047**	0.2140	**<0.0001**	0.1488	**0.0019**
C5 ACs	Unadjusted	0.3817	**<0.0001**	0.3608	**<0.0001**	0.3822	**<0.0001**	0.2159	**0.0009**
	Adjusted [2]	0.1614	**<0.0001**	0.0866	**0.0017**	0.2212	**<0.0001**	0.2181	**0.0002**
	Adjusted [3]	0.1504	**<0.0001**	0.0901	**0.0010**	0.2026	**<0.0001**	0.0466	**0.0847**

[2] Model adjusted for age, sex and total energy intakes, [3] Model adjusted for age, sex, total energy intakes and total BCAA, animal protein and red meat intakes. Significant values ($p < 0.05$) are presented in bold. Abbreviations: NW, normal weight; OW, overweight-obese; MS, metabolic syndrome; ACs, Acylcarnitines.

4. Discussion

It is not yet fully established if elevated plasma BCAA and AC levels are a cause or a consequence of IR, and if protein intakes exert an influence on their plasma concentrations. To our knowledge, we are the first to investigate the association between the individual food groups contributing the most to daily protein intakes, fasting AC and BCAA levels in normal weight and overweight/obese individuals with or without metabolic perturbations.

As expected, plasma BCAA levels were significantly greater in OW with or without MS than in NW individuals, which is consistent with the literature [22,40–43]. Worth of mention, plasma BCAAs appeared to be affected by sex, as previously reported in some studies [40–42]. However, differences in BCAA intakes between groups were not present following adjustments for age, sex and energy intake. This was expected since total protein intakes and % of energy from protein were also not different between groups after adjustments. Still, the protein's origin deserves further attention. Considering all principal protein sources, red meat seems to be driving the positive association of total animal protein intakes with plasma BCAAs since it was the only food group presenting a trend towards significance for an association with plasma BCAAs. Associations with red meat were lost in adjusted models on the whole sample, but animal protein intakes remained significant. This reflects very well the intakes of our participants: OW/MS+ consumed significantly more animal protein than

NW/MS− and OW/MS− individuals in non-adjusted and adjusted models, whereas red meat intakes were no longer different between groups after adjustments for age, sex and energy. Considering these observations, plasma BCAA levels potentially reflect the consumption of animal protein/red meat. Greater red meat intakes would have been necessary to see an effect of this food on already metabolically deteriorated individuals. These findings are concordant with recent papers reporting BCAAs consumption—correlating with animal protein and/or meat intakes—associated or correlated with plasma BCAA levels [8,17]. Still, because animal protein and red meat only explain a small portion of plasma BCAAs variance, dietary intakes might not be the main variable affecting plasma BCAA levels.

Testing the associations within the three subgroups of subjects revealed substantial differences. In OW/MS+ individuals, the association between plasma BCAAs and animal protein presented a trend toward significance that became significant after adjustments. In the model including all 12 principal protein sources, the tendency observed for red meat persisted after adjustments, but reached significance when considering animal protein sources only (not shown). Similarly to what we observed in the whole sample, red meat was the main animal protein source associated with plasma BCAA levels in metabolically disturbed individuals although the small magnitude of the relationship is probably an indicator that there are other important metabolic factors implicated in plasma BCAAs elevation in this group.

As for OW/MS−, we surprisingly did not find any association of protein intakes with plasma BCAA levels. Their intakes were more similar to NW than to OW/MS+ individuals regarding macronutrients, but were no longer significantly different after adjustments for age, sex and energy intake. Yet, compared to their MS+ counterparts, they consumed less red meat and less animal protein overall. The hypothesis that elevated plasma BCAAs is consequent to IR could explain why their levels are significantly higher than NW/MS− subjects, assuming that they are at a greater risk of developing IR. At this point, we cannot rule out the possibility that the different dietary habits of OW/MS− exert some kind of protection against elevated plasma BCAA levels. Unfortunately, the study design of the INFOGENE study does not allow the verification of this hypothesis.

What has been observed in NW/MS− individuals is quite different. All models presented different associations. In the unadjusted ones, grain products were the main protein sources positively associated with plasma BCAA levels while total animal protein, but not vegetal protein intakes, was also positively associated. This unexpected observation could rather be an indicator of a dietary pattern rich in grain products, as well as in animal protein, explaining their associations with plasma BCAAs in different models. Even more intriguing, after adjustments for confounders, red meat was negatively associated with plasma BCAA levels. Sex appeared to be a moderator of this association ($p < 0.0001$). BCAAs might be more strongly affected by sex (and other metabolic factors) than by protein sources intakes in healthy individuals. This could explain why we found very different associations depending on the model used and would corroborate with the small magnitude of the associations found with the 12 principal protein food sources intakes. Of note, a decreased predictive effect of the habitual diet on serum metabolites after sex and age adjustments was previously reported by Floegel et al [44].

Plasma AC levels were another important aspect of the present study. It appears that the association between plasma C3 and C5 ACs and plasma BCAA levels were influenced by sex but not so much by other confounders, such as age, energy intakes, animal protein, red meat or BCAA intakes, depending on the model used. Further adjustments for variables related to dietary protein intakes did not change the associations between C3 or C5 ACs and plasma BCAA levels except for the loss of the association for C5 ACs in OW/MS+. In that model, neither animal protein, red meat or BCAA intakes were significant correlates to the variance. Thus, we cannot confirm if these variables modulate the association between C5 ACs and plasma BCAA levels or if we lost the association because of a lack of statistical power, but their contribution to the variance appears to be weak. C3 and C5 ACs might be differentially associated with plasma BCAA, but literature does not report on their individual effect [25,44]. We found C3 and C5 ACs to be positively associated with plasma BCAAs as reported in a comparable study where higher levels of short-chain ACs were observed in diabetic patients compared to lean or obese individuals [45]. Since this association persisted with adjustments for confounders and animal protein, BCAA and red meat intakes in our models, there appears to be a relative independence of C3 and C5 ACs from the diet. Consequently, we propose that C3 and C5 ACs more likely represents the degree of plasma BCAAs elevation than meat consumption. For these reasons, using these short-chain ACs as a biomarker of meat consumption should be done with caution and with consideration of other metabolic markers. It would be interesting to further investigate these association in fasting and non-fasting individuals since C3 and C5 levels could be lower in fasted individuals [46].

Taken all together, these findings are in line with a study realized in a cohort of Asian Indians living in the US and at risk of CVD [47]. The investigators reported a positive association between a Western/non-vegetarian dietary pattern, characterized by higher intakes of red meat, poultry, fish, eggs and vegetables, and a metabolite signature rich in BCAAs, as well as in aromatic AAs and short-chain ACs. Participants scoring higher for that metabolite signature were also more insulin resistant, had higher fasting and 2-h insulin concentrations and had lower adiponectin levels and insulin sensitivity. Similarly, we found a metabolic signature, including BCAA leucine, C3 and C5 ACs that was associated with a Western dietary pattern in French Canadians [24]. Red meat also appeared to be an important positive loading factor for T2D risk [44]. As for our healthy volunteers, recent work found meats, sausages, meat products and eggs to be included in dietary patterns explaining variation among plasma BCAA levels in a healthy population [17]. These foods were highlighted in at least one of our models.

The mechanisms underlying the association between BCAA intakes and IR development are unclear for now and association studies reported opposite results [4,28]. The largest European prospective study found total and mostly animal protein intakes to be associated with an elevated T2D risk [48]. As observed in the present study, and in similar studies [17–20], plant-protein intakes were not inversely associated with T2D risk. Interestingly, Okekunle et al., found that a pattern rich in meat was associated with T2D risk, even if rice and wheaten foods were the main correlates of BCAAs in their study cohort [49]. These findings, alongside the higher intakes of animal protein observed in OW/MS+ individuals herein, reiterate the importance of considering the composition of the foods BCAAs are coming from. In fact, red meat does have high heme-iron content which was suggested to be associated with T2D [50–54]. Other nutrients in meats may also have an impact on IR development, including the pro-oxidant and pro-inflammatory advanced glycation end products formed by the reaction of carbonyl groups of reducing sugars with the amine groups of proteins, lipids or nucleotides [55,56]. We also cannot exclude the role of the gut microbiota (GMB) in BCAAs metabolism. Accordingly, intestinal bacteria impact AAs absorption that are used for growth or the synthesis of metabolic compounds, such as short-chain fatty acids (SCFA), including branched-chain fatty acids (BCFA), BCAA being involved in the later [57]. Finally, animal protein could have a different biodisponibility or kinetics that could predispose to IR. A small study reported that vegan, who consumed less BCAAs than omnivores at baseline, had a significant decrease in insulin sensitivity after three months of BCAA supplementation [26]. Another study found a switch to fish and plant-based protein versus meat lowered plasma BCAAs in a small sample of mainly overweight individuals [58]. Mechanisms of actions need to be the subject of future studies.

All things considered, results of the present study and a literature review lead us to two different hypotheses: First, that the protein quality has an impact on plasma BCAA levels and second, that elevated BCAAs are the consequence of a disturbed metabolism in individuals having suboptimal dietary habits. In both cases, ACs seems more likely to reflect BCAA concentrations in the plasma. If BCAA levels induce IR, the most plausible hypothesis involves the mammalian target of rapamycin (mTOR) [59,60]. BCAAs and especially leucine can activate mTORC1 through an alternative pathway ending with insulin receptor degradation. Insulin-binding to its receptor being therefore compromised, a state of insulin resistance would occur [59–66]. BCAAs could also increase the activity of p65 subunit of nuclear transcription factor Kb (NF-kβ), a pro-inflammatory pathway that could accelerate IR progression [67]. Regardless of their potential, these mechanisms might not explain the rise of plasma BCAA levels observed in our sample, granted that protein intakes and therefore amino acid pool, were not greater in OW/MS− compared to NW/MS− group. If BCAAs elevation is rather the consequence of a disturbed metabolism, it has been proposed that high fat diets, obesity, IR or insulin levels could lead to a defect in BCKD activity and expression in the liver [11]. Circulating BCAAs are transaminated into branched-chain keto acids (BCKA) by the branched-chain amino acid transferase, a reversible step, before being further oxidized by BCKD to serve as substrates in the Krebs cycle [2,11,68]. Having dysfunctional BCKD would therefore lead to BCKA and or BCAAs accumulation. BCKA being the precursors of C3 and C5 ACs, this could explain ACs elevation in conjunction with IR [2].

The present study has some limitations. As mentioned earlier, elevated BCAAs is an early predictor of IR. Individuals classified in the MS− group could be insulin resistant but without enough metabolic impairments to make it into the MS+ group and therefore dilute IR impact on our results. As previously hypothesized by Isanejad et al., the response to dietary protein might depend on metabolic health, as well as on one's degree of IR [19]. Classifying our population according to IR only could help to isolate the impact of protein intakes on BCAAs at different stages of diabetes development (healthy, insulin resistant and diabetic). Also, we considered the medication for diabetes, dyslipidemia or hypertension to define our subgroups. But taking medications artificially improve metabolic parameters, which could therefore ameliorate BCAAs metabolism and affect the associations observed. Our sample was also too small for further investigation of the effect of sex on plasma BCAA levels by subgroups based on BMI and MS presence. Finally, because we used data from a cross-sectional study, we were not able to investigate in a prospective way the associations between plasma BCAA levels and changes in consumption of plant or animal protein nor time variations in ACs. It is important to note that correction for multiple testing was not applied to data. Because of the exploratory design of this study, having applied too restrictive correction could have masked potentially interesting associations in this relatively small sample of subjects. Notwithstanding, this study has some strengths. Our decision to compare healthy and metabolically deteriorated individuals was based on the fact that plasma BCAA levels are influenced by other components of the metabolic syndrome than glycemia [2]. As such, the present work compares healthy and metabolically deteriorated individuals within a single sample allowing comparisons between groups and generalization of the results. To our knowledge, it is also the first study testing the association of BCAAs with diet between subgroups of subjects with cardiometabolic perturbations as opposed to only IR or CVD related risk factors. All measurements were standardized, including the dietary questionnaire that has been validated for our population. Finally, the detailed FFQ allowed us to explore the associations with specific subgroups of animal-derived protein sources in parallel with ACs and BCAAs, which is unique to the present study.

5. Conclusions

In summary, we found a constant tendency toward significance between plasma BCAAs and animal protein or red meat intakes in OW/MS+ individuals. In NW/MS− individuals, diverse associations were observed between models. That being said, it is likely that BCAA or animal protein/meat intakes are not the main or the sole correlate to their elevation in plasma prior to IR considering their weak contribution to the variance. Plasma ACs concentrations were also found to be associated with plasma BCAA levels. Our study cannot explain mechanisms by which plasma BCAA levels and ACs are elevated in OW/MS+ individuals, but the impact of meat, its BCAA content, the presence of other compounds in its matrix and its GMB metabolites should be further investigated.

Author Contributions: Conceptualization and design of the experiments, L.P., S.L. and M.-C.V.; data analysis, M.R., F.G., B.A.-N. and V.G.; formal analysis and writing, M.R.; supervision, M.-C.V.; review and editing, all authors.

Acknowledgments: The authors express gratitude to all participants for their much-appreciated collaboration. We recognize the contribution of Marie-Eve Bouchard, Steve Amireault, Diane Drolet, and Dominique Beaulieu for their involvement in the study coordination, recruitment of the subjects, and data collection. We would also like to thank Chenomx Inc. (Edmonton, AB, Canada) who performed the mass spectrometry analyses to measure plasma metabolite levels. Marie-Claude Vohl is Canada Research Chair in Genomics Applied to Nutrition and Metabolic Health. Michèle Rousseau received a studentship from the INITIA foundation.

References

1. Gannon Nicholas, P.; Schnuck Jamie, K.; Vaughan Roger, A. BCAA Metabolism and Insulin Sensitivity—Dysregulated by Metabolic Status? *Mol. Nutr. Food Res.* **2018**, *62*, 1700756. [CrossRef] [PubMed]
2. Gar, C.; Rottenkolber, M.; Prehn, C.; Adamski, J.; Seissler, J.; Lechner, A. Serum and plasma amino acids as markers of prediabetes, insulin resistance, and incident diabetes. *Crit. Rev. Clin. Lab. Sci.* **2018**, *55*, 21–32. [CrossRef]
3. Labonte, C.C.; Farsijani, S.; Marliss, E.B.; Gougeon, R.; Morais, J.A.; Pereira, S.; Bassil, M.; Winter, A.; Murphy, J.; Combs, T.P.; et al. Plasma Amino Acids vs Conventional Predictors of Insulin Resistance Measured by the Hyperinsulinemic Clamp. *J. Endocr. Soc.* **2017**, *1*, 861–873. [CrossRef] [PubMed]
4. Asghari, G.; Farhadnejad, H.; Teymoori, F.; Mirmiran, P.; Tohidi, M.; Azizi, F. High dietary intake of branched-chain amino acids is associated with an increased risk of insulin resistance in adults. *J. Diabetes* **2018**, *10*, 357–364. [CrossRef] [PubMed]
5. Ruiz-Canela, M.; Toledo, E.; Clish, C.B.; Hruby, A.; Liang, L.; Salas-Salvadó, J.; Razquin, C.; Corella, D.; Estruch, R.; Ros, E.; et al. Plasma branched-chain amino acids and incident cardiovascular disease in the PREDIMED trial. *Clin. Chem.* **2016**, *62*, 582–592. [CrossRef] [PubMed]
6. Song, M.; Fung, T.T.; Hu, F.B.; Willett, W.C.; Longo, V.; Chan, A.T.; Giovannucci, E.L. Animal and plant protein intake and all-cause and cause-specific mortality: Results from two prospective US cohort studies. *JAMA Intern. Med.* **2016**, *176*, 1453. [CrossRef]
7. Wang, T.J.; Larson, M.G.; Vasan, R.S.; Cheng, S.; Rhee, E.P.; McCabe, E.; Lewis, G.D.; Fox, C.S.; Jacques, P.F.; Fernandez, C.; et al. Metabolite profiles and the risk of developing diabetes. *Nat. Med.* **2011**, *17*, 448–453. [CrossRef] [PubMed]
8. Zheng, Y.; Li, Y.; Qi, Q.; Hruby, A.; Manson, J.E.; Willett, W.C.; Wolpin, B.M.; Hu, F.B.; Qi, L. Cumulative consumption of branched-chain amino acids and incidence of type 2 diabetes. *Int. J. Epidemiol.* **2016**, *45*, 1482–1492. [CrossRef]
9. Mahendran, Y.; Jonsson, A.; Have, C.T.; Allin, K.H.; Witte, D.R.; Jørgensen, M.E.; Grarup, N.; Pedersen, O.; Kilpeläinen, T.O.; Hansen, T. Genetic evidence of a causal effect of insulin resistance on branched-chain amino acid levels. *Diabetologia* **2017**, *60*, 873–878. [CrossRef]
10. Wang, Q.; Holmes, M.V.; Davey Smith, G.; Ala-Korpela, M. Genetic Support for a Causal Role of Insulin Resistance on Circulating Branched-Chain Amino Acids and Inflammation. *Diabetes Care* **2017**, *40*, 1779–1786. [CrossRef]
11. Shin, A.C.; Fasshauer, M.; Filatova, N.; Grundell, L.A.; Zielinski, E.; Zhou, J.-Y.; Scherer, T.; Lindtner, C.; White, P.J.; Lapworth, A.L.; et al. Brain insulin lowers circulating BCAA levels by inducing hepatic BCAA catabolism. *Cell Metab.* **2014**, *20*, 898. [CrossRef] [PubMed]
12. Lynch, C.J.; Adams, S.H. Branched-chain amino acids in metabolic signalling and insulin resistance. *Nat. Rev. Endocrinol.* **2014**, *10*, 723–736. [CrossRef] [PubMed]
13. Fernstrom, J.D. Branched-Chain Amino Acids and Brain Function. *J. Nutr.* **2005**, *135*, 1539S–1546S. [CrossRef] [PubMed]
14. Brosnan, J.T.; Brosnan, M.E. Branched-Chain Amino Acids: Enzyme and Substrate Regulation. *J. Nutr.* **2006**, *136*, 207S–211S. [CrossRef]

15. Platell, C.; Kong, S.E.; McCauley, R.; Hall, J.C. Branched-chain amino acids. *J. Gastroenterol. Hepatol.* **2001**, *15*, 706–717. [CrossRef]
16. López, A.M.; Noriega, L.G.; Diaz, M.; Torres, N.; Tovar, A.R. Plasma branched-chain and aromatic amino acid concentration after ingestion of an urban or rural diet in rural Mexican women. *BMC Obes.* **2015**, *2*, 8. [CrossRef]
17. Merz, B.; Frommherz, L.; Rist, M.J.; Kulling, S.E.; Bub, A.; Watzl, B. Dietary Pattern and Plasma BCAA-Variations in Healthy Men and Women—Results from the KarMeN Study. *Nutrients* **2018**, *10*, 623. [CrossRef] [PubMed]
18. Pan, A.; Sun, Q.; Bernstein, A.M.; Schulze, M.B.; Manson, J.E.; Willett, W.C.; Hu, F.B. Red meat consumption and risk of type 2 diabetes: 3 cohorts of US adults and an updated meta-analysis. *Am. J. Clin. Nutr.* **2011**, *94*, 1088–1096. [CrossRef]
19. Isanejad, M.; LaCroix, A.Z.; Thomson, C.A.; Tinker, L.; Larson, J.C.; Qi, Q.; Qi, L.; Cooper-DeHoff, R.M.; Phillips, L.S.; Prentice, R.L.; et al. Branched-Chain Amino Acid, Meat Intake and Risk of Type 2 Diabetes in the Women's Health Initiative. Available online: /core/journals/british-journal-of-nutrition/article/branchedchain-amino-acid-meat-intake-and-risk-of-type-2-diabetes-in-the-womens-health-initiative/2706233DCEB0422B3DCCA9D9925CCB3F (accessed on 10 April 2018).
20. Malik, V.S.; Li, Y.; Tobias, D.K.; Pan, A.; Hu, F.B. Dietary Protein Intake and Risk of Type 2 Diabetes in US Men and Women. *Am. J. Epidemiol.* **2016**, *183*, 715–728. [CrossRef] [PubMed]
21. Schooneman, M.G.; Vaz, F.M.; Houten, S.M.; Soeters, M.R. Acylcarnitines. *Diabetes* **2013**, *62*, 1–8. [CrossRef]
22. Newgard, C.B.; An, J.; Bain, J.R.; Muehlbauer, M.J.; Stevens, R.D.; Lien, L.F.; Haqq, A.M.; Shah, S.H.; Arlotto, M.; Slentz, C.A.; et al. A Branched-Chain Amino Acid-Related Metabolic Signature that Differentiates Obese and Lean Humans and Contributes to Insulin Resistance. *Cell Metab.* **2009**, *9*, 311–326. [CrossRef]
23. Roe, D.S.; Roe, C.R.; Brivet, M.; Sweetman, L. Evidence for a short-chain carnitine-acylcarnitine translocase in mitochondria specifically related to the metabolism of branched-chain amino acids. *Mol. Genet. Metab.* **2000**, *69*, 69–75. [CrossRef]
24. Bouchard-Mercier, A.; Rudkowska, I.; Lemieux, S.; Couture, P.; Vohl, M.-C. The metabolic signature associated with the Western dietary pattern: A cross-sectional study. *Nutr. J.* **2013**, *12*, 158. [CrossRef]
25. Cheung, W.; Keski-Rahkonen, P.; Assi, N.; Ferrari, P.; Freisling, H.; Rinaldi, S.; Slimani, N.; Zamora-Ros, R.; Rundle, M.; Frost, G.; et al. A metabolomic study of biomarkers of meat and fish intake. *Am. J. Clin. Nutr.* **2017**, *105*, 600–608. [CrossRef]
26. Gojda, J.; Rossmeislová, L.; Straková, R.; Tůmová, J.; Elkalaf, M.; Jaček, M.; Tůma, P.; Potočková, J.; Krauzová, E.; Waldauf, P.; et al. Chronic dietary exposure to branched chain amino acids impairs glucose disposal in vegans but not in omnivores. *Eur. J. Clin. Nutr.* **2017**, *71*, 594–601. [CrossRef]
27. Iwasaki, M. Validity of a Self-Administered Food-Frequency Questionnaire for Assessing Amino Acid Intake in Japan: Comparison with Intake From 4-Day Weighed Dietary Records and Plasma Levels. *J. Epidemiol.* **2016**, *26*, 36–44. [CrossRef]
28. Jennings, A.; MacGregor, A.; Pallister, T.; Spector, T.; Cassidy, A. Associations between branched chain amino acid intake and biomarkers of adiposity and cardiometabolic health independent of genetic factors: A twin study. *Int. J. Cardiol.* **2016**, *223*, 992–998. [CrossRef]
29. Nagata, C.; Nakamura, K.; Wada, K.; Tsuji, M.; Tamai, Y.; Kawachi, T. Branched-chain Amino Acid Intake and the Risk of Diabetes in a Japanese CommunityThe Takayama Study. *Am. J. Epidemiol.* **2013**, *178*, 1226–1232. [CrossRef]
30. Pallottini, A.C.; Sales, C.H.; Vieira, D.A.D.S.; Marchioni, D.M.; Fisberg, R.M. Dietary BCAA Intake Is Associated with Demographic, Socioeconomic and Lifestyle Factors in Residents of São Paulo, Brazil. *Nutrients* **2017**, *9*, 449. [CrossRef]
31. Paradis, A.-M.; Pérusse, L.; Godin, G.; Vohl, M.-C. Validity of a self-reported measure of familial history of obesity. *Nutr. J.* **2008**, *7*, 27. [CrossRef]
32. Paradis, A.-M.; Godin, G.; Pérusse, L.; Vohl, M.-C. Associations between dietary patterns and obesity phenotypes. *Int. J. Obes.* **2009**, *33*, 1419–1426. [CrossRef] [PubMed]
33. Paradis, A.-M.; Godin, G.; Pérusse, L.; Vohl, M.-C. Interaction between Familial History of Obesity and Fat Intakes on Obesity Phenotypes. *Lifestyle Genom.* **2009**, *2*, 37–42. [CrossRef] [PubMed]

34. Cormier, H.; Thifault, É.; Garneau, V.; Tremblay, A.; Drapeau, V.; Pérusse, L.; Vohl, M.-C. Association between yogurt consumption, dietary patterns, and cardio-metabolic risk factors. *Eur. J. Nutr.* **2016**, *55*, 577–587. [CrossRef]
35. Allam-Ndoul, B.; Guénard, F.; Garneau, V.; Cormier, H.; Barbier, O.; Pérusse, L.; Vohl, M.-C. Association between Metabolite Profiles, Metabolic Syndrome and Obesity Status. *Nutrients* **2016**, *8*, 324. [CrossRef]
36. Goulet, J.; Nadeau, G.; Lapointe, A.; Lamarche, B.; Lemieux, S. Validity and reproducibility of an interviewer-administered food frequency questionnaire for healthy French-Canadian men and women. *Nutr. J.* **2004**, *3*, 13. [CrossRef] [PubMed]
37. Johnson-Down, L.; Ritter, H.; Starkey, L.J.; Gray-Donald, K. Primary Food Sources of Nutrients In the Diet of Canadian Adults. *Can. J. Diet. Pract. Res.* **2006**, *67*, 7–13. [CrossRef]
38. Callaway, C.W.; Chumlea, W.C.; Bouchard, C.; Himes, J.H.; Lohman, T.G.; Martin, A.D.; Mitchell, C.D.; Mueller, W.H.; Roche, A.F.; Seefeldt, V.D. Standardization of Anthropometric Measurements. In *The Airlie (VA) Consensus Conference*; Human Kinetics Publisher: Champaign, IR, USA, 1988; pp. 29–80.
39. Friedewald, W.T.; Levy, R.I.; Fredrickson, D.S. Estimation of the Concentration of Low-Density Lipoprotein Cholesterol in Plasma, Without Use of the Preparative Ultracentrifuge. *Clin. Chem.* **1972**, *18*, 499–502. [PubMed]
40. Guevara-Cruz, M.; Vargas-Morales, J.M.; Méndez-García, A.L.; López-Barradas, A.M.; Granados-Portillo, O.; Ordaz-Nava, G.; Rocha-Viggiano, A.K.; Gutierrez-Leyte, C.A.; Medina-Cerda, E.; Rosado, J.L.; et al. Amino acid profiles of young adults differ by sex, body mass index and insulin resistance. *Nutr. Metab. Cardiovasc. Dis.* **2018**, *28*, 393–401. [CrossRef] [PubMed]
41. Takashina, C.; Tsujino, I.; Watanabe, T.; Sakaue, S.; Ikeda, D.; Yamada, A.; Sato, T.; Ohira, H.; Otsuka, Y.; Oyama-Manabe, N.; et al. Associations among the plasma amino acid profile, obesity, and glucose metabolism in Japanese adults with normal glucose tolerance. *Nutr. Metab.* **2016**, *13*, 5. [CrossRef]
42. Würtz, P.; Mäkinen, V.-P.; Soininen, P.; Kangas, A.J.; Tukiainen, T.; Kettunen, J.; Savolainen, M.J.; Tammelin, T.; Viikari, J.S.; Rönnemaa, T.; et al. Metabolic Signatures of Insulin Resistance in 7098 Young Adults. *Diabetes* **2012**, *61*, 1372.
43. Boulet, M.M.; Chevrier, G.; Grenier-Larouche, T.; Pelletier, M.; Nadeau, M.; Scarpa, J.; Prehn, C.; Marette, A.; Adamski, J.; Tchernof, A. Alterations of plasma metabolite profiles related to adipose tissue distribution and cardiometabolic risk. *Am. J. Physiol.-Endocrinol. Metab.* **2015**, *309*, E736–E746. [CrossRef]
44. Floegel, A.; von Ruesten, A.; Drogan, D.; Schulze, M.B.; Prehn, C.; Adamski, J.; Pischon, T.; Boeing, H. Variation of serum metabolites related to habitual diet: A targeted metabolomic approach in EPIC-Potsdam. *Eur. J. Clin. Nutr.* **2013**, *67*, 1100–1108. [CrossRef] [PubMed]
45. Mihalik, S.J.; Goodpaster, B.H.; Kelley, D.E.; Chace, D.H.; Vockley, J.; Toledo, F.G.S.; DeLany, J.P. Increased Levels of Plasma Acylcarnitines in Obesity and Type 2 Diabetes and Identification of a Marker of Glucolipotoxicity. *Obes. Silver Spring Md* **2010**, *18*, 1695. [CrossRef] [PubMed]
46. Strand, E.; Pedersen, E.R.; Svingen, G.F.T.; Olsen, T.; Bjørndal, B.; Karlsson, T.; Dierkes, J.; Njølstad, P.R.; Mellgren, G.; Tell, G.S.; et al. Serum Acylcarnitines and Risk of Cardiovascular Death and Acute Myocardial Infarction in Patients with Stable Angina Pectoris. *J. Am. Heart Assoc.* **2017**, *6*, e003620. [CrossRef]
47. Bhupathiraju, S.N.; Guasch-Ferré, M.; Gadgil, M.D.; Newgard, C.B.; Bain, J.R.; Muehlbauer, M.J.; Ilkayeva, O.R.; Scholtens, D.M.; Hu, F.B.; Kanaya, A.M.; et al. Dietary Patterns among Asian Indians Living in the United States Have Distinct Metabolomic Profiles That Are Associated with Cardiometabolic Risk. *J. Nutr.* **2018**, *148*, 1150–1159. [CrossRef] [PubMed]
48. van Nielen, M.; Feskens, E.J.M.; Mensink, M.; Sluijs, I.; Molina, E.; Amiano, P.; Ardanaz, E.; Balkau, B.; Beulens, J.W.J.; Boeing, H.; et al. Dietary Protein Intake and Incidence of Type 2 Diabetes in Europe: The EPIC-InterAct Case-Cohort Study. *Diabetes Care* **2014**, *37*, 1854–1862. [CrossRef]
49. Okekunle, A.P. Dietary Intakes of Branched-Chained Amino Acid and Risk for Type 2 Diabetes in Adults: The Harbin Cohort Study on Diet, Nutrition and Chronic Non-Communicable Diseases Study. *Can. J. Diabetes* **2018**, *42*, 484–492.e7. [CrossRef] [PubMed]
50. White, D.L.; Collinson, A. Red Meat, Dietary Heme Iron, and Risk of Type 2 Diabetes: The Involvement of Advanced Lipoxidation Endproducts. *Adv. Nutr.* **2013**, *4*, 403. [CrossRef]
51. Kunutsor Setor, K.; Apekey Tanefa, A.; Walley, J.; Kain, K. Ferritin levels and risk of type 2 diabetes mellitus: An updated systematic review and meta-analysis of prospective evidence. *Diabetes Metab. Res. Rev.* **2013**, *29*, 308–318. [CrossRef]

52. Bao, W.; Rong, Y.; Rong, S.; Liu, L. Dietary iron intake, body iron stores, and the risk of type 2 diabetes: A systematic review and meta-analysis. *BMC Med.* **2012**, *10*, 119. [CrossRef]
53. Zhao, Z.; Li, S.; Liu, G.; Yan, F.; Ma, X.; Huang, Z.; Tian, H. Body Iron Stores and Heme-Iron Intake in Relation to Risk of Type 2 Diabetes: A Systematic Review and Meta-Analysis. *PLoS ONE* **2012**, *7*, e41641. [CrossRef] [PubMed]
54. Talaei, M.; Wang, Y.-L.; Yuan, J.-M.; Pan, A.; Koh, W.-P. Meat, Dietary Heme Iron, and Risk of Type 2 Diabetes MellitusThe Singapore Chinese Health Study. *Am. J. Epidemiol.* **2017**, *186*, 824–833. [CrossRef] [PubMed]
55. O'Brien, J.; Morrissey, P.A.; Ames, J.M. Nutritional and toxicological aspects of the Maillard browning reaction in foods. *Crit. Rev. Food Sci. Nutr.* **1989**, *28*, 211–248. [CrossRef] [PubMed]
56. Calder, P.C.; Ahluwalia, N.; Brouns, F.; Buetler, T.; Clement, K.; Cunningham, K.; Esposito, K.; Jönsson, L.S.; Kolb, H.; Lansink, M.; et al. Dietary factors and low-grade inflammation in relation to overweight and obesity. *Br. J. Nutr.* **2011**, *106*, S1–S78. [CrossRef] [PubMed]
57. Neis, E.P.J.G.; Dejong, C.H.C.; Rensen, S.S. The Role of Microbial Amino Acid Metabolism in Host Metabolism. *Nutrients* **2015**, *7*, 2930–2946. [CrossRef]
58. Elshorbagy, A.; Jernerén, F.; Basta, M.; Basta, C.; Turner, C.; Khaled, M.; Refsum, H. Amino acid changes during transition to a vegan diet supplemented with fish in healthy humans. *Eur. J. Nutr.* **2017**, *56*, 1953–1962. [CrossRef]
59. Zoncu, R.; Efeyan, A.; Sabatini, D.M. mTOR: From growth signal integration to cancer, diabetes and ageing. *Nat. Rev. Mol. Cell Biol.* **2011**, *12*, 21–35. [CrossRef]
60. Jewell, J.L.; Russell, R.C.; Guan, K.-L. Amino acid signalling upstream of mTOR. *Nat. Rev. Mol. Cell Biol.* **2013**, *14*, 133–139. [CrossRef]
61. Yoon, M.-S. The Emerging Role of Branched-Chain Amino Acids in Insulin Resistance and Metabolism. *Nutrients* **2016**, *8*, 405. [CrossRef]
62. Krebs, M.; Krssak, M.; Bernroider, E.; Anderwald, C.; Brehm, A.; Meyerspeer, M.; Nowotny, P.; Roth, E.; Waldhäusl, W.; Roden, M. Mechanism of Amino Acid-Induced Skeletal Muscle Insulin Resistance in Humans. *Diabetes* **2002**, *51*, 599–605. [CrossRef]
63. Tremblay, F.; Krebs, M.; Dombrowski, L.; Brehm, A.; Bernroider, E.; Roth, E.; Nowotny, P.; Waldhäusl, W.; Marette, A.; Roden, M. Overactivation of S6 Kinase 1 as a Cause of Human Insulin Resistance During Increased Amino Acid Availability. *Diabetes* **2005**, *54*, 2674–2684. [CrossRef]
64. Laplante, M.; Sabatini, D.M. mTOR Signaling in Growth Control and Disease. *Cell* **2012**, *149*, 274–293. [CrossRef]
65. Zick, Y. Insulin resistance: A phosphorylation-based uncoupling of insulin signaling. *Trends Cell Biol.* **2001**, *11*, 437–441. [CrossRef]
66. Um, S.H.; D'Alessio, D.; Thomas, G. Nutrient overload, insulin resistance, and ribosomal protein S6 kinase 1, S6K1. *Cell Metab.* **2006**, *3*, 393–402. [CrossRef]
67. Zhenyukh, O.; Civantos, E.; Ruiz-Ortega, M.; Sanchez, M.S.; Vazquez, C.; Peiro, C.; Egido, J.; Mas, S. High concentration of branched-chain amino acids promotes oxidative stress, inflammation and migration of human peripheral blood mononuclear cells via mTORC1 activation. *Free Radic. Biol. Med.* **2017**, *104*, 165–177. [CrossRef]
68. Adeva, M.M.; Calviño, J.; Souto, G.; Donapetry, C. Insulin resistance and the metabolism of branched-chain amino acids in humans. *Amino Acids* **2012**, *43*, 171–181. [CrossRef]

Permissions

All chapters in this book were first published by MDPI; hereby published with permission under the Creative Commons Attribution License or equivalent. Every chapter published in this book has been scrutinized by our experts. Their significance has been extensively debated. The topics covered herein carry significant findings which will fuel the growth of the discipline. They may even be implemented as practical applications or may be referred to as a beginning point for another development.

The contributors of this book come from diverse backgrounds, making this book a truly international effort. This book will bring forth new frontiers with its revolutionizing research information and detailed analysis of the nascent developments around the world.

We would like to thank all the contributing authors for lending their expertise to make the book truly unique. They have played a crucial role in the development of this book. Without their invaluable contributions this book wouldn't have been possible. They have made vital efforts to compile up to date information on the varied aspects of this subject to make this book a valuable addition to the collection of many professionals and students.

This book was conceptualized with the vision of imparting up-to-date information and advanced data in this field. To ensure the same, a matchless editorial board was set up. Every individual on the board went through rigorous rounds of assessment to prove their worth. After which they invested a large part of their time researching and compiling the most relevant data for our readers.

The editorial board has been involved in producing this book since its inception. They have spent rigorous hours researching and exploring the diverse topics which have resulted in the successful publishing of this book. They have passed on their knowledge of decades through this book. To expedite this challenging task, the publisher supported the team at every step. A small team of assistant editors was also appointed to further simplify the editing procedure and attain best results for the readers.

Apart from the editorial board, the designing team has also invested a significant amount of their time in understanding the subject and creating the most relevant covers. They scrutinized every image to scout for the most suitable representation of the subject and create an appropriate cover for the book.

The publishing team has been an ardent support to the editorial, designing and production team. Their endless efforts to recruit the best for this project, has resulted in the accomplishment of this book. They are a veteran in the field of academics and their pool of knowledge is as vast as their experience in printing. Their expertise and guidance has proved useful at every step. Their uncompromising quality standards have made this book an exceptional effort. Their encouragement from time to time has been an inspiration for everyone.

The publisher and the editorial board hope that this book will prove to be a valuable piece of knowledge for researchers, students, practitioners and scholars across the globe.

List of Contributors

Maximilien Franck, Charles Couillard and Marie-Claude Vohl
Centre Nutrition, Santé et Société (NUTRISS) and Institut sur la Nutrition et les Aliments Fonctionnels (INAF), Université Laval, Québec, QC G1V 0A6, Canada
School of Nutrition, Université Laval, Québec, QC G1V 0A6, Canada

Juan de Toro-Martín, Valérie Guay, Michèle Kearney and Denis Roy
Centre Nutrition, Santé et Société (NUTRISS) and Institut sur la Nutrition et les Aliments Fonctionnels (INAF), Université Laval, Québec, QC G1V 0A6, Canada

Geneviève Pilon and André Marette
Centre Nutrition, Santé et Société (NUTRISS) and Institut sur la Nutrition et les Aliments Fonctionnels (INAF), Université Laval, Québec, QC G1V 0A6, Canada
Quebec Heart and Lung Institute (IUCPQ) Research Center, 2725 Chemin Sainte-Foy, Québec, QC G1V 4G5, Canada

Patrick Couture
Centre Nutrition, Santé et Société (NUTRISS) and Institut sur la Nutrition et les Aliments Fonctionnels (INAF), Université Laval, Québec, QC G1V 0A6, Canada
Endocrinology and Nephrology Unit, CHU de Québec-Université Laval, Québec, QC G1V 4G2, Canada
CHU Research Center, Québec, QC G1V 0A6, Canada

Hyun-E Yeom
College of Nursing, Chungnam National University, Munhwaro 266, Junggu, Daejeon 35015, Korea

Vladimir Lj. Jakovljevic
Department of Physiology, Faculty of Medical Sciences, University of Kragujevac, Svetozara Markovica 69, 34 000 Kragujevac, Serbia
Department of Human Pathology, I.M. Sechenov First Moscow State Medical University, Trubetskaya Street 8, 119991 Moscow, Russia

Vladimir I. Zivkovic and Ivan M. Srejovic
Department of Physiology, Faculty of Medical Sciences, University of Kragujevac, Svetozara Markovica 69, 34 000 Kragujevac, Serbia

Slobodanka Lj. Mitrovic
Department of Pathology, Faculty of Medical Sciences, University of Kragujevac, Svetozara Markovica 69, 34 000 Kragujevac, Serbia

Nemanja U. Jovicic
Department of Histology and Embryology, Faculty of Medical Sciences, University of Kragujevac, Svetozara Markovica 69, 34 000 Kragujevac, Serbia

Sergey B. Bolevich
Department of Human Pathology, I.M. Sechenov First Moscow State Medical University, Trubetskaya Street 8, 119991 Moscow, Russia

Andrey A. Svistunov
Research Institute of Pharmacy, I.M. Sechenov First Moscow State Medical University, Trubetskaya Street 8-2, 119991 Moscow, Russia

Suresh C. Tyagi
Department of Physiology, School of Medicine, University of Louisville, 500 S Preston Street, Louisville, KY 40202, USA

Nevena S. Jeremic
Department of Pharmacy, Faculty of Medical Sciences, University of Kragujevac, Svetozara Markovica 69, 34 000 Kragujevac, Serbia
Department of Physiology, School of Medicine, University of Louisville, 500 S Preston Street, Louisville, KY 40202, USA

Jovana N. Jeremic, Jovana V. Bradic and Isidora M. Milosavljevic
Department of Pharmacy, Faculty of Medical Sciences, University of Kragujevac, Svetozara Markovica 69, 34 000 Kragujevac, Serbia

Jungmin Lee
Youth Independence & Competencies Research Office, National Youth Policy Institute, Social Policy BLDG, Sejong National Research Complex, 370, Sicheong-daero, Sejong-si 30147, Korea

Amjad H. Jarrar, Ala Z. Ahmad, Asma A. Alnoaimi, Latifa S. Al Khaili, Najah H. Allowch, Fatima T. Al Meqbaali, Usama Souka and Ayesha S. Al Dhaheri
Food, Nutrition and Health Department, College of Food and Agriculture, United Arab Emirates University, Al Ain 15551, UAE

Lily Stojanovska
Food, Nutrition and Health Department, College of Food and Agriculture, United Arab Emirates University, Al Ain 15551, UAE
Institute for Health and Sport, Victoria University, Melbourne 14428, Australia

Vasso Apostolopoulos
Institute for Health and Sport, Victoria University, Melbourne 14428, Australia

Leila Cheikh Ismail
Clinical Nutrition and Dietetics Department, College of Health Sciences, University of Sharjah 27272, UAE
Nuffield Department of Women's & Reproductive Health, University of Oxford, Oxford OX1 2JD, UK

Jack Feehan
Institute for Health and Sport, Victoria University, Melbourne 14428, Australia
Department of Medicine—Western Health, The University of Melbourne, Melbourne 3021, Australia

Eric O. Ohuma
Maternal, Adolescent, Reproductive & Child Health (MARCH) Centre, London School of Hygiene & Tropical Medicine (LSHTM), London WC1E 7HT, UK
Centre for Tropical Medicine and Global Health, Nuffield Department of Medicine, University of Oxford, Oxford OX3 7LG, UK

Stéphanie Harrison and Benoît Lamarche
Centre Nutrition, santé et société (NUTRISS), Institut sur la nutrition et les aliments fonctionnels (INAF), Université Laval, Québec, QC G1V 0A6, Canada
School of Nutrition, Université Laval, Québec, QC G1V 0A6, Canada

Javier S. Perona
Instituto de la Grasa-CSIC, Campus Universidad Pablo de Olavide, Edificio 46, 41013 Seville, Spain

Ángel Fernández-Aparicio and María Correa-Rodríguez
Department of Nursing, University of Granada, Av. Ilustración, 60, 18016 Granada, Spain

Robinson Ramírez-Vélez
Department of Health Sciences, Public University of Navarra, Navarrabiomed- IdiSNA, Pamplona, 31006 Navarra, Spain

Mark D. DeBoer
Department of Pediatrics, University of Virginia, Charlottesville, VA 22908, USA

Mercedes Sotos-Prieto
Department of Preventive Medicine and Public Health, School of Medicine, Universidad Autónoma de Madrid, IdiPaz (Instituto de Investigación Sanitaria Hospital Universitario La Paz), Calle del Arzobispo Morcillo 4, 28029 Madrid, Spain
Biomedical Research Network Centre of Epidemiology and Public Health (CIBERESP), Carlos III Health Institute, 28029 Madrid, Spain
Department of Environmental Health, Harvard T.H. Chan School of Public Health, Boston, MA 02115, USA

Miguel Ruiz-Canela
Department of Preventive Medicine and Public Health, IdiSNA, University of Navarra, 31009 Pamplona, Spain
Biomedical Research Network Centre for Pathophysiology of Obesity and Nutrition (CIBEROBN), Carlos III Health Institute, 28029 Madrid, Spain

Yiqing Song
Department of Epidemiology, Richard M. Fairbanks School of Public Health, Indiana University, Indianapolis, IN 46202, USA

Costas Christophi
Department of Environmental Health, Harvard T.H. Chan School of Public Health, Boston, MA 02115, USA
Cyprus International Institute for Environmental and Public Health, Cyprus University of Technology, 30 Archbishop Kyprianou Str., 3036 Lemesos, Cyprus

Steven Mofatt
National Institute for Public Safety Health, Indianapolis, IN 46204, USA

Fernando Rodriguez-Artalejo
Department of Preventive Medicine and Public Health, School of Medicine, Universidad Autónoma de Madrid, IdiPaz (Instituto de Investigación Sanitaria Hospital Universitario La Paz), Calle del Arzobispo Morcillo 4, 28029 Madrid, Spain
Biomedical Research Network Centre of Epidemiology and Public Health (CIBERESP), Carlos III Health Institute, 28029 Madrid, Spain
IMDEA-Food Institute, CEI UAM+CSIC, 28049 Madrid, Spain

Stefanos N. Kales
Department of Environmental Health, Harvard T.H. Chan School of Public Health, Boston, MA 02115, USA
Department of Occupational Medicine, Cambridge Health Alliance, Harvard Medical School, Cambridge, MA 02145, USA

Peter Clifton
School of Pharmacy and Medical Sciences, University of South Australia, Adelaide SA 5000, Australia

Jiao Wang, Yajun Chen and Jin Jing
Department of Maternal and Child Health Care, School of Public Health, Sun Yat-Sen University, Guangzhou 510080, China

Jacqueline Schmidt-RioValle and Emilio González-Jiménez
Departamento de Enfermería, CTS-436 Adscrito al Centro de Investigación Mente, Cerebro y Comportamiento (CIMCYC), University of Granada, Av/Ilustración 60, 18016 Granada, Spain
Department of Nursing, University of Granada, Av. Ilustración, 60, 18016 Granada, Spain

Robert Ross, Simrat Soni and Sarah Houle
School of Kinesiology and Health Studies, Department of Endocrinology and Metabolism, Queen's University, Kingston, ON K7L 3N6, Canada

Vincenzo Di Marzo
École de nutrition, Université Laval, Québec, QC G1V 0A6, Canada
Institut sur la nutrition et les aliments fonctionnels, Université Laval, Québec, QC G1V 0A6, Canada
Canada Excellence Research Chair on the Microbiome-Endocannabinoidome Axis in Metabolic Health, Université Laval, Québec, QC G1V 0A6, Canada
Centre de recherche de l'Institut universitaire de cardiologie et de pneumologie de Québec, Québec, QC G1V 4G5, Canada
Department de médecine, Université Laval, Québec, QC G1V 0A6, Canada
Institute of Biomolecular Chemistry, Consiglio Nazionale delle Ricerche, 80078 Pozzuoli, Italy

Cristoforo Silvestri
Canada Excellence Research Chair on the Microbiome-Endocannabinoidome Axis in Metabolic Health, Université Laval, Québec, QC G1V 0A6, Canada
Centre de recherche de l'Institut universitaire de cardiologie et de pneumologie de Québec, Québec, QC G1V 4G5, Canada
Department de médecine, Université Laval, Québec, QC G1V 0A6, Canada

Luigi Barrea, Giovanna Muscogiuri, Daniela Laudisio, Giulia de Alteriis, Annamaria Colao and Silvia Savastano
Dipartimento di Medicina Clinica e Chirurgia, Unit of Endocrinology, Federico II University Medical School of Naples, Via Sergio Pansini 5, 80131 Naples, Italy

Giuseppe Annunziata, Maria Maisto and Gian Carlo Tenore
Department of Pharmacy, University of Naples "Federico II", Via Domenico Montesano 49, 80131 Naples, Italy

Carolina Di Somma
IRCCS SDN, Napoli Via Gianturco 113, 80143 Naples, Italy

Hitoshi Nishizawa and Iichiro Shimomura
Department of Metabolic Medicine, Graduate School of Medicine, Osaka University, 2-2-B5, Yamada-oka, Suita, Osaka 565-0871, Japan

Marja-Riitta Taskinen
Research Program for Clinical and Molecular Medicine Unit, Diabetes and Obesity, University of Helsinki, 00029 Helsinki, Finland

Chris J Packard
Institute of Cardiovascular and Medical Sciences, University of Glasgow, Glasgow G12 8QQ, UK

Jan Borén
Department of Molecular and Clinical Medicine, University of Gothenburg and Sahlgrenska University Hospital, 41345 Gothenburg, Sweden

Michèle Rousseau, Frédéric Guénard, Véronique Garneau, Bénédicte Allam-Ndoul and Simone Lemieux
Institute of Nutrition and Functional Foods (INAF), Laval University, Quebec City, QC G1V 0A6, Canada
School of Nutrition, Laval University, Quebec City, QC G1V 0A6, Canada

Louis Pérusse
Institute of Nutrition and Functional Foods (INAF), Laval University, Quebec City, QC G1V 0A6, Canada
Department of Kinesiology, Laval University, Quebec City, QC G1V 0A6, Canada

Index

www.ingramcontent.com/pod-product-compliance
Lightning Source LLC
LaVergne TN
LVHW081036210926
848485LV00004B/1034